Landmark Papers
in Rheumatology

Landmark Papers in... series

Titles in the series:

Landmark Papers in Rheumatology
Edited by Richard A. Watts and David G. I. Scott

Landmark Papers in Cardiovascular Medicine
Edited by Aung Myat, Tony Gershlick

Landmark Papers in General Surgery
Edited by Graham MacKay, Richard Molloy, and Patrick O'Dwyer

Landmark Papers in Allergy
Edited by Aziz Sheikh, Thomas Platts-Mills, and Allison Worth
Advisory Editor Stephen Holgate

Landmark Papers in Nephrology
Edited by John Feehally, Christopher McIntyre, and J. Stewart Cameron

Landmark Papers in Anaesthesia
Edited by Nigel R. Webster and Helen F. Galley

Landmark Papers in Neurosurgery
Second Edition
Edited by Reuben D. Johnson and Alexander L. Green

Landmark Papers in Rheumatology

Edited by

Dr. Richard A. Watts

Consultant Rheumatologist
Department of Rheumatology
Ipswich Hospital NHS Trust
Ipswich UK;
Honorary Senior Lecturer Norwich Medical School,
University of East Anglia, Norwich UK

Professor David G. I. Scott

Honorary Consultant Rheumatologist,
Norfolk and Norwich University Foundation NHS Trust;
Honorary Professor of Rheumatology Norwich Medical School,
University of East Anglia, Norwich UK

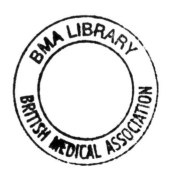

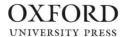

OXFORD
UNIVERSITY PRESS

OXFORD
UNIVERSITY PRESS

Great Clarendon Street, Oxford, OX2 6DP,
United Kingdom

Oxford University Press is a department of the University of Oxford.
It furthers the University's objective of excellence in research, scholarship,
and education by publishing worldwide. Oxford is a registered trade mark of
Oxford University Press in the UK and in certain other countries

First Edition published in 2015
Impression: 1

Published in the United States of America by Oxford University Press
198 Madison Avenue, New York, NY 10016, United States of America

British Library Cataloguing in Publication Data
Data available

Library of Congress Control Number: 2015932388

ISBN 978–0–19–968837–1

Printed and bound by
CPI Group (UK) Ltd, Croydon, CR0 4YY

Preface

The rheumatism is a common name for many aches and pains, which have yet got no peculiar appellation, though owing to very many different causes.

(William Heberden (1710–1801) *Commentaries on the History and Cure of Disease*, Chapter 79 (1802)).

William Heberden in many respects summarized the state of rheumatic disease nomenclature and classification in 1802 with the statement quoted above. At that time, probably only gout was clearly distinguished from many types of aches and pains. In the commentaries he also gives the first description of the bony nodes over the distal interphalangeal joints—'What are those little hard knobs, about the size of a small pea, which are *frequently seen upon the fingers, particularly a little below the top, near the joint?*' He does not understand their aetiology but recognizes them not to be linked with psoriasis. During the late eighteenth and nineteenth centuries, descriptions of disease patterns that we now recognize began to be made. Sir Archibald Garrod in 1859 gave the name 'rheumatoid arthritis' to a disease that, although around for many years, had no nomenclature and up until that stage had been described as 'rheumatic gout', 'chronic rheumatism', and 'rheumalgia'. The first steps in the scientific investigation of arthritis were also made around this time; for example, Garrod differentiated gouty arthritis using the presence of serum hyperuricaemia. This process has continued up to the present day, with differentiation of further types of arthritis, using both traditional methods of clinical pattern recognition combined with improved investigative techniques, for example, the clear differentiation of inflammation due to synovitis from that due to enthesial inflammation using MRI, and better understanding of causation, for example, the recognition that a certain form of inflammatory arthritis of children is due to borrelia infection. As the study of rheumatic disease has become more scientific simple descriptions of disease patterns have become inadequate for clinical studies and this has led to the development of validated diagnostic and classification systems for many of the rheumatic diseases.

Treatment in Heberden's day was limited and primarily consisted bleeding or purging, although the antipyretic properties of cinchona bark were recognized. The only specific therapy for a form of arthritis then was colchicine for gout, which had been used since the time of Hippocrates. Garrod suggested that hyperuricaemia could be controlled by limiting dietary intake of purines. The nineteenth century saw the development of aspirin and early analgesics. The twentieth century saw the introduction of corticosteroids—for which Hench won the Nobel prize—immunosuppressive drugs, and most recently the products of the biotechnology revolution, monoclonal antibodies and fusion proteins.

The aim of this book is to provide both practising and trainee rheumatologists with an overview of the history of their specialty by presenting some of the key papers, together with brief commentary as to why the paper is important. The authors were asked to select up to ten papers in their field covering in their opinion key developments. The papers range from initial descriptions of disease up to very recent innovations in our scientific understanding of aetiopathogenesis and therapy.

Richard A. Watts

David G. I. Scott

Acknowledgements

We are grateful to Eloise Moir-Ford and James Oates of Oxford University Press for all their unstinting help and enthusiasm during the production of this book. Without them, it would never have happened.

Our families, particularly Lesley and Dee, have been very supportive during the editing process and we are indebted to them.
Richard A. Watts
David G. I. Scott

Contents

Contributors

Nicola Ambrose
Adolescent and Adult Rheumatologist
University College Hospital,
London, UK

Tehseen Ahmed
Royal National Hospital for Rheumatic
Diseases,
Bath, UK

Ashok Bhalla
Royal National Hospital for Rheumatic
Diseases,
Bath, UK

Fraser Birrell
Institute of Cellular Medicine,
Musculoskeletal Research Group,
Newcastle University, UK

James Bluett
Centre for Musculoskeletal Research,
Institute of Inflammation
and Repair,
The University of Manchester,
Manchester Academic Health
Science Centre, UK

Ian N. Bruce
Arthritis Research UK Centre for
Epidemiology,
Centre for Musculoskeletal Research
Institute of Inflammation and Repair,
The University of Manchester,
Manchester Academic Health Science
Centre, UK

Lorna Clarson
Arthritis Research UK Primary
Care Centre,
Keele University, UK

Despina Eleftheriou
Arthritis Research UK Centre for
Adolescent Rheumatology,
Institute of Child Health,
University College London, London, UK

Asma Fikree
Queen Mary University of London, UK

Hill Gaston
Department of Medicine,
University of Cambridge, UK

Iain Goff
Department of Rheumatology
Northumbria Healthcare NHS Foundation
Trust, UK

Alan Hakim
Barts Health NHS Trust,
London, UK
Queen Mary University of London, UK

John Ioannou
Arthritis Research UK Centre for
Adolescent Rheumatology University
College London, London, UK

Haroon Khan
Department of Rheumatology,
Ipswich Hospital NHS Trust, UK

Elena Nikiphorou
Department of Rheumatology,
Addenbrooke's Hospital,
Cambridge University Hospitals NHS
Foundation Trust, UK

Benjamin Parker
Kellgren Centre for Rheumatology,
Central Manchester University
Hospitals Foundation Trust, UK

Edward Roddy
Arthritis Research UK Primary Care
Centre,
Primary Care Sciences,
Keele University, UK

David G. I. Scott
Norfolk and Norwich University
Foundation NHS Trust
Honorary Professor
Norwich Medical School,
University of East Anglia, UK

Carmel Stober
Department of Medicine,
University of Cambridge School of
Clinical Medicine, UK

Deborah Symmons
Centre for Musculoskeletal Research,
Institute of Inflammation
and Repair,
The University of Manchester,

Manchester Academic Health Science
Centre, UK

Suzanne Verstappen
Centre for Musculoskeletal Research,
Institute of Inflammation and Repair,
The University of Manchester,
Manchester Academic Health Science
Centre, UK

Adam Young
Department of Rheumatology,
City Hospital,
St Albans, UK

Richard A. Watts
Consultant Rheumatologist,
Ipswich Hospital NHS Trust
Honorary Clinical Senior Lecturer,
Norwich Medical School,
University of East Anglia,
Department of Rheumatology,
The Ipswich Hospital NHS Trust, UK

Chapter 1

Epidemiology and genetics

James Bluett, Suzanne Verstappen,
and Deborah Symmons

Introduction

Epidemiology

Epidemiology is the study of the distribution and determinants of disease in human populations. It is applied to describe the prevalence and incidence of a disease, to identify predictors (genetic and environmental) of the development of disease, and to describe the consequences of a disease. Understanding the distribution and the burden of diseases helps health policy makers and the general public to understand the impact of diseases and injuries across different regions of the world and the need for specific intervention programmes and better distribution of health care resources. We selected Paper 1.4 as an excellent example of the estimation of the occurrence/burden of rheumatic and musculoskeletal disorders (RMDs). It was published in *The Lancet* in 2012 as one of a number of papers on the global burden of disease, and possible risk factors. This paper showed that, over the last two decades, the disability-adjusted life years (DALYs) for rheumatoid arthritis, neck and back pain, and osteoarthritis have increased, whereas the death rate for rheumatoid arthritis has decreased by ~10%.

Although the Global Burden of Disease study provides the best available estimate of disease occurrence, these papers also illustrate the challenges epidemiologists face when estimating the impact of a disease in different countries, and amalgamating data from a variety of sources, often without case validation. Ideally, to determine prevalence and incidence of a disease, it is important to use validated tools for case definition. We selected two key papers (Papers 1.1 and 1.2) which demonstrate the development of case definitions for RMDs. The Kellgren and Lawrence radiological scoring system for osteoarthritis is one of the first examples of a validated tool in rheumatology. Although the scoring system has undergone a few minor changes since its introduction 50 years ago, it is often still used to estimate and compare prevalence rates for osteoarthritis and to assess radiographic damage over time in populations with osteoarthritis in different settings. For rheumatoid arthritis patients, a series of classification criteria sets have been developed by the American Rheumatism Association/American College of Rheumatology. The 1987 criteria set have been used extensively, not only to estimate the incidence and prevalence of rheumatoid arthritis but also as part of the entry criteria to clinical trials and observational studies. In the last decade there has been a shift towards earlier classification and treatment of rheumatoid arthritis. Because of their increased specificity in early rheumatoid arthritis, the 2010 American College of Rheumatology/European League Against Rheumatism criteria for rheumatoid arthritis are beginning to replace the 1987 criteria in this setting.

Epidemiology studies are also suitable to describe the occurrence and predictors of long-term consequences of a disease (e.g. co-morbidities, disability, and mortality). Standardized mortality ratios (SMRs) or standardized incidence ratios (SIRs) are often calculated, using data from the general population as the reference, to quantify the excess risk of co-morbidities. Paper 1.3 illustrates one of the first examples of the use of population registers and record linkage in RMDs. It examined the risk of lymphoma, leukaemia, and myeloma in patients with rheumatoid arthritis compared to the general population. To date, this remains one of the largest observational studies showing an increased risk of lymphoproliferative malignancies in patients with rheumatoid arthritis.

Genetic epidemiology

A genetic basis underlying a number of RMDs has been established using twin and family studies. Using rheumatoid arthritis as an exemplar, we have selected and go on to discuss the milestones that have produced step changes in our knowledge of the genetics underlying the development of disease.

Paper 1.5, published in 1987 by Gregerson et al., described the shared epitope hypothesis to explain the association of the human leukocyte antigen (HLA) *DRB1* alleles as the major risk factor for rheumatoid arthritis; the paper is still widely cited and, until very recently, no other hypotheses could better explain the association observed. The next major milestone did not occur until 2004, when Begovich et al. (Paper 1.6) discovered the second-largest genetic risk for the development of rheumatoid arthritis: a protein-coding change in the PTPN22 gene. Their research not only identified this genetic variant but also investigated its biological impact and determined that there is a genetic difference between seropositive and seronegative rheumatoid arthritis, a potential clue in the disease pathogenesis.

As technological capabilities advanced, in 2007 a consortium of scientists from all over the UK came together to test genetic variants spanning the whole genome (a genome-wide association study) in order to establish which genetic markers are associated with a number of autoimmune diseases, including rheumatoid arthritis. The study (Paper 1.7) validated previous research findings and revealed nine new genetic variants associated with rheumatoid arthritis, greatly expanding our knowledge of the disease. The results from the Wellcome Trust Case Control Consortium represented a major advance in the genetic understanding of disease, confirmed the importance of large sample sizes to enhance power to detect modest genetic effects, and demonstrated how a large group of scientists and clinicians can work together to enhance our understanding of disease.

From whole genome scanning, genetic studies have returned to focusing on particular sections of the genome. In 2012, technology and expanding cohort numbers enabled the investigation of the HLA region with fine mapping to determine the true disease-causing variants. Raychaudhuri et al. (Paper 1.8) discovered three genetic variants within the *HLA DRB1* gene that increase the risk of rheumatoid arthritis independently of each other and together and explain the association observed better than the previous shared epitope hypothesis. The variants lie within the peptide-binding grove of the HLA molecule, giving a vital clue to the importance of antigen presentation in the development of seropositive rheumatoid arthritis. Outside the shared epitope region, researchers have fine-mapped areas of previous interest, and in 2012 Eyre et al. (Paper 1.9) characterized, by fine mapping, over 40% of the known susceptibility areas to rheumatoid arthritis in one analysis. This paper was among the first to demonstrate, in rheumatoid arthritis, how genetic studies can identify novel targets for disease treatment.

Gene–environment interaction

The paradigm for the development of RMDs is that one or more environmental risk factors act in a genetically predisposed host to produce the disease phenotype. This paper (Paper 1.10) was the first to illustrate, statistically, that a genetic risk factor (the shared epitope) and an environmental risk factor (smoking) interact to enhance disease susceptibility for rheumatoid arthritis.

Paper 1.1: Radiological assessment of osteoarthritis— the Kellgren and Lawrence score

Reference

Kellgren JH, Lawrence JS. Radiological assessment of osteo-arthrosis. *Ann Rheum Dis* 1957;16(4):494–502.

Purpose

To develop and validate a system for scoring X-rays for the presence and severity of osteoarthritis.

Study design

The authors selected standard radiographs to represent 5 grades of osteoarthritis: none (0), doubtful (1), mild (2), moderate (3), and severe (4) for 11 joint areas. The standard radiographs for Grades 1–4 for the distal interphalangeal (DIP) joints, proximal interphalangeal (PIP) joints, metacarpophalangeal (MCP) joints, first carpometacarpal (CMC) joints, wrist, cervical spine, hip, and knee are reproduced in this paper—a forerunner of the much used Atlas of Standard Radiographs [1]. The other joint areas assessed were the dorsal and lumbar spine and the feet. Verbal definitions of the radiological features and the grading criteria are shown in Table 1.1.

Table 1.1 Kellgren and Lawrence grading system of osteoarthritis

Radiological features
- Formation of osteophytes on the joint margins or, in case of the knee joint, on the tibial spines.
- Periarticular ossicles; these are found chiefly in relation to the distal and proximal interpharangeal joints.
- Narrowing of joint cartilage associated with sclerosis of subchondral bone.
- Small pseudocystic areas with sclerotic walls situated usually in the subchondral bone.
- Altered shape of the bone ends, particular in the head of the femur.
Grading system:
- *Grade 0 (none):* No features of osteoarthritis.
- *Grade 1 (doubtful):* Minute osteophyte, doubtful significance.
- *Grade 2 (minimal):* Definite osteophyte, unimpaired joint space.
- *Grade 3 (moderate):* Moderate diminution of joint space.
- *Grade 4 (severe):* Joint space greatly impaired with sclerosis of subchondral bone.

Source data from Kellgren JH, Lawrence JS. Radiological assessment of osteo-arthrosis. *Ann Rheum Dis* 1957 Dec;16(4):494–502.

The inter-observer and intra-observer reliability of this scoring system was evaluated by Kellgren and Lawrence themselves using X-rays from a survey of rheumatic diseases in the Leigh, Lancashire, population, UK. X-rays of a random sample of 85 people aged 55–64 were read by the two observers by comparing these with the standard radiographs. Eleven joint areas were evaluated and the intervals between the combined and the independent readings were two months and one month, respectively, after the independent reading.

Results

Inter-observer agreement ranged from 0.10 for the wrist to 0.83 for the knee. Intra-observer agreement was higher and ranged from 0.42 for the dorso-lumbar spine to 0.88 for the MCP joints. Although, for most joints, the agreement was high, the estimated prevalence of the disease varied widely because of the cumulative effect of observer bias (±31%).

Critique of the Kellgren and Lawrence scoring system

Although the scoring system has been extensively used to define osteoarthritis, it has also been criticized. First, there are some inconsistencies in the description of the radiographic features leading to discrepancies in study results [2, 3]. Second, there is quite a large emphasis on osteophytes. Third, the scoring system is ordinal, and the lower end of the scale represents different pathological processes involving different tissues from those at the higher end of the scale. In more recent years, therefore, based on the Kellgren and Lawrence system, further subcategorization of specific features of individual joints (i.e. hand joints, knees, and hips) has been established. In addition, new atlases including standard radiographs and better descriptions of the radiographic features have increased the accuracy to grade osteoarthritis and have helped to improve the internal and external validity [4].

Significance and importance of the paper

After 50 years the Kellgren and Lawrence scoring system, albeit with some minor modifications, is still used to estimate incidence and prevalence rates and to assess radiographic progression in osteoarthritis. In the USA, incidence rates (Kellgren and Lawrence ≥2) of symptomatic hand, hip, and knee osteoarthritis were obtained among members of the Fallon Community Health Plan, a health maintenance organization in central Massachusetts [5]. Incident cases had joint symptoms at the time or up to one year before the radiographs and did not have a history of osteoarthritis. The age- and sex-standardized incidence rate of hand osteoarthritis was 100 per 100,000 person-years (95% confidence interval (CI), 86–115), for hip osteoarthritis, 88 per 100,000 person-years (95% CI, 75–101), and for knee osteoarthritis, 240 per 100,000 person-years (95% CI, 218–262). Prevalence rates of radiographic osteoarthritis have been reported in a few studies. In a Dutch study including 6,585 randomly selected inhabitants of Zoetermeer, gender- and age-specific osteoarthritis prevalence rates of 22 joints were calculated [6]. The prevalence of radiological osteoarthritis was highest for the cervical spine and increased from 0.3% in women aged

20–24 to 84.3% in women aged 75–79. In men a similar increase was observed, from 0.7% to 84.8%. Seventy-five per cent of the women had osteoarthritis (grade ≥2) of their DIP joints. Severe osteoarthritis was most common in those aged >45 years, and the prevalence rate exceeded the 20% for the cervical spine and lumbar spine, DIP joints of hands, and, in women only, MCP joints, first CMC joints, first metatarsophalangeal joints, and knees.

Since the Kellgren and Lawrence score is based on an ordinal scoring system, it is more difficult to determine annual progression than to assess changes in joint space narrowing over time. In a systematic review, the annual radiographic progression was calculated as percentage with change of at least one grade [7]. Including both data from observational studies and clinical trials, the overall mean risk of Kellgren and Lawrence annual progression of at least one grade was 5.6 ± 4.9%, with a higher risk associated with shorter disease duration, and with cohorts that included both incident and prevalent cases. This overview also showed that patients with a Kellgren and Lawrence score ≥2 at inclusion into a study have a higher risk of progression than those recruited with a Kellgren and Lawrence score ≥1 (6.2% vs 3.3%).

References

1 **Kellgren JH., Lawrence JS.** The epidemiology of chronic rheumatism. Atlas of standard radiographs. Oxford: Blackwell Scientific;1963.

2 **Spector TD, Cooper C.** Radiographic assessment of osteoarthritis in population studies: whither Kellgren and Lawrence? *Osteoarthr Cartil* 1993;**1**(4):203–6.

3 **Arden N, Nevitt MC.** Osteoarthritis: epidemiology. *Best Pract Res Clin Rheumatol* 2006;**20**(1):3–25.

4 **Altman RD, Gold GE.** Atlas of individual radiographic features in osteoarthritis, revised. *Osteoarthr Cartil* 2007;**15**(Suppl A):A1–56.

5 **Oliveria SA, Felson DT, Reed JI, Cirillo PA, Walker AM.** Incidence of symptomatic hand, hip, and knee osteoarthritis among patients in a health maintenance organization. *Arthritis Rheum* 1995;**38**(8):1134–41.

6 **van Saase JL, van Romunde LK, Cats A, Vandenbroucke JP, Valkenburg HA.** Epidemiology of osteoarthritis: Zoetermeer survey. Comparison of radiological osteoarthritis in a Dutch population with that in 10 other populations. *Ann Rheum Dis* 1989;**48**(4):271–80.

7 **Emrani PS, Katz JN, Kessler CL, et al.** Joint space narrowing and Kellgren-Lawrence progression in knee osteoarthritis: an analytic literature synthesis. *Osteoarthr Cartil* 2008;**16**(8):873–82.

Paper 1.2: The association between rheumatoid arthritis and lymphoma

Reference

Isomäki HA, Hakulinen T, Joutsenlahti U. Excess risk of lymphomas, leukemia and myeloma in patients with rheumatoid arthritis. *J Chron Dis* 1978;**31**(2):691–6.

Purpose

To compare the incidence of malignancy in patients entitled to free medication for rheumatoid arthritis in Finland with that in the general Finnish population matched for age and gender.

Population studied

The population studied comprised patients on the Finnish Social Insurance Institution's Population Data Register (started in 1965) as being entitled to reimbursable medication for 'rheumatoid arthritis'. The term 'rheumatoid arthritis' included systemic connective tissue disease until 1970 (1.7% of cases) and ankylosing spondylitis since 1970 (2.2% of all cases).

Study design

This paper describes a longitudinal observational study using population registers. Details of patients entitled to reimbursable medication for 'rheumatoid arthritis' from 1967–1973 were linked to the Finnish Cancer Registry in order to identify all new cancer cases diagnosed from 1 January 1967 or the date of the first rheumatoid arthritis prescription until 31 December 1967 or death. The numbers of various types of malignancy observed were compared with those expected in the general Finnish population matched for age and sex.

Results

The study follows 11,483 men and 34,618 women with 'rheumatoid arthritis' for 213,911 years. The authors report 1,202 incident malignancies as compared to the 1,137.89 expected.

The authors report that the incidence of cancer of the respiratory organs, lymphoma, myeloma, and leukaemia was increased in men with rheumatoid arthritis (Table 1.2). Although the overall incidence of malignancy was not increased in women, the incidence of Hodgkin's disease, lymphoma, and myeloma was increased.

Critique of the paper

There are two weaknesses in the composition of the rheumatoid arthritis cohort: (i) no case definition was used beyond the requirement of medication for a condition labelled as rheumatoid arthritis by the physician in charge of the case, and (ii) there was 'contamination' of the cohort with cases of connective tissue disorder and ankylosing spondylitis.

Table 1.2 Occurrence of malignancies by site

Sex	Primary site	Observed number	Expected number	P value	SIR (95% CI)*
Male	All	407	354.11	<0.01	1.14 (1.04–1.27)
	Respiratory organs	171	132.75	<0.01	1.28 (1.10–1.50)
	Hodgkin's disease	5	2.28	NS	2.10 (0.71–5.12)
	Lymphoma	13	4.84	<0.01	2.69 (1.43–4.59)
	Myeloma	7	3.26	<0.05	2.15 (0.86–4.42)
	Leukaemia	18	7.10	<0.01	2.54 (1.50–4.01)
Female	All	795	783.78	NS	1.01 (0.94–1.09)
	Hodgkin's disease	14	4.54	<0.01	3.08 (1.69–5.17)
	Lymphoma	25	9.34	<0.01	2.68 (1.73–3.95)
	Myeloma	21	9.49	<0.01	2.21 (1.37–3.38)
	Leukaemia	27	18.74	NS	1.44 (0.95–2.10)

* CI, confidence interval; SIR, standardized incidence ratio. Calculated using a Poisson distribution around the observed number. Not presented in the original paper.

In addition, the paper was published before the widespread calculation of relative risk and 95% CI. We have included these in Table 1.2 for completeness. In addition the authors do not address the possible reasons for the link beyond speculating that in some way patients are susceptible to both rheumatoid arthritis and lymphoproliferative malignancies.

Significance and importance of the paper

This is one of the earliest examples in rheumatology of the use of population registers and record linkage to address an important epidemiological question. The Scandinavian countries are ideally placed to conduct such studies as the use of a unique identification number, and the existence of a large number of population-based registers makes linkage relatively straightforward. This was the first study to use this design to address the hypothesis of an increased risk of lymphoproliferative malignancies in patients with rheumatoid arthritis and remains the second largest study conducted to date [1]. A meta-analysis published in 2008 of 14 studies published between 1990 and 2007 found an overall twofold increase risk of lymphoma in rheumatoid arthritis (SIR: 2.08; 95% CI, 1.80 –2.39)—very similar to that reported by Isomäki [2]. In recent years we have seen an elegant demonstration that the risk of lymphoma in rheumatoid arthritis is associated with cumulative disease activity and exposure to immunosuppressive medications such as azathioprine [3, 4]. There was considerable concern at the time of their introduction that anti-tumour necrosis factor therapy might further increase the risk of lymphoma—but this has not been borne out with time. The Isomäki paper continues to provide a useful benchmark with which to compare more recent studies conducted in an era when treatment of rheumatoid arthritis has improved dramatically and one might therefore expect the excess risk of lymphoma to diminish.

References

1 **Parikh-Patel A, White RH**. Risk of cancer among rheumatoid arthritis patients in California. *Cancer Causes Control* 2009;**20**(6):1001–10.

2 **Smitten AL, Simon TA, Hochberg M, Suissa S**. A meta-analysis of the incidence of malignancy in adult patients with rheumatoid arthritis. *Arthritis Res Ther* 2008;**10**(2):45.

3 **Baecklund E, Iliadou A, Askling J, et al**. Association of chronic inflammation, not its treatment, with increased lymphoma risk in rheumatoid arthritis. *Arthritis Rheum* 2006;**54**(3):692–701.

4 **Asten P, Barrett J, Symmons D**. Risk of developing certain malignancies is related to duration of immunosuppressive drug exposure in patients with rheumatic diseases. *J Rheumatol* 1999;**26**(8):1705–14.

Paper 1.3: The American Rheumatism Association 1987 revised criteria for the classification of rheumatoid arthritis

Reference

Arnett FC, Edworthy SM, Bloch DA, et al. The American Rheumatism Association 1987 revised criteria for the classification of rheumatoid arthritis. *Arthritis Rheum* 1988;31(3):315–24.

Purpose

The 1987 American Rheumatism Association/American College of Rheumatology criteria for rheumatoid arthritis were developed in order to improve specificity and sensitivity and additionally to improve simplicity, as compared to the 1958 American Rheumatism Association criteria. [1–4]

Participants and patients

In this study, 262 consecutive patients with rheumatoid arthritis and 262 control patients with a rheumatic disease other than rheumatoid arthritis (e.g. osteoarthritis, systemic lupus erythematosus, psoriatic arthritis, or other), including both new and established patients, were selected by the nine rheumatologist members of a subcommittee of the Diagnostic and Therapeutic Criteria Committee of the American College of Rheumatology and 32 other rheumatologists. The certainty of the patient having rheumatoid arthritis was estimated by the rheumatologist on a 10 cm visual analogue scale.

Study design

The evaluated criteria set included the individual items of the old American Rheumatism Association and New York criteria (Table 1.3) for rheumatoid arthritis and items considered to be important by the committee following a Delphi method procedure. Two statistical approaches were applied to develop the classification criteria. First, combinations of variables which were most sensitive and specific to the classification of rheumatoid arthritis were selected by means of Boolean algebra; for example, a patient would be classified as having rheumatoid arthritis if at least X out of Y criteria were present. The second method involved selecting variables which best discriminated rheumatoid arthritis patients from controls using a 'classification tree'. All analyses were repeated for patients with 'new' disease and for patients with established disease. Finally, the specificity of the two methods was tested against 137 consecutive subjects enrolled in a USA prospective study.

Results

Items selected by the committee included morning stiffness, pain on motion in joints, swelling in ≥3 joint areas, symmetric swelling, subcutaneous nodules, abnormal rheumatoid factor, and radiological findings. The accuracy, calculated as the mean of sensitivity and specificity, of these individual items varied from 50.3 for pain on motion of the distal interphalangeal joint to 87.4 for swelling of ≥3 joint areas upon physical examination. The

Table 1.3 Comparison of items included in the American Rheumatism Association criteria and the New York criteria

Item	American Rheumatism Association criteria	New York criteria
Morning stiffness	X	
Joint pain	X	X
One joint swollen	X	
Two joints swollen	X	
Symmetric swelling	X	
Joint swelling		X
Rheumatoid nodules	X	
Serum rheumatoid factor	X	X
Mucin clot	X	
Synovial biopsy	X	
Nodule biopsy	X	
Radiographic findings	X	X

Table 1.4 The 1987 revised criteria for the classification of rheumatoid arthritis (list format)*

Criterion	Definition
1. Morning stiffness	Morning stiffness in and around the joints, lasting at least one hour before maximal improvement.
2. Arthritis of three or more joint areas	At least three joint areas simultaneously have had soft tissue swelling or fluid (not bony overgrowth alone) observed by a physician. The 14 possible areas are right or left PIP, MCP < wrist, elbow, knee, ankle, and MTP joints.
3. Arthritis of hand joints	At least one area swollen in a wrist, MCP, or PIP joint.
4. Symmetric arthritis	Simultaneous involvement of the same joint areas (as defined in Criterion 2) on both sides of the body (bilateral involvement of PIP, MCP, or MTP joints is acceptable without absolute symmetry).
5. Rheumatoid nodules	Subcutaneous nodules, over bony prominences, or extensor surfaces, or in juxtaarticular regions, observed by a physician.
6. Serum rheumatoid factor	Demonstration of abnormal mounts of serum rheumatoid factor by any method for which the result has been positive in <5% of normal controls.
7. Radiographic changes	Radiographic changes typical of rheumatoid arthritis on posterior/anterior hand and wrist radiographs, which must include erosions or unequivocal bony decalcification localized in or marked adjacent to the involved joints (osteoarthritis changes alone do not qualify).

* For classification purpose, a patient shall be said to have rheumatoid arthritis if he/she has satisfied at least four of these seven criteria. Criteria 1 through 4 must have been present for at least 6 weeks. Patients with Criterion 2 clinical diagnoses are not excluded. Designation as classic, definite, or probable rheumatoid arthritis is not to be made; DIP, distal interphalangeal; PIP, proximal interphalangeal; MCP, metacarpophalangeal; MTP, metatarsophalangeal.

Source data from Arnett FC, Edworthy SM, Bloch DA, et al. The American Rheumatism Association 1987 revised criteria for the classification of rheumatoid arthritis. *Arthritis Rheum* 1988 Mar;31(3):315–24.

final seven criteria and their definitions included in the 1987 criteria for rheumatoid arthritis are shown in Table 1.4. To be classified as having rheumatoid arthritis, patients had to satisfy at least four out of these seven criteria. The criteria included in the classification tree were slightly different and did not include morning stiffness or rheumatoid nodules (Figure 1.1) [5]. Compared to the 1958 American Rheumatism Association and New York criteria, the sensitivity and specificity improved for the revised classification criteria and classification tree to 91.2% and 93.5%, respectively, for sensitivity and to 89.3% and 89.3%, respectively, for specificity.

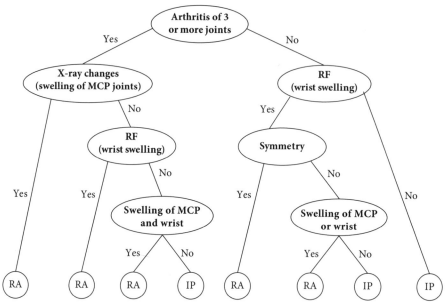

Fig. 1.1 Tree format of the American College of Rheumatology 1987 criteria for the classification of rheumatoid arthritis, as applied to patients with inflammatory polyarthritis; IP, inflammatory polyarthritis; MCP, metacarpophalangeal; RA, rheumatoid arthritis; RF, rheumatoid factor.

Critique of the 1987 criteria

The main criticism of the 1987 criteria for rheumatoid arthritis is that they were developed in a cohort of patients with established rheumatoid arthritis. The specificity of the criteria was especially low in patients with early rheumatoid arthritis. The pooled sensitivity and specificity of the 1987 criteria in early rheumatoid arthritis (<1 year disease duration) were 77% (68%–84%) and 77% (68%–84%), respectively, for the list format and 80% (72%–88%) and 33% (24%–43%), respectively, for the tree format [6]. In established rheumatoid arthritis, the pooled sensitivity and specificity were respectively 79% (71%–85%) and 90% (84%–94%), respectively, versus 80% (71%–85%) and 93% (86%–97%), respectively. In the last decade it has been shown that early and aggressive treatment of inflammatory arthritis is clinically more beneficial, resulting in less accrual joint damage and long-term disability [7–9]. If the 1987 criteria for rheumatoid arthritis are used to determine which patients should be included in treatment studies, or even as a guide in clinic for treatment decisions, those who might benefit most from early intensive treatment would be excluded. For these reasons, new criteria showing better specificity were developed and published in 2010 [10–12].

A further criticism is in the selection of the comparison cohort. Many of the patients included in the comparison cohort had non-inflammatory conditions which are easily distinguishable from rheumatoid arthritis. In studies of criteria development, the comparison group should have diseases which have features in common with the disease under study.

Finally, unlike the 1958 criteria, there are no exclusions included in the 1987 criteria. Thus it is possible, for example, for someone with classical gout to also be classified as having rheumatoid arthritis if they happen to fulfil the 1987 criteria.

Significance and importance of the paper

In the 30 years following the publication of the 1987 criteria for rheumatoid arthritis, the criteria have been used extensively as entry criteria in clinical trials and for observational studies. This has facilitated generalisability of the results of such studies. Due to a lack of diagnostic criteria for rheumatoid arthritis, the criteria have also been widely used in practice for diagnosis. Furthermore, incidence rates, based on the 1987 criteria, have been reported among different populations, ranging from 0.1 cases per 1,000 for France to 0.5 cases per 1,000 for the USA [13]. Prevalence rates range from 1.8 cases (crude rate) per 1,000 in Yugoslavia to 10.7 cases per 1,000 in the USA.

References

1 Bennett GA, Cobb S, Jacox R, Jessar RA, Ropes MW. Proposed diagnostic criteria for rheumatoid arthritis. *Bull Rheum Dis* 1956;**7**(4):121–4.

2 Cobb S, Merchant WR, Warren JE. An epidemiologic look at the problem of classification in the field of arthritis. *J Chronic Dis* 1955;**2**(1):50–4.

3 Cobb S, Thompson DJ, Rosenbaum J, Warren JE, Merchant WR. On the measurement of prevalence of arthritis and rheumatism from interview data. *J Chronic Dis* 1956;**3**(2):134–9.

4 Ropes MW, Bennett GA, Cobb S, Jacox R, Jessar RA. 1958 Revision of diagnostic criteria for rheumatoid arthritis. *Bull Rheum Dis* 1958;**9**(4):175–6.

5 Lunt M, Symmons DP, Silman AJ. An evaluation of the decision tree format of the American College of Rheumatology 1987 classification criteria for rheumatoid arthritis: performance over five years in a primary care-based prospective study. *Arthritis Rheum* 2005;**52**(8):2277–83.

6 Banal F, Dougados M, Combescure C, Gossec L. Sensitivity and specificity of the American College of Rheumatology 1987 criteria for the diagnosis of rheumatoid arthritis according to disease duration: a systematic literature review and meta-analysis. *Ann Rheum Dis* 2009;**68**(7):1184–91.

7 Combe B, Landewe R, Lukas C, et al. EULAR recommendations for the management of early arthritis: report of a task force of the European Standing Committee for International Clinical Studies Including Therapeutics (ESCISIT). *Ann Rheum Dis* 2007;**66**(1):34–45.

8 Bijlsma JW, Weinblatt ME. Optimal use of methotrexate: the advantages of tight control. *Ann Rheum Dis* 2007;**66**(11):1409–10.

9 Verstappen SM, Symmons DP. What is the outcome of RA in 2011 and can we predict it? *Best Pract Res Clin Rheumatol* 2011;**25**(4):485–96.

10 Aletaha D, Neogi T, Silman AJ, et al. 2010 Rheumatoid arthritis classification criteria: an American College of Rheumatology/European League Against Rheumatism collaborative initiative. *Ann Rheum Dis* 2010;**69**(9):1580–8.

11 Sakellariou G, Scire CA, Zambon A, Caporali R, Montecucco C. Performance of the 2010 classification criteria for rheumatoid arthritis: a systematic literature review and a meta-analysis. *PLoS One* 2013;**8**(2):e56528.

12 Vonkeman HE, van de Laar MA. The new European League Against Rheumatism/American College of Rheumatology diagnostic criteria for rheumatoid arthritis: how are they performing? *Curr Opin Rheumatol* 2013;**25**(3):354–9.

13 Alamanos Y, Voulgari PV, Drosos AA. Incidence and prevalence of rheumatoid arthritis, based on the 1987 American College of Rheumatology criteria: a systematic review. *Semin Arthritis Rheum* 2006;**36**(3):182–8.

Paper 1.4: The global burden of disease

Reference

The Global Burden of Disease Study 2010. *Lancet* 2012:380(9859): 2053–260.

Background

The Global Burden of Diseases, Injuries, and Risk Factors Study (GBD) was launched in 2007 and is a collaboration of 486 scientists from 302 institutes in 50 countries. In 2012 a summary of the methods and findings of the GBD 2010 was published in the Lancet [1–3].

Purpose

1. To assess diseases, injuries, and causes of death, including musculoskeletal disorders (MSD), across the world, and their risk factors.
2. To describe changes in the burden of disease between 1990 and 2010.

Study design

Review of all the relevant data (published and unpublished) concerning the incidence, prevalence, and burden of MSDs.

Methods

The GBD study group, with the help of experts in the field, gathered information on causes of death, diseases, and injuries and their risk factors by age, sex, and geography at specific points in time [4]. Countries were divided into 21 regions, or 7 super-regions, based on 2 criteria: epidemiological homogeneity and geographical contiguity. The burden of disease was estimated for 20 age–sex groups. The group analysed causes of death, years of life lost due to premature mortality (YLLs), years lived with disability (YLDs), and disability adjusted life years DALYs. The construct of DALYs was originally developed by the 1990 GBD group to capture both the prevalence and burden of disease and injury and premature mortality. DALYs were calculated as the sum of YLLs and YLDs. In addition, risk factors for specific diseases and causes of death were evaluated. For each analysis, a major effort was made to define the outcome and introduce a replicable scientific approach to global epidemiological research. Advanced statistical models were used to estimate DALYs, YLLs, and YLDs, and 95% uncertainty intervals were calculated to take into account the heterogeneity in empirical data, and uncertainty in the direct estimation models used when source data were scarce.

Results

Between 1970 and 2010, average life expectancy for both men and women increased from 56.4 years (55.5–57.2) to 67.5 years (66.9–68.1) for men and from 61.2 years (60.2–62.0) to 73.3 years (72.8–73.8) for women [5]. Changes in global and regional mortality rates between 1990 and 2010 from 235 causes of death were estimated for 187 countries. In 2010, there were 52.8 million deaths globally with an age-standardized death rate of 784.5

(756.3–801.6) per 100,000 [6]. The age-standardized death rate for MSDs was estimated to be 1.7 (1.1–2.2) per 100,000 in 1990 and 2.3 (1.7–3.2) per 100,000 in 2010, an increase of 37.8%. This increase was mainly attributable to MSDs other than rheumatoid arthritis, as the age-standardized death rate for rheumatoid arthritis decreased by 9.9% between 1990 and 2010 (respectively, 0.8 (0.6–1.1) vs 0.7 (0.6–1.0) per 100,000).

In addition to death rates and causes of death, it is also important to raise awareness of the prevalence and severity of non-fatal health outcomes from diseases and injuries in the general population in different regions [7]. Among 291 diseases and injuries, MSDs were very common with an estimated global prevalence for men and women of, respectively, low back pain (9.64% vs 8.70%), osteoarthritis of the knee (2.56% vs 4.74%), and other MSDs (7.56% vs 8.73%). Although all cause YLDs remained relatively stable between 1990 and 2010 (%Δ 2.5%), there was a steep increase in YLDs for all investigated MSDs: rheumatoid arthritis (%Δ 13.2%), osteoarthritis (%Δ 26.2%), low back and neck pain (%Δ 9.4%), gout (%Δ 14.9%), and other MSDs (%Δ 11.3%).

By combining YLL and YLD data, DALYs were calculated to assess the overall burden of diseases [8]. For both men and women, the impact of MSDs compared to other diseases is especially noticeable in the population aged over 40 years (Figure 1.2). MSDs accounted for 6.8 of DALYs, with low back pain accounting for about 50%, neck pain 20%, osteoarthritis 10%, and rheumatoid arthritis for approximately 3% of MSD DALYs. In the last two decades, among 291 diseases, MSDs ranked higher in 2010 compared to 1990, and the percentage increases in DALYs are as follows: low back pain (%Δ 9.7%), neck pain (%Δ 8.5%), osteoarthritis (%Δ 26.2%), and rheumatoid arthritis (%Δ 11.1%). The ranking varies by region, and MSDs are ranked higher in high-income Asia Pacific, Western Europe, Australasia, high-income North America, Central Europe, Southern Latin America, Eastern Europe, East Asia, and Central America compared to Central and East Asia and Africa.

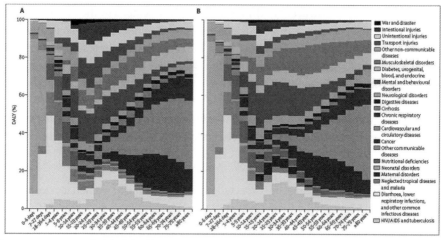

Fig. 1.2 Percentage of global disability-adjusted life years by age, sex, and cause in 2010. Distribution of disability-adjusted life years for male individuals (A) and female individuals (B); DALY, disability-adjusted life years.

Identification of risk factors for diseases will help in the development of prevention programmes [9]. In general, the most common risk factors for diseases and injuries are those associated with poverty and those that affect children. Risk factors related to MSDs were limited and included high body mass index and a diet high in sugar-sweetened beverages, both associated with osteoarthritis and low back pain. Interestingly, smoking, one of the major risk factors for developing rheumatoid arthritis, was not reported [10, 11].

Critique of the study

These estimates represent a tremendous amount of work for the scientists involved. They will have been hampered by the lack of contemporary data for many regions, and by contradictory results from studies from the same region. Then there is the challenge of developing and implementing a measure of disability and disease burden which is applicable across the whole range of human disease, the whole age span, and regions with very different health systems. This is especially challenging for diseases which are slowly progressive, as opposed to conditions which are life changing (e.g. limb trauma) but then stable.

Significance and importance of the study

The papers included in this special issue of *The Lancet* are a major contribution to researchers, health policy makers, world health organizations, and the general public in understanding the global burden of disease, injury, and its risk factors. These findings will help us to understand the impact of diseases and injuries across different regions in the world and the need of specific intervention programmes. These papers also emphasize the growing burden of MSDs. Although the death rate for rheumatoid arthritis has decreased by ~10% over the last two decades, DALYs have increased. There is also a considerable increase in DALYs for neck and back pain and osteoarthritis. The latter may partly be explained by an aging population and an increase in body mass index, especially in high-income regions.

References

1 **GBD 2010 country results: a global public good**. *Lancet* 2013;**381**(9871):965–70.

2 **Horton R**. GBD 2010: understanding disease, injury, and risk. *Lancet* 2012;**380**(9859):2053–4.

3 **Murray CJ, Ezzati M, Flaxman AD, et al**. GBD 2010: a multi-investigator collaboration for global comparative descriptive epidemiology. *Lancet* 2012;**380**(9859):2055–8.

4 **Murray CJ, Ezzati M, Flaxman AD, et al**. GBD 2010: design, definitions, and metrics. *Lancet* 2012;**380**(9859):2063–6.

5 **Salomon JA, Wang H, Freeman MK, et al**. Healthy life expectancy for 187 countries, 1990–2010: a systematic analysis for the Global Burden Disease Study 2010. *Lancet* 2012;**380**(9859):2144–62.

6 **Lozano R, Naghavi M, Foreman K, et al**. Global and regional mortality from 235 causes of death for 20 age groups in 1990 and 2010: a systematic analysis for the Global Burden of Disease Study 2010. *Lancet* 2012;**380**(9859):2095–128.

7 **Vos T, Flaxman AD, Naghavi M, et al**. Years lived with disability (YLDs) for 1160 sequelae of 289 diseases and injuries 1990–2010: a systematic analysis for the Global Burden of Disease Study 2010. *Lancet* 2012;**380**(9859):2163–96.

8 **Murray CJ, Vos T, Lozano R, et al**. Disability-adjusted life years (DALYs) for 291 diseases and injuries in 21 regions, 1990–2010: a systematic analysis for the Global Burden of Disease Study 2010. *Lancet* 2012;**380**(9859):2197–223.

9 **Lim SS, Vos T, Flaxman AD, et al**. A comparative risk assessment of burden of disease and injury attributable to 67 risk factors and risk factor clusters in 21 regions, 1990–2010: a systematic analysis for the Global Burden of Disease Study 2010. *Lancet* 2012;**380**(9859):2224–60.

10 **Sugiyama D, Nishimura K, Tamaki K, et al**. Impact of smoking as a risk factor for developing rheumatoid arthritis: a meta-analysis of observational studies. *Ann Rheum Dis* 2010;**69**(1):70–81.

11 **Lahiri M, Luben RN, Morgan C, et al**. Using lifestyle factors to identify individuals at higher risk of inflammatory polyarthritis (results from the European Prospective Investigation of Cancer-Norfolk and the Norfolk Arthritis Register—the EPIC-2-NOAR Study). *Ann Rheum Dis* 2014;**73**(1):219–26.

Paper 1.5: The shared epitope hypothesis

Reference

Gregersen PK, Silver J, Winchester RJ. The shared epitope hypothesis. An approach to understanding the molecular genetics of susceptibility to rheumatoid arthritis. *Arthritis Rheum* 1987;30(11):1205–13.

The major histocompatibility complex

The molecules of the human leukocyte antigen (HLA) interact with the immune system to discriminate self from non-self. The HLA molecules bind peptide antigens and present them to T-lymphocytes. Crucial to this role is the three-dimensional structure of the HLA molecules, as it determines peptide and T-cell binding (Figure 1.3).

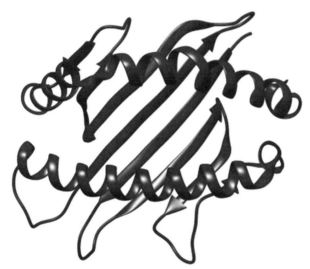

Fig. 1.3 Three-dimensional diagram of human leukocyte antigen B. This structure is based on Protein Data Bank entry 3bvp. This figure was prepared using UCSF Chimera.

The HLA molecules are encoded in a gene-rich region of chromosome 6 known as the major histocompatibility complex (MHC). There is a vast amount of genetic variation (polymorphism) within the MHC, enabling the HLA molecules to bind to a variety of peptides; the *MHC* genes are among the most polymorphic human genes.

There are two subgroups of HLA molecules: Class I includes HLA-A, B, and C. They bind to the membrane of all nucleated cells. Class II molecules include HLA-DR, DQ, and DP and are present on the cell surface of antigen-presenting cells predominantly (including B lymphocytes, macrophages, and dendritic cells). Class II molecule expression can also be induced during inflammation on cell types that normally have little or no expression. A Class II molecule is composed of an α chain and a β chain. Class I molecules contain an α chain encoded within the MHC and a β_2 microglobulin which is encoded elsewhere (Figure 1.4). Class II molecules present processed peptide fragments to CD4 T-lymphocytes, a process which, in health, causes both activation and proliferation of T-lymphocytes if non-self is presented, or anergy, whereby the T-lymphocyte is functionally inactivated if self is presented.

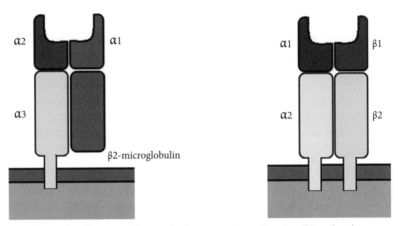

Fig. 1.4 Two-dimensional image of human leukocyte antigen Class I and II molecules.

HLA Class II genetics

Genes (such as *HLA-DRA* and *HLA-DRB*) within the MHC code for both the α (heavy) and β (light) chains. The DQ and DP antigens have highly variable (polymorphic) α and β chains which can unite in numerous combinations. The DR antigens share an essentially non-polymorphic α chain, while the β chain remains highly polymorphic. The number of *DR* genes that are expressed can also vary between individuals. In some cases, two DR molecules are expressed; both will express the same non-polymorphic DR-α chain but one will express the β chain encoded by the *DRB1* gene and the other will express a β chain encoded by a second *DR* locus, called *DRB3, DRB4, DRB5*, etc.

As the technology used to classify *HLA* genes has evolved over the years, so has the nomenclature for the different alleles at individual *HLA* genes. The original nomenclature was based upon immunological techniques. With the advent of gene sequencing methods, it was possible to further classify *HLA* genes into subtypes which required revision of the nomenclature.

HLA association with rheumatoid arthritis

With respect to HLA and rheumatoid arthritis, much focus has been on the *HLA-DR* locus. Astorga et al. first suggested that HLA subtypes may be associated with rheumatoid arthritis in 1969 [1]. They established that the lymphocytes from two different individuals with rheumatoid arthritis were frequently nonstimulatory and therefore expressed similar HLA Class II molecules. Further work established that *HLA-DR4* alleles are associated with rheumatoid arthritis [2, 3]. Within the HLA-DRβ chain, there are three highly variable regions (hypervariable regions) which distinguish between the DR subtypes. The third hypervariable region is located between amino acids 68–77 and is a major site of variation defining the *DR4* allele (Figure 1.5), and sequence differences in this region affect T-cell function [4].

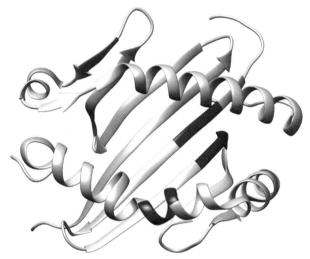

Fig. 1.5 Three-dimensional diagram of the human leukocyte antigen DRB chain illustrating the three hypervariable regions (dark coloured). This structure is based on Protein Data Bank entry 3pdo. This figure was prepared using UCSF Chimera.

However, *HLA-DR4* is neither necessary nor sufficient for the development of rheumatoid arthritis. Other alleles such as *HLA-DR1* also confer an increased susceptibility to rheumatoid arthritis. This has led to the shared epitope hypothesis [5].

Significance and importance of this paper

The shared epitope hypothesis aims to explain the association of multiple *HLA* alleles with rheumatoid arthritis. Gregersen et al. described the results of previous research as evidence for their shared epitope hypothesis. Three subtypes of *HLA-DR4* (historically named *Dw4*, *Dw6*, and *Dw14*) were strongly associated with rheumatoid arthritis, whereas a fourth subtype (*Dw10*) was not. Gregersen et al. compared the sequences of HLA alleles associated with rheumatoid arthritis and discovered a region of shared amino acid sequence in the third hypervariable region (Figure 1.5). This led to the shared epitope hypothesis, which proposed that this shared amino acid sequence conferred a proportion of risk for the development of rheumatoid arthritis.

The shared epitope hypothesis provides a vital clue to the pathogenesis of rheumatoid arthritis. The epitope is vital in binding specific peptides which may stimulate the development of inappropriate T-lymphocyte activation leading to rheumatoid arthritis.

References

1 **Astorga GP, Williams RC Jr.** Altered reactivity in mixed lymphocyte culture of lymphocytes from patients with rheumatoid arthritis. *Arthritis Rheum* 1969;**12**(6):547–54.

2 **Stastny P.** Association of the B-cell alloantigen DRw4 with rheumatoid arthritis. *N Engl J Med* 1978;**298**(16):869–71.

3 **Gibofsky A, Winchester RJ, Patarroyo M, Fotino M, Kunkel HG.** Disease associations of the Ia-like human alloantigens. Contrasting patterns in rheumatoid arthritis and systemic lupus erythematosus. *J Exp Med* 1978;**148**(6):1728–32.

4 **Mengle-Gaw L, Conner S, McDevitt HO, Fathman CG.** Gene conversion between murine class II major histocompatibility complex loci. Functional and molecular evidence from the bm 12 mutant. *J Exp Med* 1984;**160**(4):1184–94.

5 **Legrand L, Lathrop GM, Marcelli-Barge A, et al.** HLA-DR genotype risks in seropositive rheumatoid arthritis. *Am J Hum Genet* 1984;**36**(3):690–9.

Paper 1.6: The association between protein tyrosine phosphatase 22 and rheumatoid arthritis

Reference

Begovich AB, Carlton VEH, Honigberg LA, et al. A missense single-nucleotide polymorphism in a gene encoding a protein tyrosine phosphatase (*PTPN22*) is associated with rheumatoid arthritis. *Am J Genet* 2004;75(2);330–7.

Background

Until 2004, *HLA-DRB1* was the only genetic variant known to be consistently associated with rheumatoid arthritis.

Hypothesis

Genetic variants (single-nucleotide polymorphisms (SNPs)) outside the HLA region are associated with rheumatoid arthritis and explain some of the heritability of the disease.

Study design

This report describes a genetic case–control association study comparing the genotype frequency of 87 candidate SNPs between rheumatoid arthritis cases and controls.

Study participants

In Phase 1, 475 patients with rheumatoid arthritis, who fulfilled the 1987 American Rheumatism Association/American College of Rheumatology criteria and who were exclusively rheumatoid factor (RF) positive, were recruited. Patients were matched 1:1 to healthy controls according to sex, age, and ethnicity (grandparental country/region of origin). In Phase 2, the replication cohort, 463 patients with rheumatoid arthritis fulfilling the 1987 criteria and who were RF positive or negative were recruited. Patients were matched 1:2 to healthy controls according to sex, age, and ethnicity (grandparental country/region of origin). DNA was extracted from both patients and controls and was analysed for 87 candidate SNPs. All participants were Caucasian and North American.

Results

A candidate SNP (rs2476601) located in the gene *PTPN22* was significantly associated with rheumatoid arthritis in Phase 1 (P = 6.6×10^{-4}). The SNP encodes for an amino acid change from arginine (R) to tryptophan (W) at amino acid position 620 (R620W). There are therefore two forms of the PTPN22 protein (620R and 620W). The 620W SNP was associated with an increased risk of rheumatoid arthritis (P = 6.6×10^{-4}, odds ratio (OR) 1.65, 95% CI, 1.23–2.20). In Phase 2, the replication phase, the association was much stronger (P = 5.6×10^{-8}, OR 1.97, 95% CI 1.55–2.50). The SNP was not associated with rheumatoid arthritis in the RF-negative cohort. Having two copies of 620W more than doubled the risk of rheumatoid arthritis. The analysis adjusted for the presence/absence of the *HLA-DRB1* genotype and showed that the association of *PTPN22* with rheumatoid arthritis remained, thus demonstrating an independent effect.

The R620W SNP alters the amino acid code of the PTPN22 protein. This may significantly affect protein folding and therefore the function of the protein and its ability to bind to any substrate. In health, PTPN22 binds to the tyrosine kinase Csk and is responsible for transmitting signals from outside the cell to the nucleus to help control the activity of T-lymphocytes [1]. The authors showed that PTPN22 is present in other haematopoietic cells, including cells of the immune system such as B-lymphocytes, monocytes, neutrophils, dendritic cells, and natural killer cells.

Using Jurkat cells (immortalized T-lymphocytes), the authors also showed that T-lymphocytes with reduced PTPN22 levels have increased levels of stimulation, confirming that PTPN22 is a negative regulator of T-lymphocyte activation. In a further experiment, the authors found that PTPN22 620W had lower affinity for Csk than the 620R form did, demonstrating that the SNP affects binding to Csk and therefore function.

Critique of the paper

This study, published in 2004, was an exceptionally well-conducted genetic study which included an independent validation cohort to ensure the results were robust. The study linked the genetic association with independent functional results showing that PTPN22 is central to T-lymphocyte activation. The study controlled for confounding factors such as ethnicity and the presence of *HLA-DRB1*.

Significance and importance of the paper

The authors demonstrated the first significant genetic association, outside the HLA region, with rheumatoid arthritis. The study showed that the 620W SNP affects PTPN22 function and protein binding and that PTPN22 is present in cells of the immune system. The results excitingly showed that 620W is not associated with RF-negative disease, suggesting that RF-positive and RF-negative diseases are genetically dissimilar and may have important differences in pathogenesis. Since the publication of this paper, genetic variants in *PTPN22* have been found to be associated with Grave's disease, myasthenia gravis, and Addison's disease, suggesting a strong role in autoimmunity [2–4].

References

1 Hill RJ, Zozulya S, Lu Y-L, Ward K, Gishizky M, Jallal B. The lymphoid protein tyrosine phosphatase Lyp interacts with the adaptor molecule Grb2 and functions as a negative regulator of T-cell activation. *Exp Hematol* 2002;**30**(3):237–44.

2 Skorka A, Bednarczuk T, Bar-Andziak E, Nauman J, Ploski R. Lymphoid tyrosine phosphatase (PTPN22/LYP) variant and Graves' disease in a Polish population: association and gene dose-dependent correlation with age of onset. *Clin Endocrinol (Oxf)* 2005;**62**(6):679–82.

3 Vandiedonck C, Capdevielle C, Giraud M, et al. Association of the PTPN22*R620W polymorphism with autoimmune myasthenia gravis. *Ann Neurol* 2006;**59**(2):404–7.

4 Skinningsrud B, Husebye ES, Gervin K, et al. Mutation screening of PTPN22: association of the 1858T-allele with Addison's disease. *Eur J Hum Genet* 2008;**16**(8):977–82.

Paper 1.7: The Wellcome Trust genome-wide association study of rheumatoid arthritis

Reference

Wellcome Trust Case Control Consortium. Genome-wide association study of 14,000 cases of seven common diseases and 3,000 shared controls. *Nature* 2007;447 (7145):661–78.

Background

Prior to this study, genetic investigations were largely limited to candidate gene studies—representing a best guess for hypothesis generation. By 2007, there had been a major technological advance, allowing association testing across the whole of the genome in a hypothesis-free investigation. The Affymetrix GeneChip 500K Mapping Array Set can genotype over 500,000 genetic variants across the genome. Recognizing the importance of large cohorts to detect genetic variants with low effect sizes, collaborations were formed to increase cohort size. The Wellcome Trust Case Control Consortium (WTCCC) was formed by over 50 research groups in the UK to investigate the genetics of human disease. The WTCCC simultaneously investigated seven diseases, including rheumatoid arthritis, to determine the genetic differences and similarities to susceptibility in these diseases. This study represents the first genome-wide association study in rheumatoid arthritis.

Purpose

To identify which, out of 500,000 SNPs tested, were associated with rheumatoid arthritis.

Study design

Hypothesis-free case–control genetic association testing was carried out, comparing the genotype frequencies of more than 500,000 SNPs between 2,000 cases and 3,000 controls. The study had an 80% power to detect a relative risk of 1.5 at significance level $P < 5 \times 10^{-7}$.

Study participants

Cases comprised 2,000 Caucasian individuals who were over the age of 18 years old and who satisfied the 1987 criteria for rheumatoid arthritis. Controls comprised 1,500 participants who were derived from the 1958 British Birth Cohort. This cohort represents a subset of samples from all births in England, Wales, and Scotland during one week in 1958 and contains those who are of self-reported white ethnicity. Participants were aged 44–45 years at the time of venepuncture. Another 1,500 anonymized controls aged 18–69 years were derived from blood donors recruited from the UK Blood Transfusion Service.

Results

This study confirmed the association of *PTPN22* variants and *HLA-DRβ1* with rheumatoid arthritis at genome-wide significance levels ($P = 4.9 \times 10^{-26}$ and 2.6×10^{-27}, respectively). The study also revealed nine novel SNPs associated with rheumatoid arthritis at significance levels between 1×10^{-5} and 5×10^{-7}.

Critique of the paper

A concern of the study design is that the controls from the 1958 British Birth Cohort were aged 44–45 at the time of DNA extraction. It is therefore possible that a significant number of controls may go on to develop rheumatoid arthritis over time, reducing the power of the study to detect association. The authors attempted to control for this by recruiting control groups from two different sources to reduce the potential of misclassification bias. This reduces the number of people likely to develop rheumatoid arthritis by including those with a range of ages, limiting the impact misclassification bias would have.

A further disadvantage of the study is the lack of an independent replication cohort confirming the novel associations. However, since its publication, association has been replicated for the majority of variants associated with rheumatoid arthritis [1–3]. The lack of separation of rheumatoid arthritis into seropositive disease and seronegative disease is a weakness, as it has previously been shown that the genetics of seropositive disease and seronegative disease are different, such as with respect to *PTPN22* variants [4].

The quality control of the genetic data was commendable. The risk of contamination of samples was reduced by excluding samples with a high genotype failure rate. Rare variants were excluded from the analysis; as the study was not powered to detect a difference between cases and controls for variants which are rare, including these in the study would have increased the risk of a false-positive result (Type 1 statistical error). Individuals who were detected as being related to each other through genetic analysis were excluded from the study. The authors also confirmed that there was no significant genetic variation between the two control groups and so controlled for any undetected population stratification.

Significance and importance of the paper

This paper represents a major advance in the discovery of the genetic causes of rheumatoid arthritis. The authors recruited the largest cohort for its time and utilized genome-wide scanning for hypothesis-free testing to establish SNPs associating with rheumatoid arthritis. The quality control methods used in this paper are still employed today.

References

1 Thomson W, Barton A, Ke X, et al. Rheumatoid arthritis association at 6q23. *Nat Genet* 2007;**39**(12):1431–3.

2 Stahl EA, Raychaudhuri S, Remmers EF, et al. Genome-wide association study meta-analysis identifies seven new rheumatoid arthritis risk loci. *Nat Genet* 2010;**42**(6):508–14.

3 Terao C, Yamada R, Ohmura K, et al. The human AIRE gene at chromosome 21q22 is a genetic determinant for the predisposition to rheumatoid arthritis in Japanese population. *Hum Mol Genet* 2011;**20**(13):2680–5.

4 Begovich AB, Carlton VEH, Honigberg LA, et al. A missense single-nucleotide polymorphism in a gene encoding a protein tyrosine phosphatase (PTPN22) is associated with rheumatoid arthritis. *Am J Hum Genet* 2004;**75**(2):330–7.

Paper 1.8: Five amino acids in three proteins encoded by MHC genes explain most of the association between the MHC locus and seropositive rheumatoid arthritis

Reference

Raychaudhuri S, Sandor C, Stahl EA, et al. Five amino acids in three HLA proteins explain most of the association between MHC and seropositive rheumatoid arthritis. *Nat Genet* 2012;44(3):291–6.

Background

The shared epitope is a five amino acid sequence located within HLA-DRβ1 [1]. This region explains a large proportion of genetic susceptibility to anti-citrullinated protein antibody (ACPA)-positive rheumatoid arthritis, contributing to up to 50% of the genetic component for rheumatoid arthritis [2]. Further investigation of other variants within the MHC locus has been slow due to technological constraints. Direct genotyping of HLA genes is expensive, and variants are often inherited together (linkage disequilibrium), thereby masking the true disease-causing variant. Imputation is a statistical technique designed to indirectly genotype samples, thus reducing costs. Data from a reference cohort can be used to infer or impute missing genotypes in a population under investigation through calculations based on the likelihood of a particular set of genotypes or haplotype, thereby determining the most likely HLA alleles.

Hypothesis

Other variants within the MHC locus, outside the shared epitope, contribute to disease susceptibility in ACPA-positive rheumatoid arthritis.

Study design

A genetic case–control association study imputing the likely HLA alleles and comparing the frequencies between cases and controls.

Study participants

In Phase 1, genotype data were obtained from six independent genome-wide association studies from the UK, Sweden, Canada, and the USA. All cases were ACPA positive and fulfilled the 1987 criteria for rheumatoid arthritis. The total sample size was 19,992 individuals of self-reported European descent, comprising 5,018 ACPA-positive cases and 14,974 controls. Missing HLA alleles were imputed from a reference panel collected by the Type 1 Diabetes Genetics Consortium (T1DGC) [3]. Phase 2 consisted of a replication group of 616 South Korean ACPA-positive rheumatoid arthritis samples and 675 South Korean healthy controls.

Results

The accuracy of the imputation procedure was assessed by comparing the imputed *HLA-DRβ1* alleles in a subset that had been previously directly genotyped. The results demonstrated a 95.8% accuracy of the imputation procedure within this subset of individuals. This validates imputation as a cost-effective measure to indirectly genotype individuals across the MHC region.

Comparison of the frequencies of HLA alleles showed that five amino-acid sequence changes in three HLA proteins were strongly associated with the risk of developing ACPA-positive rheumatoid arthritis when controlling for the strongest associated effect, indicating an independent effect, as shown in Table 1.5.

Table 1.5 Strongest independent associations between *HLA* genes and rheumatoid arthritis

Class	*HLA gene*	Amino-acid position	Amino acid	Odds ratio	P value
2	DRβ1	11	Valine	3.7	$<10^{-526}$
		71	Lysine	2.0	5.6×10^{-38}*
		74	Alanine	2.1	1.5×10^{-11}†
1	B	9	Aspartic acid	2.1	$<2 \times 10^{-37}$‡
2	DPβ1	9	Phenylalanine	1.4	$<10^{-20}$§

* Conditioning for the effects of amino acid 11.

† Conditioning for the effects of amino acids 11 and 71.

‡ Conditioning for the effects of amino acids 11, 71, and 74.

§ Conditioning for the effects of HLA-DRβ1 and HLA-β.

Source data from Raychaudhuri S, Sandor C, Stahl EA et al. Five amino acids in three HLA proteins explain most of the association between MHC and seropositive rheumatoid arthritis. *Nat Genetics* 2012; 44 (3): 291–6.

Amino acid 11 maps away from the shared epitope positions that were previously discovered (amino-acid position 71–74). The results validate that genetic variants within the shared epitope are independently associated with disease susceptibility.

In Phase 2, the authors used genome-wide SNP data and *HLA-DRβ1* genotypes that were derived from direct resequencing and confirmed that amino acid 11 was significantly associated with ACPA-positive rheumatoid arthritis ($P = 6.1 \times 10^{-36}$).

Interestingly, the amino acids associated with rheumatoid arthritis are located within the peptide-binding grooves of HLA-DRβ, HLA-β, and HLA-DPβ, as shown in Figure 1.6. This region of the HLA molecule is vital in antigen presentation; thus, this observation implies that the genetic variants have a significant functional impact.

Critique of the paper

The major strength of this paper is the use of a large cohort of cases and controls, with independent replication of results. The paper confirmed associations at amino-acid positions 71 and 74 which had originally been described over two decades ago.

The study utilized imputation in order to reduce the cost of direct genotyping. Crucially, the authors validated this procedure by determining its accuracy in a subset of individuals who had been previously directly genotyped for *HLA-DRβ1* alleles.

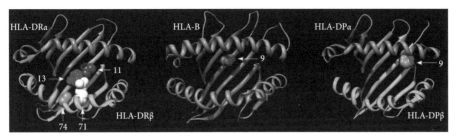

Fig. 1.6 Three-dimensional diagram of HLA-DR, HLA-B, and HLA-DP proteins. Key amino-acid positions associated with rheumatoid arthritis are highlighted.

Reprinted by permission from Macmillan Publishers Ltd: Nature Genetics, Soumya Raychaudhuri et al, Five amino acids in three HLA proteins explain most of the association between MHC and seropositive rheumatoid arthritis, Vol 44, Copyright 2012.

While the paper discusses the location of the amino acids and their importance in antigen presentation, no functional impact was explored or investigated to determine if the genotype affected the observed phenotype.

Significance and importance of the paper

This paper has renewed interest in the shared epitope hypothesis, which was first suggested over two decades ago. The study demonstrated significant association, not just within the shared epitope, but also outside this region, demonstrating multiple independent effects, some of which were stronger than that of the shared epitope. Of the genetic variants discovered, all lie within the peptide-binding groove of the HLA molecule, an observation implying that antigen presentation is a significant component of pathogenesis involved in the development of ACPA-positive rheumatoid arthritis.

References

1 Gregersen PK, Silver J, Winchester RJ. The shared epitope hypothesis. An approach to understanding the molecular genetics of susceptibility to rheumatoid arthritis. *Arthritis Rheum* 1987;**30**(11):1205–13.
2 Bowes J, Barton A. Recent advances in the genetics of RA susceptibility. *Rheumatology* 2008;**47**(4):399–402.
3 Brown WM, Pierce J, Hilner JE, et al. Overview of the MHC fine mapping data. *Diabetes Obes Metab* 2009;**11**(Suppl 1):2–7.

Paper 1.9: High-density genetic mapping identifies new susceptibility loci for rheumatoid arthritis

Reference

Eyre S, Bowes J, Diogo D, et al. High-density genetic mapping identifies new susceptibility loci for rheumatoid arthritis *Nat Genet* 2012;44(3):291–6.

Background

Prior to this study, 32 regions of the genome (loci) had been shown to be associated with rheumatoid arthritis. Most of these loci were discovered through genome-wide association studies using commercially available genotyping chips. However, current commercial genotyping chips can only highlight regions that are associated with disease—the denser the genotype markers, the more sensitive the chip is to find genetic variants associated with disease. There is therefore a need for fine-mapping studies, to focus on regions of interest and densely genotype these regions to discover the true disease-causing variants. Autoimmune diseases can cluster in families or even in an individual [1]. This phenomenon suggests that there are genetic markers that increase the overall risk of autoimmune diseases rather than there being disease-specific loci. Testing for these genetic markers in a cohort of individuals with rheumatoid arthritis may identify new variants associated with rheumatoid arthritis.

Purpose

1. To conduct a fine-mapping study to define more precisely the genetic regions of association to rheumatoid arthritis.

2. To genotype markers known to increase risk of other autoimmune diseases in a cohort of patients with rheumatoid arthritis, in order to investigate if there are polymorphisms that increase the overall risk of autoimmune disease.

3. To investigate the genetics of ACPA-positive and ACPA-negative rheumatoid arthritis.

Study design

A customized Illumina genotyping array was designed that contained all known SNPs from resequencing studies in order to fine-map regions of association, and SNPs associated with 12 autoimmune diseases.

Study participants

Samples from 11,475 rheumatoid arthritis cases from 6 cohorts were utilized (UK, USA, The Netherlands, Spain, and two Swedish cohorts). The ACPA status of all rheumatoid arthritis cases was known. Samples from 15,870 healthy controls served as the comparison group. DNA of the cases and controls was tested for 129,464 SNPs, and the results were combined with previous genotyping results from genome-wide association study data in a meta-analysis.

Results

Fourteen new loci associated with rheumatoid arthritis were discovered. These new loci accounted for 4% of the heritability of rheumatoid arthritis, increasing the estimated heritability of rheumatoid arthritis to 51%. The authors confirmed the association of amino acid position 11 of HLA-DRB1 through imputation in ACPA-positive patients (P < 1 × 10^{-677}), amino acid positions 71 and 74, and HLA-DPB1 amino acid position 9 (P = 1 × 10^{-17}), as associated with ACPA-positive rheumatoid arthritis independently, validating the work by Raychaudhuri et al. [2].

Five loci were found to have significantly stronger association with ACPA-positive disease than with ACPA-negative disease (*PTPN22*, *CCR6*, *CD40*, *RASGRP1*, and *TAGAP*), indicating that there are substantial genetic differences between ACPA-negative rheumatoid arthritis and ACPA-positive rheumatoid arthritis. Fine-mapping of the previously associated SNPs revealed that 12 loci positions shifted and, for 19 loci, association was refined to a single gene, specifically implicating these genes in the pathogenesis of rheumatoid arthritis.

Excitingly, a non-synonymous SNP in the *IL-6R* gene which alters the amino acid sequence was associated with rheumatoid arthritis (P = 1.3×10^{-8}). IL-6R is a target for the drug tocilizumab, which is already licensed for use in the treatment of rheumatoid arthritis. This work provides proof of concept that studying the genetics of complex diseases may lead to novel targets of treatment.

Critique of the paper

A disadvantage of Immunochip genotyping is the lack of coverage of the whole genome. As a fine-mapping experiment, it is designed to characterize regions of previous association. However, the genotyping is not genome wide and only targets regions previously known to be associated with autoimmune diseases; this approach may therefore miss novel regions that are associated with disease.

Significance and importance of the paper

This pioneering paper characterized over 40% of the known susceptibility loci to rheumatoid arthritis, in one analysis. The work has validated the multiple associations at the *HLA-DR* and *DP* loci and has fine-mapped disease loci, implicating certain gene products in the susceptibility to rheumatoid arthritis and giving us vital clues to the pathogenesis of disease. Importantly, the results of this paper demonstrate that adequately powered genetic studies of complex diseases may, in the future, lead to novel targets for treatment.

References

1 **Anaya JM, Corena R, Castiblanco J, Rojas-Villarraga A, Shoenfeld Y**. The kaleidoscope of autoimmunity: multiple autoimmune syndromes and familial autoimmunity. *Expert Rev Clin Immunol* 2007;**3**(4):623–35.

2 **Raychaudhuri S, Sandor C, Stahl EA, et al**. Five amino acids in three HLA proteins explain most of the association between MHC and seropositive rheumatoid arthritis. *Nat Genet* 2012;**44**(3):291–6.

Paper 1.10: Gene–environment interaction in the aetiology of rheumatoid arthritis

Reference

Padyukov L, Silva C, Stolot P, et al. A gene–environment interaction between smoking and shared epitope genes in HLA-DR provides a high risk of seropositive rheumatoid arthritis. *Arthritis Rheum* 2004;50(10):3085–92.

Background

With time, an increasing number of genetic markers and environmental factors which increase an individual's risk of rheumatoid arthritis have been identified.

Purpose

1. To investigate whether there is an interaction between the genes which confer the highest risk for rheumatoid arthritis (the genes encoding the shared epitope in HLA-DR) and cigarette smoking, a known environmental risk factor for rheumatoid arthritis [1].

2. To establish whether any interaction between the shared epitope genes and smoking varies between RF-positive rheumatoid arthritis cases and RF-negative rheumatoid arthritis cases.

Study design

This report describes a population-based case–control study.

Study participants

Between May 1996 and February 2001, all newly diagnosed cases of rheumatoid arthritis (who satisfied the 1987 criteria for rheumatoid arthritis and were aged 18–70 years) in mid- and southern Sweden were invited to participate in a study of early rheumatoid arthritis. This analysis includes 858 cases (612 women) who completed a questionnaire covering demographic and lifestyle factors and gave a blood sample for DNA and RF analysis. Sixty-four per cent of the women and 66% of the men were RF positive. For each potential case, a control, matched for age, sex, and residential area, was selected at random from the national population register. Controls were asked to complete the same questionnaire and give a blood sample. Controls who declined to participate were replaced. A total of 1,048 controls (736 women) were included in the analysis. The DNA samples were tested for the *HLA-DRB1*0101* and *HLA-DRB4* alleles.

Logistic regression was used to compare the odds of RF-positive rheumatoid arthritis, RF-negative rheumatoid arthritis, and total rheumatoid arthritis, in subjects with different genotypes and smoking status (current vs never). The study design permitted the ORs to be interpreted as relative risks (RRs). Matched and unmatched analyses were conducted but only the unmatched analysis (adjusted for age, sex, and residential area) is presented in the paper. Interaction between genotype and smoking status was assessed using departure from additivity of effects as the criterion of interaction [2]. This was quantified by estimating the attributable proportion (AP) of incidence due to the interaction between the risk factors (i.e. smoking and the shared epitope) in individuals exposed to both risk factors [3].

Results

Twenty-seven per cent of the rheumatoid arthritis cases and 23% of the controls were current smokers. The adjusted RR of developing rheumatoid arthritis was 1.5 (95% CI, 1.2–2.0) in current smokers versus 'never smokers'. This risk was confined to RF-positive rheumatoid arthritis; the adjusted RR for RF-positive rheumatoid arthritis was 2.2 (96% CI, 1.7–3.0) and the adjusted RR for RF-negative rheumatoid arthritis was 0.8 (95% CI, 0.6–1.2).

Both a single and a double copy of the shared epitope were associated with the development of RF-positive but not of RF-negative rheumatoid arthritis, in both men and women. Overall, being positive for the shared epitope was associated with an RR of 2.8 (95% CI, 2.1–3.8) of RF-positive rheumatoid arthritis in women, and 4.8 (95% CI, 2.9–7.8) in men.

Among current smokers with one or more shared epitope genes, the RR of developing RF-positive rheumatoid arthritis was 7.5 (95% CI, 4.2–13.1; i.e. higher than either risk factor alone, or the two added together; Table 1.6). The AP for interaction was 0.4 (95% CI, 0.2–0.7). The interaction was even more pronounced in smokers with two copies of the shared epitope. The same pattern was seen in men and women. Smoking, the shared epitope, or the combination did not increase the risk of RF-negative rheumatoid arthritis.

Critique of the paper

The response rate for this study among both cases (95%) and controls (83%) for completion of the questionnaire was high. Most of the cases (98%) but only 60% of the controls provided a blood sample—raising the possibility of selection bias among the controls. Only controls who completed the questionnaire were asked to provide a blood sample and there was no difference in smoking status between controls who did and did not provide a blood sample. It is difficult to see that shared epitope status could have influenced response among the controls. The analysis was restricted to current smokers versus never smokers. The authors had previously explored the effect of prior smoking and cumulative smoking exposure on rheumatoid arthritis risk in this same cohort but not in the context of genetic stratification [4].

Significance of the paper

This is the first study to show an interaction between genetic and environmental factors—thus bringing together two different areas of enquiry in the aetiology of rheumatoid arthritis. It is of interest that the interaction is demonstrated statistically rather than in the test tube. Further laboratory work will be required to establish the underlying mechanism whereby smoking can trigger RF production and rheumatoid arthritis in genetically susceptible individuals. The observation provides further support for the hypothesis that RF-positive rheumatoid arthritis and RF-negative rheumatoid arthritis have different genetic and environment risk factors, and it has important implications for targeted disease prevention.

Table 1.6 Relative risk of developing rheumatoid arthritis and rheumatic factor-positive rheumatoid arthritis and rheumatic factor-negative rheumatoid arthritis among all male and female subjects exposed to different combinations of cigarette smoking habits and shared epitope genes, and attributable proportion due to interactions between cigarette smoking and shared epitope genes (single, double, or any)*

	No SE		Single SE		Double SE		Any SE	
	Cases/controls	RR(95% CI)	Cases/controls	RR(95% CI)	Cases/controls	RR(95% CI)	Cases/controls	RR(95% CI)
RF-positive RA†								
Never smokers	26/86	1.0	68/104	2.4 (1.4–4.2)	35/31	4.2 (2.1–8.3)	103/135	2.8 (1.6–4.8)
Current smokers	40/60	2.4 (1.3–4.6)	77/57	5.5 (3.0–10.0)	53/14	15.7 (7.2–34.2)	130/71	7.5 (4.2–13.1)
AP				0.3 (0.0–0.7)		0.6 (0.4–0.9)		0.4 (0.2–0.7)
RF-negative RA†								
Never smokers	53/86	1.0	59/104	0.9 (0.6–1.5)	14/31	0.7 (0.4–1.6)	73/135	0.9 (0.6–1.4)
Current smokers	20/60	0.6 (0.3–1.1)	30/57	0.9 (0.5–1.7)	10/14	1.2 (0.5–3.0)	40/71	1.0 (0.6–1.7)

*Values are the relative risk (RR) and 95% confidence interval (95% CI) as compared with 'never smokers' without shared epitope genes. Cases/controls are the number of exposed cases/number of exposed controls; AP, attributable proportion; RA, rheumatoid arthritis; RF, rheumatic factor; SE, shared epitope.

† RR adjusted for age (10 strata), sex, and residential area.

Source data from Padyukov L, Silva C, Stolot P et al. A gene-environment interaction between smoking and shared epitope genes in HLA-DR provides a high risk of seropositive rheumatoid arthritis *Arthritis Rheum* 2004; 50: 3085–92.

References

1 **Sugiyama D, Nishimura K, Tamaki K, et al**. Impact of smoking as a risk factor for developing rheumatoid arthritis: a meta-analysis of observational studies. *Ann Rheum Dis* 2010;**69**(1):70–81.

2 **Rothman KJ, Greenland S, Walker AM**. Concepts of interaction. *Am J Epid* 1980;**112**(4):467–70.

3 **Hosmer DW, Lemeshow S**. Confidence interval estimation of interaction. *Epidemiology* 1992;**3**(5):452–6.

4 **Stolt P, Bengtsson C, Nordmark B, et al**. Quantification of the influence of cigarette smoking on rheumatoid arthritis: results from a population based case-control study, using incident cases. *Ann Rheum Dis* 2003;**62**(9):835–41.

Chapter 2

Rheumatoid arthritis

Elena Nikiphorou and Adam Young

Introduction

In 1859, Alfred Baring Garrod (1819–1907), a physician at University College London, made one of his major contributions to rheumatology: in his treatise he gave the name 'rheumatoid arthritis' to a disease that, although had been around for many years, had no nomenclature and up until that stage had been described as 'rheumatic gout', 'chronic rheumatism', and 'rheumalgia' [1]. He divided rheumatoid arthritis into acute, chronic, and irregular forms of generalized and localized type.

Rheumatoid arthritis as we know it today can be a chronic, destructive, deforming disease of the joints that needs prompt diagnosis and treatment in order to prevent or at least slow down its progression. This is now possible, as a result of a number of therapeutic advances made over time.

Right from the years of Hippocrates, there were historical records of pain-relieving treatments, including powders and extracts made from plants. Since then and especially in the last century, there have been several landmark dates relating to the treatment of this debilitating disease, treatment which in the early days focused predominantly on symptom control. Starting from 1897, when the German chemist Felix Hoffman isolated aspirin [3], which has been used for 'rheumatic' pains, through to 1951, when the Nobel Prize winner Philip Hench, an American physician, discovered cortisone and its application in the treatment of rheumatoid arthritis [2], we have subsequently entered three important landmark eras. First, in the 1970s–1980s, a large number of non-steroidal anti-inflammatory drugs (NSAIDs) were discovered that had effects similar to those of aspirin but with fewer adverse events, in the short term at least. Second, over a 50-year period in the 1980s–1990s, a series of disease-modifying anti-rheumatic drugs (DMARDs), starting with gold, were discovered, including the discovery of what is now the most commonly used DMARD, methotrexate; and third, in the twentieth century, we entered the era of biologic DMARDs, heralded by the discovery of anti-tumour necrosis factor agents.

The remarkable progress made in the understanding of rheumatoid arthritis as a disease, as well as its treatment, has revolutionized the specialty as a whole, resulting in tremendous benefits to our patients. This chapter aims to give a historical perspective of landmark discoveries around the diagnosis and treatment of rheumatoid arthritis, discoveries which have contributed significantly to changing the face of this disease, converting it from a devastating, debilitating, chronic condition to one that can be fully managed and put into remission.

Landmark paper selection

This chapter discusses ten papers that have resulted in landmark developments in the diagnosis, assessment, and treatment of rheumatoid arthritis. These are presented in chronological order under two main areas, covering measures of disease and therapeutics. We believe that the papers presented here have had a significant worldwide impact on the understanding of disease, its presentation, and, importantly, its treatment. The selected papers on therapeutics cover not only individual types of compounds but also changes in treatment approaches that have had proven benefits on disease outcomes.

The first three papers focus on measures of disease; Paper 2.1 discusses diagnostic criteria, Paper 2.2 addresses the clinical assessment as measured by the Disease Activity Score, and Paper 2.3 addresses the clinical assessment as measured by the Health Assessment Questionnaire (HAQ). The therapeutics papers are subdivided into individual treatment compounds and therapeutic strategies. The papers on individual treatments centre on steroids (Paper 2.4), methotrexate (Paper 2.5), and biologics (Paper 2.6). Papers on therapeutic strategies include severity and mortality in rheumatoid arthritis (Paper 2.7), C-reactive protein/erythrocyte sedimentation rate and X-ray changes (Paper 2.8), tight control of rheumatoid arthritis activity (Paper 2.9), and early intensive and combination therapeutic regimens (Paper 2.10).

References

1 **Garrod AB**. Treatise on nature and treatment of gout and rheumatic gout. London: Walton and Maberly; 1859.
2 **Hench PS**. Cortisone, hydrocortisone and corticotropin; some facts and speculations with special reference to rheumatoid arthritis. *Trans Assoc Life Insur Med Dir Am* 1951;**35**:5–33.
3 **Sneader W**. The discovery of aspirin: a reappraisal. *BMJ* 2000;**321**(7276):1591–4.

Paper 2.1: Rheumatoid arthritis in a population sample

Reference

Kellgren JH, Lawrence JS: Rheumatoid arthritis in a population sample. *Ann Rheum Dis* 1956;15(1):1–11.

Purpose

To study radiological, serological, and clinical findings in a general population sample, recording all forms of rheumatic disease in defined grades of severity.

Patients

The patients in this study comprised adult inhabitants of a one-in-ten sample of houses in Leigh, an industrial town in Lancashire with a population of approximately 48,000. All study participants belonged to a group with ages ranging from 50 to 59 years. A second survey was carried out in 1954, when the individuals studied were five years older.

Study design

This study comprised a survey involving house visits by investigators who collected information about past and present rheumatic complaints and any resulting disability. Participants were also invited to attend an examination centre, where a more detailed clinical and occupational history was taken.

The examiner's impression of the individual's personality was recorded, along with the patient's height and weight. A sample of blood was taken for a differential sheep-cell agglutination test as well as antero-posterior radiographs of hands, feet, knees, and pelvis, and lateral radiographs of the lumbar and cervical spine. Individuals who were unable or unwilling to come to the centre were examined and X-rayed in their own homes but, in these cases, only radiographs of the hands and feet were performed.

Trial end points measured

Clinical, serological, and radiological findings were determined in patients with rheumatic complaints.

Results

Clinical findings

Concurrent rheumatoid arthritis and generalized osteoarthritis were only noted in eight women but the investigators concluded that this could be due to the fact that only a highly selected sample of the population attended hospital.

Serological findings

Positive agglutination (occurring in a dilution of 1:32 at 18 hours) in the sheep-cell agglutination test (differential agglutination test (DAT)) was seen in 5% of men and 6% of women. The investigators suggest a prevalence of 4% in this age group in the Leigh population, based on an assumption that all those not tested were negative. The investiga-tors accept though that this is almost certainly not a safe assumption and suggest that the true prevalence is likely to be nearer to 5%.

Radiological findings

Based on a composite score from three readings, a score of 5 or over was taken as positive. Radiological changes of this grade or above were recorded in the hands and/or feet in 8% of women and 7% of men. Assuming that all those not X-rayed were negative, the authors suggest that the minimal prevalence rates would be 6% for each of the two sexes. As far as X-rays of the larger limb joints and cervical spine are concerned, moderate or severe changes were recorded in seven individuals in whom the films of hands and feet had a composite score of less than 5 and were therefore classed as negative. Their X-rays showed destruction of discs and irregularity of the interfacetal joints in the cervical spine which were thought to be rheumatoid in nature. On rereading these spinal films, two were discarded as prob-ably nonrheumatoid, leaving five individuals with positive films of the cervical spine. Two were men and, of these, one had a positive DAT and the other had borderline changes in the hand films and a past history of severe polyarthritis in adult life. Of the three women with moderate changes in the cervical spine, all three had borderline changes in the hand films, and one had a positive DAT and 'clinical rheumatoid of slight severity', the second gave a history of polyarthritis, and the third showed no other evidence of rheumatoid arthritis.

These additional 5 cases were considered radiologically positive, bringing the final figure up to 20 women (10%) and 14 men (8%). The distribution of the X-ray changes of rheuma-toid arthritis would therefore also appear to be similar in the two sexes in this age group. On the other hand, osteoporosis, when read separately, appeared to be largely confined to women.

Summary of main results

+ Clinical rheumatoid arthritis at all grades of severity was found twice as frequently among women but the titre values in the sheep-cell agglutination test were distributed equally between the sexes.

+ Radiological evidence of rheumatoid arthritis was also found equally in men and women.

+ In nine out of ten individuals with severe clinical rheumatoid arthritis, the diagnosis was confirmed by a positive X-ray and/or agglutination test. With lesser degrees of clin-ical disease, such confirmation became less frequent and there were 20 individuals with positive X-rays and/or agglutination tests among 283 who were considered to be free from clinical rheumatoid arthritis.

+ The estimated prevalence rates ranged from 1% for men and 3% for women with severe clinical rheumatoid arthritis confirmed by X-ray and/or agglutination test to 11% for men and 27% for women with all grades of clinical disease, including a past history of polyarthritis.

Critique of the paper

The population studied was confined to the group aged 55–64 and was drawn exclusively from one town in Lancashire; therefore, the data presented are not representative of overall prevalence rates at the time and no general conclusions can be drawn. In terms of the methodology, this was a survey-based study and yet the questions asked were not based on validated questionnaires; therefore, the initial screening process may have been biased. Also, the lack of precision in diagnostic definition may also have affected the results. Furthermore, there was no control group involved and no screening tests performed on patients who gave negative responses to the questions asked, which could have been used to compare.

Significance and importance of the paper

Despite its limitations, this was an exceptional population-based study of the era and provided important UK data in the 1950s concerning the prevalence of rheumatoid arthritis and rheumatoid factor. The findings suggested that, first, self-limited polyarthritis was both more common than hitherto realized and also more common than rheumatoid arthritis in general populations; and, second, a subclinical form was identified which fulfilled the agreed diagnostic criteria for rheumatoid arthritis. This and other early population-based studies were followed by the establishment of a number of early rheumatoid arthritis cohorts in order to establish the natural course of rheumatoid arthritis, initially in the UK in the 1960–1970s [1–4]. From the late 1980s to the early 1990s, many other similar cohorts were initiated, mainly in the UK and other north European countries. From the reports of these cohorts, it became recognized that rheumatoid arthritis in the clinical setting differed from rheumatoid arthritis in population studies and had a very variable course and, although a high proportion of these patients had progressive disease, a benign form of rheumatoid arthritis was identified.

References

1 **Lawrence JS, Bennett PH**. Benign polyarthritis. *Ann Rheum Dis* 1960;**19**(1):20–30.
2 **Jacoby RK, Jayson MI, Cosh JA**. Onset, early stages, and prognosis of RA: a clinical study of 100 patients with 11-year follow-up. *BMJ* 1973;**2**(5858):96–100.
3 **Fleming A, Crown J, Corbett M**. Incidence of joint involvement in early rheumatoid arthritis. *Rheumatol Rehabil* 1976;**15**(2):92–6.
4 **Brooks A, Corbett M**. Radiographic changes in early rheumatoid arthritis. *Ann Rheum Dis* 1977;**36**(1);71–3.

Paper 2.2: Judging disease activity in clinical practice in rheumatoid arthritis: first steps in the development of a disease activity score

References

van der Heijde DMFM, van't Hof MA, van Riel PLCM, et al. Judging disease activity in clinical practice in RA: first step in the development of a disease activity score. *Ann Rheum Dis* 1990;49(11):916–20.

Smolen JS, Breedveld FC, Schiff MH, et al. A simplified disease activity index for rheumatoid arthritis for use in clinical practice. *Rheumatology* 2003;42(2):244–57.

Paper A: Development of a disease activity score in clinical practice

van der Heijde DMFM, van't Hof MA, van Riel PLCM, et al. Judging disease activity in clinical practice in RA: first step in the development of a disease activity score. *Ann Rheum Dis* 1990;49(11):916–20.

Purpose

The purpose of the study was to develop a disease activity score using clinical and laboratory variables in clinical practice.

Patients

This study involved 113 patients with early rheumatoid arthritis.

Study design

This paper describes a prospective study of up to three years' duration involving 113 patients with early rheumatoid arthritis. Two specially trained research nurses assessed all the patients every four weeks. All patients were followed up by their rheumatologists, independently of the evaluations of the research nurses, on average four to six times a year. Two groups of patients, one with high and one with low disease activity (the criterion for this decision being the need to treat with anti-rheumatic drugs) were formed.

Factor analysis resulted in five factors, which enabled easy handling of the large number of clinical and laboratory variables without loss of information.

Discriminant analysis was undertaken to determine the extent to which each factor contributed to discrimination between the two groups of differing disease activity.

Multiple regression analysis was used to determine which laboratory and clinical variables underlie the factors of the discriminant function, resulting in a 'disease activity score' consisting of the Ritchie articular index, number of swollen joints, erythrocyte sedimentation rate, and general health, in declining importance.

Treatment

The rheumatologists' policy was to start treatment with slow-acting anti-rheumatic drugs if the disease was not adequately controlled after two months' of treatment with NSAIDs. The sequence of the start of the various slow-acting anti-rheumatic drugs in this study followed a fixed schedule: first step, hydroxychloroquine or sulphasalazine; second step, intramuscular gold; thereafter, D-penicillamine, azathioprine, or methotrexate. Cortico-steroids and NSAIDs were allowed as adjuvants at all stages.

Trial end points measured

The following assessments were made every four weeks: number of tender joints, num-ber of swollen joints, Ritchie articular index, morning stiffness (minutes), fatigue (hours after rising), pain (on a visual analogue scale (VAS) of 10 cm, 0 = no pain, 10 = worst pain possible), general health (VAS of 10 cm, 0 = best possible, 10 = worst possible), grip strength with a vigorimeter (mmHg) and body weight (kg). Laboratory tests included IgM rheumatoid factor, erythrocyte sedimentation rate according to Westergren (mm in first hour), haemoglobin (g/l), leucocyte count ($10^9/1$), thrombocyte count ($10^9/1$), total protein, and other biochemical and haematological tests. Every six months, plain anterior radiographs of the hands and feet were obtained, all patients completed a ques-tionnaire on their physical and psychosocial wellbeing, and the production of tears was assessed with a Schirmer test (normal >10 mm). Serum and plasma were stored at −20°C at every visit.

The Ritchie articular index, number of swollen joints, erythrocyte sedimentation rate, and general health were the main parameters used in the calculation of the disease activ-ity score.

Follow-up

The study duration was up to three years.

Results

The study resulted in the development of a disease activity score based on the variables collected by the research nurses and composed using different statistical procedures. The variables included in the disease activity score were Ritchie score (semi-objective, clini-cal variable), number of swollen joints (objective, clinical variable), erythrocyte sedimen-tation rate (laboratory variable), and general health (subjective variable). As, in real-life practice, general health is not a variable that is always determined, a constant was calcu-lated to be added to the equation of the disease activity score with three variables so that the means of the scores based on three and four variables were equal, making the two disease activity scores interchangeable. Although not chosen for this reason, the variables are part of the whole spectrum: clinical, laboratory, objective, and subjective. The Ritchie index gives most weight to the equation. Swollen joints are important, followed by eryth-rocyte sedimentation rate and general health.

Paper B: A simplified disease activity index for rheumatoid arthritis for use in clinical practice

Reference

Smolen JS, Breedveld FC, Schiff MH et al. A simplified disease activity index for rheumatoid arthritis for use in clinical practice. *Rheumatology* 2003;42(2):244–57.

Purpose

To verify the usefulness of a simple disease activity index (SDAI) for rheumatoid arthritis.

Patients

A total of 1,839 patients with active rheumatoid arthritis were evaluated.

The SDAI was compared with the HAQ, Disease Activity Score 28 (DAS 28), and American College of Radiology (ACR) response criteria that were determined for patients enrolled in one of the three Phase III clinical trials, a multinational clinical trial of leflunomide (MN301), and validated by comparison with the HAQ, DAS 28, and ACR response in the other two Phase III clinical trials in the leflunomide database (MN302 and US301).

The study presents data from the analysis of the entire patient populations treated during the individual Phase III clinical trials: leflunomide versus placebo, versus sulphasalazine (MN301—6 months of treatment) [2]; leflunomide versus placebo, versus methotrexate (US301—12 months of treatment) [3]; and the comparative study of leflunomide versus methotrexate (MN302—12 months of treatment) [1]. Thus, data of all patients of individual trials, regardless of their treatment, were combined for this investigation.

The leflunomide database is thought to represent the largest collection of data concerning randomized controlled trials of DMARD therapy of rheumatoid arthritis patients, with over 2,241 cases randomized and 1,339 patients treated with leflunomide. Inclusion in the leflunomide trials required a diagnosis of active rheumatoid arthritis based on the revised classification criteria of the ACR w20x and was of Functional Class I, II or III.

Study design

The leflunomide patient database was used as described above.

SDAI calculation: SDAI = tender joint count + swollen joint count + patient global assessment of disease activity + physician global assessment of disease activity + C-reactive protein level.

Comparison with validated disease assessments: the SDAI was compared with the HAQ as well as the DAS 28 w11x and the ACR response criteria w12x, both of which include many of the same components.

Comparative analyses of the SDAI: disease activity was calculated using the SDAI, DAS 28 and ACR response criteria (20%, 50%, 70%, and 90% response) for each of the treated patients in the three studies (MN301, MN302, and US301) at baseline and study end point, and the change in activity at end point (intent-to-treat, last observation carried forward analysis). The SDAI was also compared with the HAQ and modified HAQ (MHAQ, assessed in US301) scores in all treated patients.

Comparison of survey results with the SDAI: the overall rank order of disease activity determined by surveyed physicians (see below), as well as their mean assessments for disease activity classified as mild, moderate, or severe, were compared with the SDAI ranking via simple linear regression to determine significant association between the assessments. Validity tests were undertaken during this process.

Rheumatologist survey: to test further the usefulness of the SDAI as a measure of disease activity, an informal survey among 21 European and North American rheumatologists selected on the basis of their clinical expertise (junior and senior rheumatologists, about 50% each) was conducted. Survey participants were provided with rheumatoid arthritis cases containing the data for the five SDAI components blinded to the SDAI derivation and its value and were asked to (i) rank the cases by disease activity (20 cases evaluated); (ii) categorize the disease activity for 20 cases in terms of mild, moderate, or severe disease (scored 1, 2, or 3, respectively); and (iii) categorize a change in disease activity as no, minimal, or major improvement (25 cases evaluated and scored on an ordinal scale of 1, 2, or 3, respectively).

Trial end points measured

SDAI, DAS 28, ACR response criteria, mean HAQ scores, and changes in total Sharp score were measured.

Follow-up

Follow-up was 12 months.

Results

The mean SDAI calculated for patients at baseline in study MN301 was 50.06 (range, 25.10–96.10). In the MN302 study it was 50.55 (range, 22.10–98.10) and in the US301 study, 43.20 (range, 12.90–78.20). In all three trials, the SDAI was correlated with a high level of statistical significance to the DAS 28 and HAQ scores at baseline, end point, and change at end point. Correlations of the SDAI with the HAQ in study MN301 using linear regression revealed a significant linear relationship of change in the SDAI and change in the HAQ between baseline and six months ($r = 0.56$, $P < 0.0001$). This correlation was validated in studies US301 and MN302 by comparing changes in the SDAI with changes in HAQ or transformed MHAQ between baseline and month 12 ($r = 0.57$ and $r = 0.48$, respectively; $P < 0.0001$). Significant correlation was confirmed at all time points (baseline and at 6 and 12 months).

When physician global assessment was replaced by patient pain, the correlations between change of this revised SDAI and change in the HAQ were almost identical (MN301: $r = 0.57$; US301: $r = 0.56$; MN302: $r = 0.49$; $P < 0.0001$ for all analyses). When the SDAI was further modified to exclude C-reactive protein, the changes of such modified SDAI were again similarly significantly correlated to changes of the HAQ/MHAQ (MN301: $r = 0.56$; US301: $r = 0.56$; MN302: $r = 0.47$; $P < 0.0001$ for all analyses).

Patients achieving the ACR 20%, 50%, 70%, or 90% response showed proportionate changes in the SDAI. Analysis of surveyed physician responses showed a significant association between the perception of disease activity and the SDAI, as well as changes in the SDAI. Qualitative analysis of radiographic progression at 6 and 12 months for patients showing either major, minor, or no improvement of the SDAI showed correspondingly larger increases of the total Sharp score at 12 months.

Treatment

The analysis presented in this study focuses on the patient populations in the leflunomide database treated during the individual Phase III clinical trials: leflunomide versus placebo, versus sulphasalazine (MN301—6 months of treatment) [2]; leflunomide versus placebo, versus methotrexate (US301—12 months of treatment) [3]; and the comparative study of leflunomide versus methotrexate (MN302—12 months of treatment) [1].

Critique of the papers

The van der Heijde paper was an important and well-designed study, which lead to the development of one of the most important and well-established clinical tools for determining disease activity in clinical practice. However, the whole study was based on the patients of six rheumatologists at one centre, in a university hospital in the Netherlands. It could therefore be argued that treatment decisions and even judgement of clinical disease parameters such as the number of tender and swollen counts, and even the patient sample could fail to reflect wider practice and population, therefore bringing into question the generalizability of results. However, as the authors clearly state, this was the very first step in the development of a disease activity score, and subsequent studies followed to test the validity of this tool and its application in the wider population.

The large patient numbers and prospective data collection in the Smolen et al. study based on randomized controlled trials comparing leflunomide with other DMARDs represents a major strength of the study [2]. This was a well-thought-out and well-designed study, difficult to fault. A couple of points that may have improved the study though, are as follows. Joint counts and global assessments were given comparable weight in the SDAI, which could have introduced some bias. Physician's global assessment had been converted from a five-point Likert to a ten-point VAS scale in two trials. This could have lessened the sensitivity to change in these trials; however, because of the similarity of the results obtained among all trials, the authors suggested that this did not confound the conclusions drawn.

Significance and importance of the papers

From the 1960s there have been many and varied clinical and laboratory measures of joint inflammation and severity of rheumatoid arthritis, one example being the Ritchie index [6, 7], making comparisons of clinical studies difficult to interpret. This study was the first step in the development of a disease activity score to be used in routine clinical practice. It marked the beginning of a new era which encouraged the use of validated and unified measures of disease activity with subsequent refinements gaining universal approval in Europe.

Studies from the 1990s suggested that clinical examination of small joints could predict with reasonable accuracy the Larsen radiographic score and that radiographic destruction in larger joints was related to small joint damage, a physical disability index, and cumulative disease activity [4, 5]. In another study, a simple measure of overall status in rheumatoid arthritis was developed known as Overall Status in Rheumatoid Arthritis, whereby the number of damaged large joints and the need for splints, other aids, and small joint surgery were used as a measure of articular damage [8].

The results of the papers discussed here demonstrated that it is possible to obtain a sensitive index by forming an arithmetic sum of core set variable data. The SDAI formulated and validated by Smolen et al. combined swollen joint counts, tender joint counts, patient global assessment, physician global assessment, and C-reactive protein levels (mg/dl) in a simple numerical summation [2]. The study demonstrated that the SDAI is significantly correlated with the DAS 28 and the HAQ, and is a simple and effective measure of disease activity. The study also showed that the ACR response at increasingly stringent levels was mirrored by proportionate changes in the SDAI and in addition, increasing improvement by the SDAI was associated with decreasing radiographic progression. SDAI was shown to be a viable supplement to the DAS 28 or ACR criteria, with suitable application in routine clinical practice. The two studies presented here were among the initial studies leading to the generation of a simplified, validated, and unified measure of disease activity, with subsequent refinements gaining universal approval in Europe.

References

1 Emery P, Breedveld FC, Lemmel EM, et al. A comparison of the efficacy and safety of leflunomide and methotrexate for the treatment of rheumatoid arthritis. *Rheumatology* 2000;**39**(6):655–665.

2 Smolen JS, Kalden JR, Scott DL, et al. European Leflunomide Study Group: efficacy and safety of leflunomide compared with placebo and sulphasalazine in active rheumatoid arthritis: a double-blind, randomised, multicentre trial. *Lancet* 1999;**353**(9149):259–66.

3 Strand V, Cohen S, Schiff M, et al. Treatment of active rheumatoid arthritis with leflunomide compared to placebo and methotrexate. *Arch Intern Med* 1999;**159**(21):2542–50.

4 Kuper HH, van Leeuwen MA, van Riel PLCM, Prevoo ML, Houtman PM, Lolkema WF, et al. Radiographic damage in large joints in early rheumatoid arthritis: relationship with radiographic damage in hands and feet, disease activity, and physical disability. *Br J Rheumatol* 1997;**36**(8):855–60.

5 Plant MJ, Saklatvala J, Jones PW, Dawes PT. Prediction of radiographic damage in hands and feet in rheumatoid arthritis by clinical evaluation. *Clin Rheumatol* 1994;**13**(3):487–91.

6 Ritchie DM, Boyle J A, McInnes J M, et al. Clinical studies with an articular index for the assessment of joint tenderness in patients with rheumatoid arthritis. *Q J Med* 1968;**37**(3):393–406.

7 Ritchie DA, Boyle JA, McInnes JM, et al. Evaluation of a simple articular index for joint tenderness in rheumatoid arthritis. *Ann Rheum Dis* 1969;**28**(2):196.

8 Symmons DPM, Hassell AB, Gunatillaka KAN, et al. Development and preliminary assessment of a simple measure of overall status in rheumatoid arthritis (OSRA) for routine clinical use. *Q J Med* 1995;**88**(6):429–37.

Paper 2.3: Measurement of patient outcome in rheumatoid arthritis

Reference

Fries JF, Spitz P, Kraines RG, Holman HR. Measurement of patient outcome in rheumatoid arthritis. *Arthritis Rheum* 1980;23(2):137–45.

Purpose

The goal of this study was to develop a questionnaire with 'good reliability, validity, conciseness, and coherence' to measure patient outcome in patients with rheumatoid arthritis in five separate dimensions: death, discomfort, disability drug (therapeutic) toxicity, and dollar cost.

Patients

For the evaluation of questionnaires (Study I), the first 20 volunteers with rheumatoid arthritis who either entered the Stanford Immunology Clinic or who were participants in the Stanford Outcome in Rheumatoid Arthritis (ORA) study were chosen. Data were collected from 18 women and 2 men. Ages ranged from 34 to 75 years old; the average age was 54 years old.

For Study II, patients in the Stanford ORA population were mailed self-administered questionnaires. 28 patients were contacted upon return of their questionnaires, and 25 agreed to a home evaluation. The patient population consisted of 18 women and 7 men. Ages ranged from 34 to 74 years old; the average age was 57 years old.

Study design

The question selection for the questionnaires was based on a variety of sources, including the Uniform Database for Rheumatic Diseases and the scales for measuring patient status developed by Convery et al. [1, 2].

A questionnaire consisting of approximately 100 questions was designed, used by a nurse-assessor in a patient interview situation. The questionnaire was revised several times, following the interviews and input from patients.

This process was followed by a self-administered format that was designed to capture the same information gathered in the nurse-assessor interview. The five principal dimensions (death, disability, discomfort, drug toxicity, and dollar costs) were broken down into several subdimensions.

In the next step of the process, the questionnaires were evaluated in two studies, conducted independently of each other:

Study I—The two instruments (assessor and self-administered) were tested with new samples of patients. This study was aimed at testing replicability or reliability.

Study II—The responses on the disability dimensions of the self-administered questionnaire were compared to the patient's ability to perform the same tasks in the home. This study was aimed at testing objectivity (or validity) by evaluating performance at standardized tasks.

Trial end points measured

Patient outcome was measured in five dimensions (Box 2.1).

Results

This study resulted in the development of a questionnaire that proved to be reliable, valid, concise, and coherent. Overall, high Spearman rank correlations were demonstrated for most components (0.56–0.85). The component of sexual activity was an example of poor correlation. Relatively few people had responded to this question and this component was subsequently reformulated, with an improved patient response rate. Inter-method correlations were also shown to be 'respectable' (0.47) to 'excellent' (0.88). Overall questionnaire/

Box 2.1 Dimensions of patient outcome

A. Death

B. Disability index

  1. Physical

- dressing
- arising
- eating
- walking
- hygiene
- reach
- grip
- outside activity
- sex

  2. Psychological

C. Discomfort index

  1. Physical

- severity
- trend

  2. Psychological

- dissatisfaction

D. Drug (therapeutic) toxicity index

  1. Medical

- surgical
- investigational

Box 2.1 Dimensions of Patient outcome *(continued)*

E. Total dollar costs

1. Medical and surgical

   ◆ medications
   ◆ laboratory tests
   ◆ X-rays
   ◆ physician visits
   ◆ paramedical visits
   ◆ devices
   ◆ hospitalizations
   ◆ surgeries
   ◆ out-of-pocket expenses
   ◆ social
   ◆ employment
   ◆ domestic
   ◆ transportation

evaluator agreement was tested in two ways. On the most detailed level, the authors report that questionnaire and evaluator agreed exactly on 59% of the responses and were within one point 93% of the time. The second way of testing questionnaire/evaluator agreement was through a weighted kappa statistic, using rank disagreement weights. The kappa statistic was calculated at 0.52.

With regards to the disability index, the first principal component consisted of a weighted sum of 15 questions. Sixty-five per cent of all interperson variability was found to be accounted for in this one dimension and therefore the authors conclude that the disability index (an equal-weight sum) is appropriate for measuring overall arthritis 'severity' and that the questionnaire is well focused for the measurement of this 'severity'.

As a result of this study, a questionnaire was designed for use in rheumatoid arthritis to measure patient outcomes. The questionnaire had been administered to over 500 patients with rheumatoid arthritis, and the authors state that it has been found well suited for use in the community.

Critique of the paper

In terms of the methodology, although there was an overall careful design of the process of questionnaire development and evaluation, the study does not clearly state the process of selection of questions and domains to be assessed. Also, the authors state that the self-administered questionnaire (following the patient interviews) was 'pretested and revised repeatedly', but the actual process of how this was done is not described. Furthermore, the authors state that 'no attempt was made to include all possible activities, but over 200 possible observations were considered' but no further details given. The questionnaire designed and used by the nurse-assessor consisted of approximately 100 questions, used by a nurse-assessor in a patient interview situation. Later on in the study description, it is mentioned that, for the evaluation of question-naires, 'in all cases the interviews were conducted by the same trained nurse-assessor'. It would have been perhaps better in terms of the validation process to involve more than one nurse-assessor to ensure that consistency was maintained and interperson variability tested for.

During the evaluation process of the questionnaire, the results obtained from the asses-sor interviews were compared to those recorded on the self-administered questionnaire (Study I). There was no consistency in the timing of the interview or questionnaire com-pletion: in ten patients, the interview was done first; in the other ten, the questionnaire was administered first. For some patients, both were done on the same day; in others, the forms were completed 10 to 12 days apart. Although the authors report that 'no signifi-cant effects were noted from the order of administration or with time between testing', it is not clear what 'significant effects' mean and this inconsistency may have been a potential source of bias.

A similar inconsistency in the methodology seems to have taken place with Study II, which involved an assessment of validity of the responses on the disability dimension of the self-administered questionnaire compared to the patient's ability to perform these tasks in the home. Although an attempt was made to schedule the home visit as soon as possible after completion of the questionnaire, this interval varied from 4 to 16 days, with the average length of time being 8 days. Again, this might have been a potential source of bias.

Finally, the process of developing the questionnaire did not involve an assessment of co-morbidity, which could have affected the ability of the questionnaire to be used as a tool to test patient outcomes. The authors reported, however, that co-morbid conditions were present in less than 10% of the subjects, with very few disabled by co-morbidities, and that their principal component analysis suggested that any such effects were minimal.

Significance and importance of the paper

Several outcome measures and health status instruments were developed and standard-ized for clinical trials and observational studies in rheumatoid arthritis in the 1980–1990s. This has been one of the pivotal studies leading to the development of a valid and easy-to-use instrument to assess function in rheumatoid arthritis. Because of its sub-jective element, unpredictable quality, and interrelationship with age and co-morbidity, functional assessment in rheumatoid arthritis has been problematic to measure. The development of HAQ in the 1980s has stood the test of time internationally and has been adapted by most countries in Europe and other parts of the world to allow for dif-ferences in normal activities. It is incorporated in nearly all clinical trials and studies, and its relative brevity allows its use in ordinary clinical settings. In the UK it is a major influence on the National Institute for Health and Care Effectiveness cost-effective assessments of new drugs.

References

1 Convery FR, Minteer MA, Amiel D, Connett KL. Polyarticular disability: a functional assessment. *Arch Phys Med Rehab* 1977;**58**(11):494–9.

2 Fries JF, Hess EV, Klinenberg J. A standard database for rheumatic disease. *Arthritis Rheum* 1974;**17**(3):327–36.

Paper 2.4: Effects of cortisone acetate and pituitary adrenocorticotropic hormone on rheumatoid arthritis, rheumatic fever, and certain other conditions

Reference

Hench PS, Kendal EC, Slocumb CH, et al. Effects of cortisone acetate and pituitary ACTH on rheumatoid arthritis, rheumatic fever and certain other conditions. *Arch Intern Med* 1950;85(4):545–666.

Purpose

The purpose of this paper was to provide preliminary results of the clinical effects of steroids in rheumatoid arthritis by the unique group of clinicians and biochemists who had recently discovered them. It is not a clinical trial nor does it have an a priori hypothesis; instead, it is presented as a study in clinical physiology of a very important topic.

Patients

The subjects of these studies were patients admitted to the Mayo Clinic, Rochester, USA, in the 1940s and who had chronic, disabling, and severe rheumatoid arthritis. Patients were selected if it was considered that improvement could be detected clinically and were excluded if clinical features were irreversible, as in permanent flexion contractures.

Study design

An experimental and observational type study design was used to assess the effects of varying doses of oral steroids and/or adrenocorticotropic hormone (ACTH) injections in patients with rheumatoid arthritis. Patients acted as their own controls and were administered an inert preparation in similar circumstances at separate times, recording the same measures.

Treatment

Any anti-rheumatic medication (e.g. acetyl acetic acid) was stopped prior to clinical and laboratory assessments, Administration of substance E (oral), the pituitary hormone ACTH (IV), or both were administered to 23 patients. Because of a shortage of supply of both preparations, dosages and length of courses depended on response and were not standardized. An inert preparation was administered in similar circumstances at separate times to all patients as their own controls.

Trial end points measured

Patients' overall symptoms, articular indices, and motion pictures were assessed before and after steroid administration, and before and after the control preparation. Detailed assessments included articular redness, tenderness, swelling, limitation of movement, and the patients' assessment of pain at rest. Grading consisted of mild, moderate, severe, ad very severe. Motion pictures recorded movements of daily living—rising from a chair, walking, using stairs, etc. Laboratory tests included haemoglobin (HB), WCC, and sedimentation rates, serum proteins, blood and urine glucose, glucose tolerance, and urinary excretion of corticosteroids. Very detailed records were made of all other unexpected and side effects reported by patients and detected clinically; seven patients had synovial biopsies prior to and during the study.

Follow-up

All patients remained in hospital under close scrutiny and remained in prolonged follow-up.

Results

Twelve patients had very marked responses to steroids, eight had marked responses, and one had a moderate response. The paper describes in detail the timing (immediate, delayed), maximal responses, length of responses, and relation of response to dosage for each course administered. Considerable attention was paid to other unexpected and adverse effects during courses and on withdrawal. These include most of the well-recognized side effects known to us today. In view of the success of these compounds and to determine how disease specific they were, the study was extended to include other conditions including rheumatic fever, SLE, psoriatic arthritis, and gout, with mixed but generally favourable effects. Synovial biopsies showed reduction in histological inflammation.

Critique of the paper

As the authors pointed out, this study was designed as an examination of the clinical physiology of steroid administration in rheumatoid arthritis and not a clinical trial, and in this sense it was exploratory. Much of the paper is purely descriptive. However, it does record in great detail the rationale behind all decisions concerning the design and process of the study and all the events that occurred. Many aspects of the study have since become required features of randomized controlled trials. None of the clinical measures were standardized but were very detailed and many have since been adapted into rheumatology randomized controlled trials and clinical practice.

Significance and importance of the paper

The discovery of steroid compounds in the 1940s was based on the astute clinical observations of a physician with an interest in inflammatory conditions like rheumatoid arthritis. At this time, rheumatoid arthritis was a progressive crippling condition with limited therapeutic options. Amelioration of the inflammatory signs of rheumatoid arthritis was first noted in coincident jaundice in 1929 and then in post-traumatic episodes like surgery. It was not until the same phenomena were seen in pregnancy in the 1930s that the group proposed that these changes were induced by normally produced hormones (hypothetical substance X) and were not disease specific. Despite concerted efforts, it proved possible to extract only small amounts of adrenal cortex hormones in order to test formally the possible beneficial effects of the now named substance E. However, enough anecdotal reports had been accumulated and sufficient amounts of substance E produced by the 1940s to investigate the possibility that the signs of rheumatoid arthritis could be reversed employing a number of experiments on a small number of willing patients.

This is the first paper to describe the events and rationale that lead to the discovery of corticosteroids, their production, and beneficial and adverse effects in inflammatory arthritis, for which Hench received the Nobel Prize. It showed for the first time that rheumatoid arthritis was not necessarily a progressive destructive disease but was reversible.

Many features in this study later became the basis of future clinical trials and in fact informed one of the first randomized controlled trials in medicine and which was designed by Hench and his colleagues to corroborate the results presented here. It took a few years before the devastating effects of long-term steroid use were recognized and subsequently steroids fell out of favour. Since the 1950s, rheumatologists' opinions and the use of steroids have varied and still vary considerably in the management of rheumatoid arthritis, because of both short- and long-term toxicity. However, steroids can be life-saving in the short term and still have an important place in a number of therapeutic strategies, mainly as the result of two more recent and important studies [1, 2].

References

1 **Kirwan JR**. The effect of glucocorticoids on joint destruction in rheumatoid arthritis. The Arthritis and Rheumatism Council Low-Dose Glucocorticoid Study Group. *N Engl J Med* 1995;**333**(3):142–6.
2 **Boers M, Verhoeven AC, Markusse HM, et al**. Randomised comparison of combined step-down prednisolone, methotrexate and sulphasalazine with sulphasalazine alone in early rheumatoid arthritis. *Lancet* 1997;**350**(9074):309–18.

Paper 2.5: Efficacy of low-dose methotrexate in rheumatoid arthritis

Reference
Weinblatt ME, Coblyn JS, Fox DA, et al. Efficacy of low-dose methotrexate in rheumatoid arthritis. *N Engl J Med* 1985;312(13):818–22.

Purpose
To assess efficacy of low-dose methotrexate (2.5–5 mg every 12 hours for three doses weekly) in rheumatoid arthritis, compared to placebo.

Patients
This study involved 35 patients with rheumatoid arthritis (based on the American Rheumatism Association criteria) and who received gold-salt therapy; of these, 28 (80%) also received penicillamine, 23 (66%) hydroxychloroquine, and 2 azathioprine. These drugs had been discontinued because of ineffectiveness or toxicity. Patients were not accepted into the trial until gold, penicillamine, and hydroxychloroquine had been withdrawn for at least two months and azathioprine for at least six months.

Other criteria included disease onset after age 18 and the presence of active disease, as indicated by at least three of the following:

- three or more swollen joints;
- six or more tender joints;
- 45 minutes or more of morning stiffness;
- a Westergren erythrocyte sedimentation rate of 28 mm per hour or higher;
- mean grip strength for both hands of 192 mmHg or less in men and 146 mm Hg or less in women, as averaged from three measurements.

Women either had no childbearing potential or were practising contraception.

The radiographic anatomic stage of disease was Stage II or greater in all patients (based on plane hand radiographs at the point of study entry).

Study design
This paper describes a randomized double-blind crossover study of low-dose oral weekly methotrexate.

Trial end points measured
Clinical trial end points included the following:

- number of swollen joints (out of 66);
- number of tender joints on pressure, pain on passive motion, or both (out of 68);
- the joint-swelling index, expressed as a sum in which each joint was graded for swelling as 0 (none), 1 (mild), 2 (moderate), or 3 (severe);

- the joint-tenderness/pain index (the sum for joints graded according to the above scale);
- mean grip strength for both hands (mmHg);
- 15 m (50 ft) walking time without assisting devices;
- duration of morning stiffness;
- physician's assessment of disease activity graded as 0 (asymptomatic), 1 (mild), 2 (moderate), 3 (severe), or 4 (very severe); and
- the patient's assessment of disease activity graded on the same scale.

Overall responses to treatment were determined to be as follows:

- therapeutic remission, as defined by the preliminary criteria of the American Rheumatism Association [1];
- marked improvement in the joint-swelling index and in the joint-tenderness/pain index, defined as a decrease of 50% or more in their values at entry or crossover;
- moderate improvement, defined as decreases of 30%–49% in these indexes;
- no change, if the value for an index remained within 30% of the original value; and
- worsening, if the value for an index increased 30% or more.

Laboratory tests: erythrocyte sedimentation rate was performed. In addition, complete blood count (including platelets and the erythrocyte sedimentation rate and liver-enzyme tests) (3-weekly), serum creatinine (6-weekly), and typing for *HLA-A*, *B*, *C*, and *D* polymorphisms were undertaken, along with immunologic tests, including that for rheumatoid factor.

Follow-up

Follow-up was for 24 weeks.

Treatment

Patients were randomly assigned in blocks of four to receive initially indistinguishable tablets consisting of either methotrexate (2.5 mg) or a placebo for 12 weeks (Period 1).

Tablets were ingested in equal numbers on three consecutive occasions at 12-hour intervals beginning on the same day of each week. Three tablets were taken weekly for the first six weeks. At six weeks, the dose could be increased to six tablets weekly if a satisfactory response was not noted by the physician–investigator.

At 12 weeks, crossover occurred; patients initially assigned to methotrexate received placebo for the final 12 weeks of the study (Period 2), and patients originally assigned to placebo received methotrexate. Elective increases in dosage were incorporated into week 6 of Period 2, with patients and their rheumatologists as well as the investigators remaining unaware of drug assignments until completion of the study.

Results

Methotrexate group

Significant reductions (P < 0.01), as compared to the placebo group, were observed in the number of tender or painful joints, the duration of morning stiffness, and disease activity at the 12-week visit. There were also significant reductions in the number of swollen joints ($P < 0.05$) and 15 m walking time ($P < 0.03$). At 24 weeks, the above variables as well as grip strength and erythrocyte sedimentation rate showed significant ($P < 0.01$) improvement in the population crossed over to methotrexate.

Eight patients had what was considered a substantial response to methotrexate and were found to have a significantly increased frequency ($P < 0.03$) of the *HLA-DR2* haplotype.

Adverse reactions during methotrexate treatment included transaminase elevation (21%), nausea (18%), and diarrhoea (12%); one patient was withdrawn from the study due to diarrhoea. One death was reported in a patient receiving placebo. Methotrexate was not found to affect measures of humoral or cellular immunity.

Critique of the paper

The small number of patients and short study duration may mean that severe adverse effects secondary to methotrexate, such as bone-marrow suppression and acute pulmonary toxicity, could have been missed. Furthermore, there was no comparison made between the patients receiving steroids at entry and those not, and this may have affected outcomes such as the time to and duration of remission. Finally, it could be argued that the splitting of the study into two periods made it difficult to determine the degree of benefit attributable to the drug in Period 2.

Significance and importance of the paper

The early/mid-1980s brought several new effective and relatively safer slow-acting disease-modifying drugs to rheumatology, drugs which had been adapted from previous use in other specialties. This study provided evidence for the short-term efficacy of methotrexate in rheumatoid arthritis. Following this study, longer trials were undertaken to investigate the safety and effectiveness of this drug, which remains the preferred first and anchor DMARD [2], although it took longer for it to be accepted in the UK than in the US and Europe.

In the UK, national guidelines recommend the use of DMARD combinations, one of which should be methotrexate at maximally tolerated doses used as first-line treatment ideally within three months of persistent symptom onset [4]. European League Against Rheumatism (EULAR) guidelines recommend reaching an optimal methotrexate dose within a few weeks and maintaining the maximal dose (25–30 mg weekly) for at least eight weeks [3].

References

1 **Pinals RS, Masi AT, Larsen RA, et al**. Preliminary criteria for clinical remission in rheumatoid arthritis. *Arthritis Rheum* 1981;**24**(10):1308–15.

2 **Pincus T, Yazici Y, Sokka T, et al**. Methotrexate as the 'anchor drug' for the treatment of early rheumatoid arthritis. *Clin Exp Rheumatol* 2003;**21**(Suppl 31):S178–85.

3 **Smolen JS, Landewé R, Breedveld FC, et al**. Recommendations for the management of rheumatoid arthritis with synthetic and biological disease-modifying antirheumatic drugs: 2013 update. *Ann Rheum Dis* 2014;**73**(3):492–509.

4 **National Institute for Health and Care Excellence**. Rheumatoid arthritis: the management of rheumatoid arthritis in adults. <http://www.nice.org.uk/guidance/CG79>, accessed 20 January 2015.

Paper 2.6: Infliximab (chimeric anti-tumour necrosis factor alpha monoclonal antibody) versus placebo in rheumatoid arthritis patients receiving concomitant methotrexate: a randomized Phase III trial

Reference

Maini R, St Clair EW, Breedveld F, et al. Infliximab (chimeric anti-tumour necrosis factor alpha monoclonal antibody) versus placebo in rheumatoid arthritis patients receiving concomitant methotrexate: a randomised phase III trial. *Lancet* 1999;354(9194):1932–9.

Purpose

To determine whether the addition of infliximab therapy at two doses every 4 or 8 weeks in patients who were inadequately controlled on methotrexate is safe and effective in relieving signs and symptoms of disease.

Patients

This study involved 428 patients with active rheumatoid arthritis despite continuous treatment with methotrexate for at least three months and at a stable dose (at 12.5 mg/week or more) for at least four weeks. Patients using oral corticosteroids (10 mg/kg or less prednisone equivalent) or NSAIDs should have been on a stable dose for at least four weeks before screening: if a patient was not using such drugs, the patient should not have received either drug for at least four weeks before screening.

Study

The study comprised an international, double-blind, placebo-controlled Phase III clinical trial.

Trial end points measured

The primary end point was prospectively defined as 20% improvement, according to ACR criteria, at the week 30 visit, without requiring a surgical joint procedure (i.e. arthrodesis and joint replacement), initiation of new drugs for rheumatoid arthritis, or increases in dose of medication for rheumatoid arthritis. Secondary measurements of response to therapy included documentation of 50% and 70% improvement, reduction in individual measurements of disease activity, and a general health assessment [1].

Follow-up

Follow-up was for 30 weeks.

Treatment

Patients were randomized to placebo (n = 88) or one of four regimens of infliximab at either 3 mg/kg or 10 mg/kg at weeks 0, 2, and 6. All patients were given intravenous infusions at weeks 0, 2, and 6. Two infliximab groups (3 mg/kg or 10 mg/kg) and the placebo group received subsequent infusions every four weeks, whereas two further groups received infliximab (3 mg/kg or 10 mg/kg) every eight weeks and placebo infusions on interim four-week visits to maintain blinding. All infusions were given over two hours. Patients remained on a background stable dose of methotrexate (median 15 mg/week for >6 months, range 10–35 mg/week) and were assessed every 4 weeks for 30 weeks.

Results

The authors report that more patients (P < 0.001) treated with infliximab, achieved the intention-to-treat primary efficacy measurement (the ACR 20 response) than in the placebo group:

> At 30 weeks, ACR 20 criteria were achieved in 53%, 50%, 58%, and 52% of patients receiving 3 mg/kg every 4 or 8 weeks or 10 mg/kg every 4 or 8 weeks, respectively, compared with 20% of patients receiving placebo plus methotrexate (P < 0.001 for each of the four infliximab regimens vs placebo). A 50% improvement was achieved in 29%, 27%, 26%, and 31% of infliximab plus methotrexate in the same treatment groups, compared with 5% of patients on placebo plus methotrexate (P < 0.001). Infliximab was well-tolerated; withdrawals for adverse events as well as the occurrence of serious adverse events or serious infections did not exceed those in the placebo group.

The results therefore provided support for up to 30 weeks of treatment of rheumatoid arthritis by combining infliximab with methotrexate without an increase in serious adverse events. The response and safety characteristics in those receiving infliximab every eight weeks suggested advantages in terms of cost, convenience, and compliance over four-weekly regimens.

Critique of the paper

The protocol in the study prespecified that pharmacokinetic data would be analysed in the first 200 subjects. However, the number of subjects with human anti-chimeric antibody (HACA) formation was not stated. The authors stated that HACA formation could not be measured in patients receiving infliximab since the drug interfered with the assay. Pharmacokinetic measurements were performed in 197 patients, and the results were consistent with the previously defined half-life of 8–12 days. However, 27 patients who discontinued treatment before 30 weeks were tested for HACA formation, and 3 patients (11%) tested positive for HACA (2 with a titre of 1/10 and 1 with a titre of 1/40). It would have been interesting to derive information on formation of HACA, especially in these patients with concurrent immunosuppression with methotrexate, and to relate this data to the rate of infliximab infusion reactions. Furthermore, serious infliximab-related complications such as lymphoma would be difficult to examine in this study, as longer follow-up would be required.

Significance and importance of the paper

Following years of intense laboratory investigation, the identification of cytokines and the understanding of pathways of inflammatory activity resulted in the development of a new breed of powerful, fast-acting, and highly effective biological agents for rheumatoid arthritis. These agents have introduced completely new standards for the management of rheumatoid arthritis, with clinical remission a realistic target. The anti-tumour necrosis factor agents demonstrated efficacy in relieving signs and symptoms of rheumatoid arthritis and provided new hope. The present study investigated infliximab, a chimeric human–mouse anti-tumour necrosis factor α monoclonal antibody, and provided evidence for its additional clinical benefit to patients with active rheumatoid arthritis despite receiving methotrexate, making this one of the landmark rheumatoid arthritis papers in the biologics era. Further studies followed, demonstrating the beneficial effects of infliximab when added to methotrexate [3–5].

The high cost of anti-tumour necrosis factor drugs restricts their use in the UK. Based on national guidelines [2], infliximab is currently one of five recommended anti-tumour necrosis factor drugs for rheumatoid arthritis, provided there is evidence of active disease (DAS 28 >5.1) and patients have failed treatment with two DMARDs, one of which being methotrexate.

References

1 **Fries JF, Spitz PW, Young DY**. The dimensions of health outcomes: the health assessment questionnaire, disability and pain scales. *J Rheumatol* 1982;**9**(5):789–93.

2 **National Institute for Health and Care Excellence**. Rheumatoid arthritis: the management of rheumatoid arthritis in adults. <http://www.nice.org.uk/guidance/CG79>, accessed 20 January 2015.

3 **Smolen JS, Han C, van der Heijde DM, et al**. Radiographic changes in rheumatoid arthritis patients attaining different disease activity states with methotrexate monotherapy and infliximab plus methotrexate: the impacts of remission and TNF-blockade. *Ann Rheum Dis* 2009;**68**(6):823–7.

4 **St Clair EW, van der Heijde DM, Smolen JS, et al**. Combination of infliximab and methotrexate therapy for early rheumatoid arthritis: a randomized, controlled trial. *Arthritis Rheum* 2004;**50**(11):3432–43.

5 **van Vollenhoven RF, Ernestam S, Geborek P, et al**. Addition of infliximab compared with addition of sulfasalazine and hydroxychloroquine to methotrexate in patients with early rheumatoid arthritis (Swefot trial): 1-year results of a randomised trial. *Lancet* 2009;**374**(9688):459–66.

Paper 2.7: Taking mortality in rheumatoid arthritis seriously—predictive markers, socio-economic status, and co-morbidity

Reference

Pincus T, Callahan L. Taking mortality in rheumatoid arthritis seriously—predictive markers, socioeconomic status and comorbidity. *J Rheumatol* 1986 13(5):841–5.

Purpose

This paper is an editorial summarizing the data available on mortality in rheumatoid arthritis from the 1960s to early 1980s, and as such no a priori hypothesis is proposed.

Patients

The study data presented comes from cross-sectional and observational studies examining clinical features and measures of disease in rheumatoid arthritis in patients attending both community-based and hospital departments.

Study design

This is an editorial supported with data from the authors' own studies. The data shown and results referred to are based on the majority of the major observational studies designed to provide information on predictive markers and outcomes in rheumatoid arthritis and which had been published in mainstream journals by the 1980s, with mortality included as an outcome. A few were on inception or prospective cohorts but the remainder and majority were cross-sectional studies. It is not a meta-analysis or a formal literature appraisal. It is an editorial representing the personal views of a rheumatologist with a track record of conducting observational studies and developing measures of rheumatoid arthritis assessment, bringing together the 13 most important available data on mortality in rheumatoid arthritis and including some recent data from the authors' work. The paper summarizes the current and speculative views on mortality in rheumatoid arthritis.

Trial end points measured

The main outcome discussed is survival and causes of death in rheumatoid arthritis, and includes predictive markers.

Follow-up

This varied considerably from study to study.

Treatment

The article covers standard therapies available in this era appropriate to the patients' condition.

Results

Predictors of survival from most previous studies were specific features of rheumatoid arthritis-like extra-articular manifestations (e.g. nodules) and X-ray erosions, and laboratory measures like rheumatoid factor and erythrocyte sedimentation rate. An important new and unexpected finding from the recent studies of this era reported here was the predictive value of several measures of function for reduced survival in rheumatoid arthritis. The important point is made that severely affected function in rheumatoid arthritis reduces survival by 50% or less, a prognosis no less severe than that for Stage IV Hodgkin's disease or three-vessel coronary artery disease.

Socio-economic status had been reported as a predictor of survival in a number of conditions, including rheumatoid arthritis. This paper reported the value of a novel assessment of socio-economic status using level of formal education as a simple measure which could be collected easily in ordinary rheumatology clinics. It is not confounded by the usual measures of socio-economic status, such as income and occupation, which can be affected by chronic disease. Co-morbidity in rheumatoid arthritis may be related to socio-economic status, as in other conditions.

Critique of the paper

Although citing most of the recognized names in this field, this is a personal view and open to considerable bias. Many of the reports referred to are cross-sectional or prospective cohorts, and there was only one inception cohort. The results from other inception cohorts started in this era had still not reached publication stages. Despite this, many of the conclusions of this paper have been corroborated subsequently by later and more robustly designed studies.

Significance and importance of the paper

Different types of studies in several different countries commonly report similar findings in medical research but may not achieve the importance they deserve unless highlighted in a major meta-analysis, literature review, or an editorial. This paper highlights the mismatch between the commonly held view of rheumatoid arthritis being a non-fatal disease and reports reduced survival, varying from 3–13 years, in rheumatoid arthritis. It is now well recognized that there is significantly higher risk of cardiovascular morbidity and mortality in patients with rheumatoid arthritis when compared to the general population [1–5]. The proportions of actual causes of death are similar to normal populations but this was one of the earlier papers to highlight the several sources of this finding and also bought attention to both socio-economic status and co-morbidity as predictors of more severe rheumatoid arthritis.

This and other papers by Pincus highlighted the severity of outcomes in rheumatoid arthritis and especially reduced survival, and also the fact that this was comparable to other more well-known medical conditions. As a result of these small prospective and cross-sectional studies of the 1980s, and clinical experience, US rheumatologists were advocating earlier and more intense interventions in an attempt to reduce by whatever means the poor prognosis of rheumatoid arthritis, although there was no evidence at this time to support such therapeutic measures. This report introduced the concept that rheumatoid arthritis was more than just a painful and deforming condition but carried a reduced life expectancy, similar to some lymphoproliferative conditions with equally ineffective therapies. This became one of the important drivers for pursuing a better understanding of the immunopathology of the condition and the development of better drugs for rheumatoid arthritis.

References

1 Maradit-Kremers H, Nicola PJ, Crowson CS, et al. Cardiovascular death in rheumatoid arthritis: a population-based study. *Arthritis Rheum.* 2005;**52**(3):722–32.

2 Meune C, Touze E, Trinquart L, et al. Trends in cardiovascular mortality in patients with rheumatoid arthritis over 50 years: a systematic review and meta-analysis of cohort studies. *Rheumatology* 2009;**48**(10):1309–13.

3 Turesson C, Jarenros A, Jacobsson L. Increased incidence of cardiovascular disease in patients with rheumatoid arthritis: results from a community based study. *Ann Rheum Dis* 2004;**63**(8):952–5.

4 Watson D, Rhodes T, Guess H. All-cause mortality and vascular events among patients with RA, OA, or no arthritis in the UK General Practice Research Database. *J Rheumatol* 2003;**30**(6):1196–202.

5 Young A, Koduri G, Batley M, et al. Mortality in rheumatoid arthritis. Increased in the early course of disease, in ischaemic heart disease and in pulmonary fibrosis. *Rheumatology* 2007;**46**(2):350–7.

Paper 2.8: Rheumatoid arthritis: treatment which controls the C-reactive protein and erythrocyte sedimentation rate reduces radiological progression

Reference

Dawes PT, Fowler PD, Clarke S, et al. Rheumatoid arthritis: treatment which controls the C-reactive protein and erythrocyte sedimentation rate reduces radiological progression. *Rheumatology* 1986;25(1):44–9.

Purpose

The purpose of the study was to examine whether radiographic progression was reduced in patients with controlled disease activity, as measured by the C-reactive protein level and erythrocyte sedimentation rate.

Patients

This study included 150 patients with active 'definite' or 'classical' rheumatoid arthritis (based on American Rheumatism Association Criteria).

Study design

Patients were initially assessed twice within a four-week interval and then allocated to one of two therapeutic groups. If patients had received a DMARD in the previous three months, they were excluded. Admission criteria included failure to respond to NSAIDs, progression of disease as shown by increasing clinical, laboratory, or radiographic features, or patients showing poor prognostic features early in the disease, for example, nodules or early erosive changes. Mandatory entry criteria for both groups were (i) painful joints and (ii) either erythrocyte sedimentation rate >30 mm/hour, or C-reactive protein >20 mg/l. The decision to allocate a patient to a particular treatment group (see 'Results') was clinical.

Trial end points measured

The trial end points measured in the study included the Larsen score, the erythrocyte sedimentation rate, and levels of C-reactive protein.

Follow-up

The study mentions that the patients were studied over a four-year period but the potential was to reach 12 months' of treatment (measurements of baseline, 6, and 12 months).

Treatment

Patients with more severe disease were treated with gold or D-penicillamine, and less severe disease was treated with chloroquine or dapsone (standard dosage regimen used).

Results

The patient groups in this study were as follows:

Group I: 60 patients who did not complete 12 months' therapy;

Group II: patients in whom the erythrocyte sedimentation rate and the C-reactive protein level fell to <30 mm/hour and 20 mg/l, respectively, and remained at these levels between 6 and 12 months;

Group III: patients who between 6 and 12 months had variable erythrocyte sedimentation rates and C-reactive protein levels; and

Group IV: patients in whom erythrocyte sedimentation rate and C-reactive protein levels fell but remained >30 mm/hour and 20 mg/l, respectively, and remained at these levels between 6 and 12 months.

The study has shown that in Groups II, III, and IV there was a significant deterioration (P < 0.01) in the hand/foot radiographs from zero to six months. Between 6 and 12 months, the radiographs in Group III continued to show significant radiological progression (P < 0.01) but those of Group II did not alter. The authors concluded that radiological deterioration continues during the first six months regardless of clinical response but thereafter, if the erythrocyte sedimentation rate and C-reactive protein levels are consistently controlled, further deterioration is less likely to occur.

Critique of the paper

The design of this study and specifically the choice of treatment may have predisposed it to confounding by indication because the initial selection of patients for specific treatment groups was based on disease severity, although in a second step there was randomization to individual treatments (see 'Study design').

Another potential source of bias is the fact that the radiographs were read by a single observer, although the authors reported a correlation of r = 0.95 of the same radiographs 'read at different times' by the single observer. The authors comment that 'because of variability in film quality' all joints were scored a minimum of 1 on the Larsen score [7] for the purpose of statistical analysis. Again, this may have affected the results.

Significance and importance of the paper

A delay in treating within the first three months results in substantially more radiographic damage at five years [1, 6, 10]. It is now widely accepted that intensive treatment strategies produce better outcomes in the management of early rheumatoid arthritis [2–5, 8, 9, 11].

This study demonstrates that this concept was raised some decades before in the 1980s, based on clinical experience and earlier clinical studies when monotherapy was standard practice, and has subsequently been confirmed with the current improved therapeutic strategies. Studies like this were 'key' in showing that anything that kept laboratory markers of inflammation low was matched by radiographic change and encouraged further studies to be undertaken to investigate the effect of various treatment strategies on disease outcomes.

References

1 **Egsmose C, Lund B, Borg G, et al**. Patients with rheumatoid arthritis benefit from early 2nd line therapy: 5-year follow-up of a prospective double blind placebo controlled study. *J Rheumatol* 1995;**22**(12):2208–13.

2 **Emery P, Breedveld FC, Dougados M, et al**. Early referral recommendation for newly diagnosed rheumatoid arthritis: evidence based development of a clinical guide. *Ann Rheum Dis* 2002;**61**(4):290–7.

3 **Goekoop-Ruiterman YP, de Vries-Bouwstra JK, Allaart CF, et al**. Comparison of treatment strategies in early rheumatoid arthritis: a randomized trial. *Ann Intern Med* 2007;**146**(6):406–15.

4 **Grigor C, Capell H, Stirling A, et al**. Effect of treatment strategy of tight control for rheumatoid arthritis (the TICORA study): a single-blind randomised controlled trial. Lancet 2004;**364**(9430):263–9.

5 **Korpela M, Laasonen L, Hannonen P, et al**. Retardation of joint damage in patients with early rheumatoid arthritis by initial aggressive treatment with Disease-Modifying Antirheumatic Drugs. Five-year experience from the FIN-RACo study. *Arthritis Rheum* 2004;**50**(7):2072–81.

6 **Lard LR, Visser H, Speyer I, et al**. Early versus delayed treatment in patients with recent-onset rheumatoid arthritis: comparison of two cohorts who received different treatment strategies. *Am J Med* 2001;**111**(6):446–51.

7 **Larsen A, Dale K, Eck M**. Radiographic evaluation of rheumatoid arthritis and related conditions by standard reference films. Acta Radiol Diagn 1977;**18**(4):481–91.

8 **Möttönen T, Hannonen P, Leirisalo-Repo M, et al**. Comparison of combination therapy with single-drug therapy in early rheumatoid arthritis: a randomised trial. *Lancet* 1999;**353**(9164): 1568–73.

9 **O'Dell JR, Haire CE, Erikson N, et al**. Treatment of rheumatoid arthritis with methotrexate alone, sulfasalazine and hydroxychloroquine, or a combination of all three medications. *N Engl J Med* 1996;**334**(20):1287–91.

10 **Tsakonas E, Fitzgerald AA, Fitzcharles MA, et al**. Consequences of delayed therapy with second-line agents in rheumatoid arthritis: a 3 year follow-up on the Hydroxychloroquine in Early Rheumatoid Arthritis (HERA) study. *J Rheumatol* 2000;**27**(3):623–9.

11 **van der Heide A, Jacobs JW, Bijlsma JW, et al**. The effectiveness of early treatment with 'second-line' antirheumatic drugs. A randomized, controlled trial. *Ann Intern Med* 1996;**124**(8):699–707.

Paper 2.9: Effect of a treatment strategy of tight control for rheumatoid arthritis (the TICORA study): a single-blind randomized controlled trial

Reference

Grigor C, Capell H, Stirling A, et al. Effect of a treatment strategy of tight control for rheumatoid arthritis (the TICORA study): a single-blind randomized controlled trial. *Lancet* 2004;364(9430):264–9.

Hypothesis

To test the hypothesis that an improved outcome can be achieved by employing a strategy of intensive outpatient management of patients with rheumatoid arthritis—for sustained, tight control of disease activity—compared with routine outpatient care.

Patients

Recruited patients belonged to the age group 18 to 75 years and had rheumatoid arthritis for fewer than 5 years. All patients had active disease, as defined by a disease activity score of more than 2.4. Patients who had previously received combination DMARD treatment, or had relevant concurrent liver (aspartate aminotransferase >80 IU/l, alkaline phosphatase >700 IU/l), renal (creatinine >0.2 mmol/l), or haematological disease (white-cell count <4.0109/l, platelet count <150,109/l) were excluded.

Study design

The study comprised a single-blind, randomized controlled trial based in two National Health Service (NHS) teaching hospitals in Glasgow, UK, between August 1999 and April 2001. One hundred and eleven patients out of 183 screened participated in the study.

Treatment

The treatment used for the intensive treatment group (n = 55) was as follows (see Figure 2.1):

> Monthly assessment, any swollen joint amenable to intra-articular steroid was injected, unless the joint had been injected within the previous 3 months or the patient declined. A maximum of three joints per assessment were injected, up to a total dose of 120 mg triamcinolone acetonide per visit. Within the first 3 months of starting a new DMARD, if 120 mg of triamcinolone acetonide was not injected intra-articularly, the balance was given by an intramuscular injection if the disease activity score remained more than 2.4. At every assessment after month 3, patients with a score of more than 2.4 received an escalation of their oral treatment according to a protocol, unless they declined or toxic effects precluded this approach.

Treatment of the routine care group (n = 55) was as follows:

> 3-Monthly review with no formal composite measure of disease activity used in clinical decision making. DMARD monotherapy was given in patients with active synovitis and failure of treatment (because of toxic effects or lack of effect) resulted in a change to alternative monotherapy, or addition of a second or third drug at the discretion of the attending rheumatologist. Intra- articular

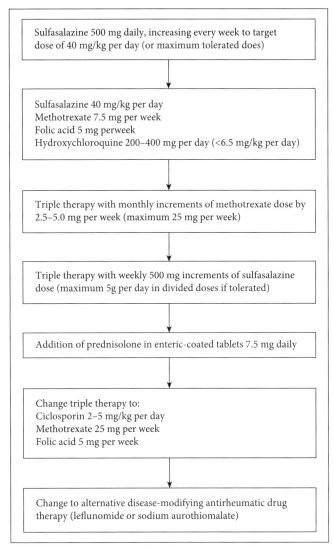

Fig. 2.1 Protocol for escalation of disease-modifying anti-rheumatic therapy in patients with persisting disease activity [1].

Reprinted from The Lancet, Vol. 364, Catriona Grigor et, Effect of a treatment strategy of tight control for rheumatoid arthritis (the TICORA study): a single-blind randomised controlled trial, 263–269, Copyright 2004, with permission from Elsevier.

injections of corticosteroid were given to patients assigned routine care with the same restrictions as those in the intensive group. Every 3 months, a metrologist assessed patients from both groups.

In both groups, no intra-articular injections were allowed in the month preceding the assessments.

The end of trial medications were as follows:

Intensive group (n = 53)

methotrexate, sulphasalazine, and hydroxychloroquine triple therapy (n = 27);

sulphasalazine or methotrexate monotherapy (n =16);

other DMARD combinations (n = 5);

methotrexate and cyclosporin (n = 2);

sodium aurothiomalate (n = 1); or

penicillamine (n = 1).

Routine group (n = 51)

DMARD monotherapy (n = 45);

other DMARD combinations (n = 4); and

triple therapy (n = 2).

Patients in the intensive group were prescribed higher doses of methotrexate than those in the routine care group (mean dose 17.6 mg/week vs 13.6 mg/week, respectively) but similar doses of sulphasalazine were given to both groups (mean dose 2.9 g/day vs 3 g/day, respectively). In addition, patients in the intensive group received more intramuscular and intra-articular injections than did patients in the routine group, with a mean triamcinolone acetonide dose of 28 mg/month (15.3 mg (54.5%) intra-articular, 12.7 mg (45.5%) intramuscular), compared with 8 mg/month (3.9 mg (49%), 4.1 mg (51%)), respectively.

Trial end points measured

Primary outcome measures

The primary outcome measures were mean fall in the Disease Activity Score (a composite of erythrocyte sedimentation rate, Ritchie articular index, joint swelling count, and patients' global assessment of disease activity) and the proportion of patients with a good response (EULAR definition—i.e. Disease Activity Score <2.4 and a fall in score from baseline by >1.2).

Secondary outcome measures

Secondary outcome measures comprised the proportion of patients in remission (EULAR definition—i.e. disease activity scores <1.6) (Prevoo et al., 1996), ACR 20, 50, and 70 response rates, and other constituents of the EULAR core measures of disease activity and outcome, namely, visual analogue pain score, assessor's global assessment of disease activity, and patient's function measured by the HAQ (at 0 and 18 months). The short form-12 questionnaire (Hurst et al., 1998) was used to measure health-related quality of life. Two radiologists scored radiographs of hands and feet at 0 and 18 months with the van der Heijde modification of the Sharp score (van der Heijde, 1999). Films were scored with the sequence of radiographs known but the radiologists masked to treatment groups.

Other

Data on resource use from case-note review and patients' diaries were recorded. Hospital resource use in terms of the number of outpatient visits, inpatient stays by specialty, and prescription costs of DMARDs or non-steroidal anti-inflammatory drugs were measured.

Community resource use (visits to the family practitioner, practice nurse, or other health professionals, and blood-test monitoring) was obtained with 1-month prospective patients' diaries at 0, 6, and 12 months. Cost calculations were undertaken from an NHS perspective. Incremental cost differences between each arm of the trial for patients who completed the trial were calculated.

Follow-up

Follow-up was performed at 18 months.

Results

At the 18-month assessment, patients in the intensive group had a higher rate of EULAR good response, remission, and ACR 70 response than the routine group (Table 2 from the article). Figure 3 from the article shows the fall in disease activity scores for both groups during the study. The mean fall in disease activity score was significantly greater in the intensive group than in the routine care group, and this difference was sustained throughout the trial (Table 3 from the article).

One patient withdrew after randomization, and seven dropped out during the study. The mean fall in Disease Activity Score was greater in the intensive group than in the routine group (-3.5 vs -1.9, difference 1.6 (95% CI, 1.1–2.1), $P < 0.0001$), with the difference sustained throughout the trial. Patients in the intensive group showed significantly greater improvements in all disease activity variables (except C-reactive protein), physical function, and quality of life. Patients in the intensive group had reduced progression of erosion scores and total Sharp scores but no difference was noted in the progression of joint-space narrowing. These patients were also more likely to be in remission than those in the routine care group (Disease Activity Score <1.6; 36/55 (65%) vs 9/55 (16%), 9.7 (3.9–23.9), $P < 0.0001$). Three patients assigned routine care and one allocated intensive management died during the study; none of the deaths was judged attributable to treatment.

Costs were lower in the intensive group than in the routine group but did not differ significantly for total hospital cost per patient or total community cost per patient. Although outpatient and prescribing costs were significantly higher in the intensive treatment group, higher inpatient costs in the routine group offset these effects.

Critique of the paper

Before every assessment, patients were sent a letter stating that they should make no mention of their drug treatment or the identity of their doctors (single-blinded study). A double-blinded study design may have strengthened the validity of the study.

In terms of the baseline characteristics and measures of disease activity in the two patient groups, these were similar, although patients randomly assigned to the intensive group had slightly higher erythrocyte sedimentation rates and C-reactive protein concentrations. This may have resulted in higher mean falls in Disease Activity Score and other disease parameters. However, the authors state that differences in baseline measures of disease activity were not deemed to be clinically significant.

In the health economic analysis part of the study, an assumption was made that the rate of resource use was constant for every subsequent month after completion of the previous patient's diary. This could be a source of bias, resulting in over or under-estimation of the results.

Significance and importance of the paper

This was one of the landmark clinical trials which demonstrated that strategies of 'tighter control' and 'targeted therapies' produced better outcomes in the management of early rheumatoid arthritis. The results of this study had major implications in the treatment of rheumatoid arthritis and form a core part of recommendations in guidelines as standard practice [4–6]. As discussed by the authors of this paper, it is noteworthy that, in this era of targeted biological therapies, this tight control in the TICORA study was achieved with standard DMARDs without the use of biologics (i.e. anti-tumour necrosis factor during the particular study period).

The TICORA study supported the findings of the earlier FIN-RACo trial (Finnish Rheumatoid Arthritis Combination Therapy) and demonstrated that the increase in the Larsen scores in the combination DMARD group was approximately twofold that in a patient group receiving monotherapy [2].

To date, there is a wealth of research data supporting attenuation of the disease process with early intensive therapy, and this approach along with a 'treat to target' approach forms a core part to the current management of rheumatoid arthritis [3].

References

1 Grigor C, Capell H, Stirling A, et al. Effect of a treatment strategy of tight control for rheumatoid arthritis (the TICORA study): a single-blind randomised controlled trial. *Lancet* 2004;**364**(9430): 264–9.

2 Möttönen T, Hannonen P, Leirisalo-Repo M, et al. Comparison of combination therapy with single-drug therapy in early rheumatoid arthritis: a randomised trial. *Lancet* 1999; **353**(9164):1568–73.

3 Quinn MA, Emery P. Window of opportunity in early rheumatoid arthritis: possibility of altering the disease process with early intervention. *Clin Exp Rheumatol* 2003;**21**(5):S154–7.

4 Smolen JS, Landewé R, Breedveld FC, et al. Recommendations for the management of rheumatoid arthritis with synthetic and biological disease-modifying antirheumatic drugs: 2013 update. *Ann Rheum Dis* 2014;**73**(3):492–509.

5 The British Society for Rheumatology. Current BSR guidelines. <http://www.rheumatology.org.uk/ resources/guidelines/bsr_guidelines.aspx>, accessed 20 January 2015.

6 National Institute for Health and Care Excellence. Rheumatoid arthritis: the management of rheumatoid arthritis in adults. <http://www.nice.org.uk/guidance/CG79>, accessed 20 January 2015.

7 Prevoo ML, van Gestel AM, van T Hof MA, van Rijswijk MH, van de Putte LB, van Riel PL. Remission in a prospective study of patients with rheumatoid arthritis: American Rheumatism Association preliminary remission criteria in relation to the disease activity score. Br J Rheumatol 1996; **35**:1101–15.

8 Hurst NP, Ruta DA, Kind P. Comparison of the MOS short form-12 (SF12) health status questionnaire with the SF36 in patients with rheumatoid arthritis. Br J Rheumatol 1998; **37**:862–69.

9 Van der Heijde D. How to read radiographs according to the Sharp/van der Heijde method. J Rheumatol 1999; **26**:743–45.

Paper 2.10: Clinical and radiographic outcomes of four different treatment strategies in patients with early rheumatoid arthritis (the BeSt study): a randomized, controlled trial

Reference

Goekoop-Ruiterman YP, de Vries-Bouwstra JK, Allaart CF, et al. Clinical and radiographic outcomes of four different treatment strategies in patients with early rheumatoid arthritis (the BeSt study): a randomized, controlled trial. *Arthritis Rheum* 2005;52(11):3381–90.

Purpose

To compare clinical and radiographic outcomes of four different treatment strategies in patients with early rheumatoid arthritis (the BeSt study).

Patients

Patients with early rheumatoid arthritis, as defined by the ACR 1987 revised criteria [1], with disease duration of ≤2 years, age ≥18 years with active disease with ≥6 of 66 swollen joints, ≥6 of 68 tender joints, and either an erythrocyte sedimentation rate ≥28 mm/hour or a global health score of ≥20 mm on a 0–100 mm VAS, where 0 = best and 100 = worst.

Study design

Multicentre, randomized clinical trial of 508 patients allocated one of four treatment strategies.

Trial end points measured

The primary end points were Disease Activity Score 44 (DAS 44), functional ability, measured by the Dutch version of the HAQ (D-HAQ), and radiographic joint damage according to the modified Sharp/Van der Heijde score (SHS) [3], with a range of 0–448 [4], assessed on radiographs of the hands and feet obtained at baseline and after one year of follow-up.

Follow-up

The follow-up was for 1 year.

Treatment

The study involved four treatment groups, with treatment adjustments made every three months in an effort to obtain low disease activity (a disease activity score <2.4 in 44 joints). If the clinical response was consistently adequate (DAS 44 ≤2.4 for at least six months), medication was gradually tapered until one drug remained at a maintenance dose.

Group 1

Sequential disease-modifying anti-rheumatic drug monotherapy was used, starting with methotrexate 15 mg/week and increased to 25–30 mg/week if the DAS 44 was >2.4.

Subsequent steps for patients with an insufficient response were sulphasalazine (SSZ) monotherapy, leflunomide monotherapy, methotrexate with infliximab, gold with methyl-prednisolone, and, finally, methotrexate with cyclosporin A (CSA) and prednisone.

Group 2

Step-up combination therapy was used, starting with 15 mg/week methotrexate, which was increased to 25–30 mg/week if the DAS 44 was >2.4. If response to therapy was still insufficient, SSZ was added, followed by the addition of hydroxychloroquine (HCQ) and then by prednisone. Patients whose disease failed to respond to the combination of these four drugs were subsequently switched to methotrexate with infliximab, methotrexate with CSA and prednisone, and, finally, to leflunomide.

Group 3

An initial combination therapy with tapered high-dose prednisone was used. Patients started with the combination of 7.5 mg/week methotrexate, 2,000 mg/day SSZ, and 60 mg/day prednisone (the last of which was tapered in seven weeks to 7.5 mg/day). In the case of a DAS 44 of >2.4, methotrexate was augmented to 25–30 mg/week and, if the response was still insufficient, the combination was replaced subsequently by a combination of metho-trexate with CSA and prednisone, followed by methotrexate with infliximab, leflunomide monotherapy, gold with methylprednisolone, and, finally, by azathioprine (AZA) with prednisone. In the case of a persistent DAS 44 of ≤2.4, first, prednisone was tapered to zero after 28 weeks and then methotrexate was tapered to zero after 40 weeks.

Group 4

An initial combination therapy with the tumour necrosis factor antagonist infliximab was used. The patients started with 25–30 mg/week methotrexate with 3 mg/kg infliximab at weeks 0, 2, and 6 and every eight weeks thereafter. After three months, the dose of in-fliximab was increased to 6 mg/kg/every eight weeks if the DAS 44 was >2.4. Extra DAS 44 calculations for dose adjustments were performed every eight weeks within one week before the next infusion of infliximab. If the DAS 44 was >2.4, the dose of the next infusion was increased to 7.5 mg/kg/every eight weeks and finally to 10 mg/kg/every eight weeks. If patients still had a DAS 44 of >2.4 while receiving methotrexate with 10 mg/kg infliximab, medication was subsequently switched to SSZ, then to leflunomide, then to the combina-tion of methotrexate, CSA, and prednisone, then to gold with methylprednisolone, and, finally, to AZA with prednisone. In the case of a persistent good response (DAS 44 of ≤2.4 for at least six months), the dose of infliximab was reduced (from 10 to 7.5, 6, and then 3 mg/kg) every next infusion until stopped.

Results

Initial combination therapy including either prednisone (Group 3) or infliximab (Group 4) resulted in earlier functional improvement than did sequential monotherapy (Group 1) and step-up combination therapy (Group 2), with mean scores at three months on the D-HAQ of 1.0 in Groups 1 and 2 and 0.6 in Groups 3 and 4 (P < 0.001). After one year, mean D-HAQ scores were 0.7 in Groups 1 and 2 and 0.5 in Groups 3 and 4 (P = 0.009). The median increases in total Sharp/Van der Heijde radiographic joint score were 2.0, 2.5, 1.0, and 0.5 in Groups 1–4, respectively (P < 0.001). There were no significant differences in the number of adverse events and withdrawals between the groups.

Critique of the paper

The study showed that 'by the end of the first year, there was a marked improvement in all groups, with 32% of all patients having clinical remission of their disease (DAS 44 of <1.6).' The authors comment that 'presumably, this result after 1 year was due to close monitoring with immediate treatment adjustments made in all patients who had a DAS 44<2.4.'

Almost a third of all patients going into remission are a high number compared to real-life clinical practice and although the explanation for this observation could be as given in the discussion by the authors, there could also be other reasons, for example, milder rheumatoid arthritis.

Significance and importance of the paper

The study supported the results of the TICORA study but this time showing the impact of intensive treatment involving the newer biologic DMARDs [2]. It showed that patients with early rheumatoid arthritis, initial combination therapy including either prednisone or infliximab resulted in earlier functional improvement and less radiographic damage after one year than did sequential monotherapy or step-up combination therapy.

All new therapies licensed for use in rheumatoid arthritis demonstrate acceptable safety profiles but also suppression of inflammation, to varying degrees. Complete 'cure' and prolonged drug free remission have not been demonstrated. This was one of the first studies to show that it was possible to halt structural damage as seen on X-ray with the currently available agents in combination and has been a major achievement of contemporary treatment strategies for rheumatoid arthritis. Understandably, studies like this one have revolutionized the treatment and changed the face of this once devastating and destructive joint disease.

References

1 **Arnett FC, Edworthy SM, Bloch DA, et al**. The American Rheumatism Association 1987 revised criteria for the classification of rheumatoid arthritis. *Arthritis Rheum* 1988;**31**(3):315–24.

2 **Grigor C, Capell H, Stirling A, et al**. Effect of a treatment strategy of tight control for rheumatoid arthritis (the TICORA study): a single-blind randomised controlled trial. *Lancet* 2004;**364**(9430):264–69.

3 **Siegert CE, Vleming LJ, Vandenbroucke JP, et al**. Measurement of disability in Dutch rheumatoid arthritis patients. *Clin Rheumatol* 1984;**3**(3):305–9.

4 **Van der Heijde DM, van Riel PL, Gribnau FW, et al**. Effects of hydroxychloroquine and sulphasalazine on progression of joint damage in rheumatoid arthritis. *Lancet* 1989;**1**(8646):1036–8.

Chapter 3

Spondyloarthropathies

Carmel Stober and Hill Gaston

Introduction

The choice of landmark papers in spondyloarthritis (SpA) has been influenced by several considerations. The first is the delineation of the disorders themselves, and the classic papers, now more than 50 years old, which used clinical observation to group together certain otherwise disparate forms of inflammatory arthritis and separate them from rheumatoid arthritis; hence, the inclusion of the papers by Wright, and by Moll et al. (again from the Leeds school), on, first, the recognition of psoriatic arthritis and, later, the broader concept of spondyloarthritis. The paper from Rosenberg and Petty shows one extension of the concept into paediatric rheumatology. It is possible for the modern reader to assume that SpA has always been recognized as a condition and it is important to be aware of the history and basis of the classification. These papers also highlight how good clinical observation can be the basis for classification which later receives support from genetics and investigations into pathogenesis. Of course, the classic genetic finding undergirding the SpA concept was the discovery of the association with *HLA-B27* by Brewerton et al. and it is impossible to ignore a paper which in many ways set the agenda for speculation on the pathogenesis of SpA over succeeding decades, and still remains a hot topic today. The most modern paper chosen, by Evans et al., is really an extension of this approach using the power of modern genetics—though it is hard not to prefer the early study which made a critical finding on 75 patients as compared to the recent one which required more than 5,000! The crucial demonstration of the ability of *HLA-B27* itself (and not a linked gene) to cause SpA pathology came with the generation of the B27 transgenic rat by Hammer et al., and subsequent work with this rat has clarified many aspects of the likely involvement of HLA-B27 in pathogenesis, while not producing definitive answers.

Other approaches consolidated the SpA concept; Mielants et al. drew attention to gut involvement in the non-psoriatic forms of SpA, a finding which is now being vigorously pursued with our ability to characterize the gut (and indeed skin) microbiome in health and disease. In reactive arthritis, the form of SpA self-evidently related to infection, the findings by Granfors et al. on the traffic of bacterial antigens to the joint, and the later demonstration of potent T-cell mediated responses to these antigens within affected joints, cast light on one aspect of SpA pathogenesis, although not helping to solve the B27 puzzle. McGonagle et al. made a telling contribution to understanding of SpA by drawing attention to the enthesis as the primary site of pathology, an idea which has received substantial support recently from various animal models of SpA.

This collection of papers may differ from those chosen in other forms of arthritis in having a paucity of papers on treatment, and in particular no classic double-blind placebo-controlled clinical trials. The single trial included, by Brandt et al., was a small (tiny) open label trial, but nevertheless established beyond reasonable doubt the major role of TNF inhibition in treatment of AS—later confirmed in formal trials and extended to other forms of SpA. Arguably, this has been the only significant advance in treatment of SpA in the last three to four decades (discounting the necessary testing of various novel NSAIDs over the years). Many other biologics and small molecules are of course being investigated currently for SpA treatment, and while this is an exciting time in SpA treatment research, it has not yet generated any 'classic' papers. Perhaps a future edition will incorporate some of these!

Paper 3.1: Recognition of psoriatic arthritis

Reference

Wright, V. Psoriasis and arthritis. *Ann Rheum Dis* 1956;15(4):348–56.

Purpose

Clinical description of arthritis in patients with psoriasis, and differentiation of psoriatic arthritis from rheumatoid disease.

Patients

A retrospective series of 42 patients with psoriasis and arthritis, of whom 34 had erosive disease. These were compared with 55 rheumatoid factor (Rose-Waaler) seropositive patients without psoriasis and 310 patients with psoriasis and no arthritis.

Study design

The study carefully documented clinical features and carried out a number of relevant laboratory investigations.

Results

The paper made a good case for the recognition of an erosive inflammatory arthritis which was clinically distinguishable from rheumatoid arthritis. Among the distinguishing features was the lack of rheumatoid factor; only 2 of the 34 patients with erosive disease were rheumatoid factor positive; one of these had rheumatoid nodules, no nail involvement, and was almost certainly a true case of coincidence of the two diagnoses. Other features noted were the near equal sex incidence compared to the female preponderance in rheumatoid arthritis (this had been previously reported), a tendency for less severe joint damage (though the subset with arthritis mutilans was seen), the common involvement of DIP joints, and more patients presenting in adolescence. Interestingly 50% of the population achieved long-lasting remission in their disease, some apparently spontaneous rather than related to use of the limited therapies available at that time.

A high incidence of ankylosing spondylitis (3 of 34) was also noted. Of the eight patients with arthritis other than erosive disease, one had gout, one rheumatic fever, and six osteoarthritis, and these were all judged to be co-occurrence of these conditions with psoriasis.

Critique of the paper

The patient series is relatively small; it lacked power to show for instance that the observed difference in sex incidence between psoriatic arthritis and rheumatoid arthritis was statistically significant despite being striking (53% male in psoriatic arthritis vs 25% in rheumatoid arthritis). Nevertheless, careful documentation established features which have been confirmed in subsequent studies and effectively addressed and refuted some of the prevailing ideas on psoriatic arthritis at that time [1–3].

Significance and importance of the paper

Prior to this paper, an increased prevalence of 'atrophic' inflammatory arthritis (i.e. what would now be termed erosive or osteopenic disease) was recognized by dermatologists within their psoriasis population: ~5%–8%. Likewise, rheumatologists estimated that around 3% of their population with this form of arthritis had psoriasis as compared to the general population prevalence for psoriasis of 0.7%. No such increase in psoriasis prevalence was seen in osteoarthritis patients. However, among rheumatologists there was considerable discussion whether there was a true entity of psoriatic arthritis, rather than the co-occurrence of RA and psoriasis—two relatively common diseases—with the higher incidence of 'RA' perhaps relating a predisposition to inflammatory disease in both skin and joints. In addition, if psoriatic arthritis were to be considered a distinct entity, what were its characteristics? Again, there were several ideas being put forward:

- that psoriatic arthritis was a form of arthritis in which the skin and joint disease 'marched in parallel', that is, when one disease was active, so was the other;
- that treatment of the skin was effective in controlling arthritis;
- that 'true' psoriatic arthritis is restricted to the DIP joints; and
- that 'arthritis mutilans' is the typical form of the disease.

All of these notions were clearly addressed by the paper and either refuted or clarified. The idea that skin and joint disease followed parallel courses was firmly rejected; 23% of patients had the onset of arthritis prior to skin involvement. In these the importance of a family history of psoriasis was emphasized—this was present in 35% of arthritis patients compared to 2% of those with rheumatoid arthritis. Around half could not identify any relationship between the activity of their skin disease and arthritis, with a further 25% claiming an inverse relationship. Treatment of skin disease did not appear to be effective for arthritis.

The paper made interesting and important observations on the relationship between psoriatic nail disease and arthritis; these take on new significance with the emergence of the idea that the structure of nail bed may have some entheseal features, as proposed by McGonagle and Benjamin [4]. Wright noted that 77% of arthritis patients had nail disease compared to 10%–25% in the general psoriasis population (in two patients, psoriasis was confined to nails). While, in general, psoriasis and arthritis activity did not align, this was not the case with nail disease, where exacerbations were often synchronous in nails and joints. The involvement of the DIP adjacent to the affected nail was noted and nicely illustrated (Figure 3.1). In this series, even though DIP involvement was frequent, no patient had disease completely confined to these joints; subsequent larger surveys have identified some patients of this kind. However, the concept that 'psoriatic arthritis' was essentially a DIP arthropathy was dismissed, since involvement of joints other than DIPs showed a similar pattern to rheumatoid arthritis (Figure 3.2). Psoriatic arthritis was more commonly monoarticular at onset than rheumatoid disease (62% vs 41%—although Figure 3.2 was derived from a separate published study, not the series being reported). DIP disease was commonly present initially (~50%).

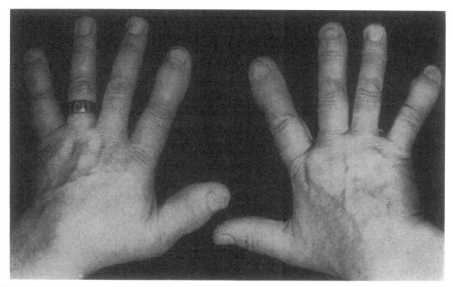

Fig. 3.1 Topographical association of DIP and nail lesions in erosive arthritis with psoriasis. The index and middle fingers of the left hand show a contrast between affected and unaffected nails.

Reproduced from Annals of the Rheumatic Diseases, Psoriasis and Arthritis, V. Wright, Volume 15, copyright 1956, with permission from BMJ Publishing Group Ltd.

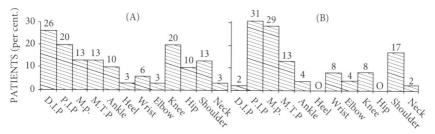

Fig. 3.2 Joints involved initially: A. in patients with arthritis and psoriasis; B. in patients with rheumatoid arthritis.

Reproduced from Annals of the Rheumatic Diseases, Psoriasis and Arthritis, V. Wright, Volume 15, copyright 1956, with permission from BMJ Publishing Group Ltd.

Laboratory investigations showed similar elevations in inflammatory markers (ESR, CRP, immunoglobulins) as in rheumatoid arthritis. Psoriatic arthritis patients had raised serum cholesterol, an early indication of the metabolic syndrome which often accompanies psoriasis; this measurement was not made in the rheumatoid patients.

In summary the paper clearly delineated a seronegative arthritis associated with psoriasis and also pointed towards its classification as a spondyloarthritis or even enthesopathy, with its recognition of nail disease, a high prevalence of ankylosing spondylitis, and interestingly the predominance of stiffness as the most troublesome symptom—nearly a quarter rated stiffness rather than pain as their principal complaint.

References

1 **Gladman DD**. Psoriatic arthritis. *Rheum Dis Clin North Am* 1998;**24**(4):829–44, x.

2 **Gladman DD, Antoni C, Mease P, et al**. Psoriatic arthritis: epidemiology, clinical features, course, and outcome. *Ann Rheum Dis* 2005;**64**(Suppl 2):ii14–7.

3 **Helliwell PS, Taylor WJ**. Classification and diagnostic criteria for psoriatic arthritis. *Ann Rheum Dis* 2005;**64**(Suppl 2):ii3–8.

4 **McGonagle D, Lories RJU, Tan AL, et al**. The concept of a "synovio-entheseal complex" and its implications for understanding joint inflammation and damage in psoriatic arthritis and beyond. *Arthritis Rheum* 2007;**56**(8):2482–91.

Paper 3.2: Associations between ankylosing spondylitis, psoriatic arthritis, Reiter's disease, the intestinal arthropathies, and Behçet's syndrome

Reference

Moll JM, Haslock I, Macrae IF, Wright V. Associations between ankylosing spondylitis, psoriatic arthritis, Reiter's disease, the intestinal arthropathies, and Behçet's syndrome. *Medicine* 1974;53(5):343–64.

Purpose

The objective of the paper was to review evidence from the literature, and from the author's own institutions, to support classification criteria for '*seronegative spondarthritides*' (SpA).

Results

Prior to this manuscript, diseases such as psoriatic arthritis (PsA) and ankylosing spondylitis (AS) had been considered by many rheumatologists as atypical forms of rheumatoid arthritis (RA) [1]. In this landmark paper, the authors presented six classification criteria to define the SpA as a unique group of disorders distinct from RA (Table 3.1). Note that the authors favoured the term spondarthritis but later usage has preferred spond**ylo**arthritis or occasionally spond**yl**arthritis.

Table 3.1 Criteria for member of the Seronegative Spondarthritis Group

1	Negative test for rheumatoid factor
2	Absence of subcutaneous ('rheumatoid') nodules
3	Presence of inflammatory peripheral arthritis
4	Radiological sacroiliitis with or without ankylosing spondylitis
5	Evidence of clinical overlap between members of the group*
6	Tendency to familial aggregation

*Defined as ≥2 of psoriasiform skin or nail lesions, ocular inflammation, buccal ulceration, ulceration of small or large intestine, genital ulceration, genito-urinary infection, erythema nodosum, pyoderma gangrenosum, and thrombophlebitis.

The clinical entities the authors included in the classification were those currently regarded as members of the SpA family (AS, PsA, arthritis associated with ulcerative colitis (UC) or Crohn's disease, and reactive arthritis) together with Whipple's disease and Behçet's syndrome. This selection was based on information provided from surveys, observations of previous workers, and personal study at the Rheumatism Research Unit in Leeds [2]. Evidence was also provided for interrelationships between members of the group.

First, the authors presented evidence that an alternative diagnosis to RA should be sought in the presence of a persistently negative rheumatoid factor. In a series of 346 patients with inflammatory polyarthritis, only 17% showed a fluctuation in rheumatoid factor over 3 years [3], demonstrating that once serological status is established it remains stable. Second, while skin lesions complicate SpA, these differ histologically from rheumatoid nodules. With respect to the third criterion, approximately 60% of patients with AS [4], 6.8% of 548 patients with psoriasis [5], 11.5% with UC [6], and 4.5% of 600 individuals with Crohn's disease [7] have peripheral arthritis. Bilateral sacroiliitis has been found in 20% of patients with PsA [8–10], 50% of those with ReA of >5 years duration [11], and 18% of those with UC [6]. In terms of spondylitis, there were previous claims of radiologically unique features for forms of SpA other than AS. However, the authors contested the previous observation of atypical paravertebral ossification described by Bywaters and Dixon in PsA and the distribution of syndesmophytes in PsA and ReA by McEwan et al. [12, 13]. The prevalence of radiological sacroiliitis and spondylitis in PsA, UC, and Crohn's disease observed by the authors was comparable to published data [2].

In support of the fourth criterion, there are many clinical features that overlap in the diseases which they wished to group together, as demonstrated by Wright and Reed comparing PsA and ReA [14]. UC and Crohn's disease share many features, including the pattern of arthropathy and extra-articular manifestations. In addition, Behçet's syndrome also demonstrates overlap with the UC and Crohn's disease, while a prevalence of inflammatory bowel disease in 17.5% of patients with AS had been reported [15].

The final criterion concerned familial aggregation. Kellgren reported a 40-fold increase in AS in the relatives of probands with disease [16]. Familial association was also found for psoriasis, PsA, UC, Crohn's, and ReA. In addition, the authors documented and referenced the increased prevalence of different forms of SpA among family members.

Critique of the paper

The paper was the first to draw together classification criteria for the SpA, and these have formed the basis for more recent classifications including those of Amor (1990) [17], the European Spondylarthropathy Study Group (ESSG; 1991) [18], the Berlin criteria (2004) [19], and the Assessment of Spondylarthritis international Society (ASAS) criteria for axial SpA (2009) [20, 21]. Evidence was derived from previous studies (Criteria 1–6) in addition to the personal experiences of the authors (Criteria 4–6). Of note is the exclusion of HLA-B27 in the classification criteria, even though the association with AS had been described the previous year by Brewerton et al. [22]. The authors also declined to say how many of the criteria were required to fulfil the classification and did not evaluate the specificity or sensitivity of their criteria against another gold standard.

Two conditions initially included within the SpA classification were Behçet's syndrome and Whipple's disease. The former has recently been re-evaluated by the International Criteria for Behçet's Disease (ICBD), a consortium of 27 countries submitting data on 2,556 patients diagnosed with BD, and 1,163 controls [23]. A unique set of criteria was proposed, with 93.9% sensitivity and 92.1% specificity. BD is now considered a miscellaneous condition rather than a form of SpA. Whipple's disease is now known to be caused by the Gram-positive bacterium *Tropheryma whipplei* and, although it can result in arthritis and sacroiliitis and may possibly be associated with HLA-B27, it is no longer considered a form of SpA but rather an unusual form of joint infection, since the organism can be demonstrated in inflamed synovia.

Significance and importance of the paper

More recent classification systems for SpA have been developed using a scoring system, and then comparing the results to those obtained from some form of gold standard (e.g. expert opinion) to evaluate sensitivity and specificity. The Amor criteria were developed from data from 1,219 SpA patients and 157 other rheumatic disease controls and combine 12 items, including clinical elements, pelvic radiographs, HLA-B27, family history, and response to non-steroidal anti-inflammatory drugs [17]. ESSG criteria are based on data from 403 SpA patients and 674 control rheumatology patients, with patient entry criteria including inflammatory spinal pain or synovitis plus one minor criterion from a list of seven; HLA-B27 was not included [18]. Examination of the Amor criteria revealed a sensitivity of 90% and specificity of 86.6% when evaluated prospectively, while evaluation of the ESSG criteria revealed a sensitivity of 78.4% and specificity of 89.6%. In addition to the diseases included by Moll et al., the Amor and ESSG criteria also define undifferentiated SpA as a specific entity.

In 2009, ASAS developed criteria sets tested against a cohort of 649 patients from 25 centres in 16 countries [21]. The criteria for axial SpA are summarized in Table 3.2. Sensitivity was 82.9%, and specificity 84.4%; the specificity of the imaging arm alone was 97.3%. Interestingly, the application of Amor or ESSG criteria to the ASAS cohort significantly reduced the specificity and sensitivity of the respective classifications, which was improved when MRI data were included [24].

Table 3.2 ASAS criteria for axial SpA (in patients with ≥ 3 months back pain and aged <45 years) [21]

Sacroiliitis on imaging plus ≥1 SpA feature	HLA-B27 plus ≥2 other SpA features
SpA features	
1. Dactylitis	6. Inflammatory back pain
2. Psoriasis	7. Crohn's/Colitis
3. Enthesitis (heel)	8. Elevated CRP
4. Arthritis	9. Family history SpA
5. Uveitis	10. Good response to NSAIDs
	11. HLA-B27

Source data from Rudwaleit M, van der Heijde D, Landewe R, Listing J, Akkoc N, Brandt J, et al. The development of Assessment of SpondyloArthritis International Society classification criteria for axial spondyloarthritis (part II): validation and final selection. *Annals of the Rheumatic Diseases*. 2009 Jun;68(6):777–83.

The establishment of classification criteria for the SpA has facilitated awareness of the condition and thus earlier and more accurate diagnosis of disease. It has also led to the development of assessment tools for disease severity and outcomes, including BASDAI and

ASDAS [25, 26], and the implementation of ASAS improvement and remission criteria for the purposes of clinical trials [27]. Thus, the paper may be seen as seminal in defining a 'non-RA' group of inflammatory arthritides; this basic idea has now received enormous support from studies of the genetics, pathogenesis, and response to treatment of these conditions.

References

1 Copeman WSC, ed. Textbook of the rheumatic diseases. London: E & S Livingstone Ltd; 1969.

2 Moll JM, Haslock I, Macrae IF, et al. Associations between ankylosing spondylitis, psoriatic arthritis, Reiter's disease, the intestinal arthropathies, and Behcet's syndrome. *Medicine* 1974;**53**(5):343–64.

3 Alexander WRM. Laboratory aspects of polyarthritis. In: The Royal College of Physicians of Edinburgh Symposium on Polyarthritis, 1964.

4 Sharp J. Differential diagnosis of ankylosing spondylitis. *BMJ* 1957;**1**(5025):975–8.

5 Leczinsky CG. The incidence of arthropathy in a 10 year series of psoriasis cases. *Acta Derm Venereol* 1948;**28**(5):483–7.

6 Wright V, Watkinson G. Sacro-iliitis and ulcerative colitis. *BMJ* 1965;**2**(5463):675–80.

7 Van Patter WN, Bargen JA, Dockerty MB, et al. Regional enteritis. *Gastroenterology* 1954;**26**(3):347–450.

8 Baker H. Epidemiological aspects of psoriasis and arthritis. *Br J Dermatol* 1966;**78**(5):249–61.

9 Reed WB. Psoriatic arthritis. A complete clinical study of 86 patients. *Acta Derm Venereol* 1961;**41**:396–403.

10 Wright V. Psoriatic arthritis: a comparative radiographic study of rheumatoid arthritis and arthritis associated with psoriasis. *Ann Rheum Dis* 1961;**20**(2):123–32.

11 Mason RM, Murray RS, Oates JK, et al. A comparative radiological study of Reiter's disease, rheumatoid arthritis and ankylosing spondylitis. *J Bone Joint Surg Br* 1959;**41**(1):137–48.

12 Bywaters EG, Dixon AS. Paravertebral ossification in psoriatic arthritis. *Ann Rheum Dis* 1965;**24**(4):313–31.

13 McEwen C, DiTata D, Lingg C, et al. Ankylosing spondylitis and spondylitis accompanying ulcerative colitis, regional enteritis, psoriasis and Reiter's disease. A comparative study. *Arthritis Rheum* 1971;**14**(3): 291–318.

14 Wright V, Reed WB. The link between Reiter's syndrome and psoriatic arthritis. *Ann Rheum Dis* 1964;**23**(1):12–21.

15 Jayson MI, Bouchier IA. Ulcerative colitis with ankylosing spondylitis. *Ann Rheum Dis* 1968;**27**(3):219–24.

16 Kellgren JH. The epidemiology of rheumatic diseases. *Ann Rheum Dis* 1964;**23**(2):109–22.

17 Amor B, Dougados M, Mijiyawa M. [Criteria of the classification of spondylarthropathies]. *Rev Rhum Mal Osteoartic* 1990;**57**(2):85–9.

18 Dougados M, van der Linden S, Juhlin R, et al. The European Spondylarthropathy Study Group preliminary criteria for the classification of spondylarthropathy. *Arthritis Rheum* 1991;**34**(10):1218–27.

19 Rudwaleit M, van der Heijde D, Khan MA, et al. How to diagnose axial spondyloarthritis early. *Ann Rheum Dis* 2004;**63**(5):535–43.

20 Rudwaleit M, Landewe R, van der Heijde D, et al. The development of Assessment of SpondyloArthritis International Society classification criteria for axial spondyloarthritis (part I):

classification of paper patients by expert opinion including uncertainty appraisal. *Ann Rheum Dis* 2009;**68**(6):770–6.

21 **Rudwaleit M, van der Heijde D, Landewe R, et al**. The development of Assessment of SpondyloArthritis International Society classification criteria for axial spondyloarthritis (part II): validation and final selection. *Ann Rheum Dis* 2009;**68**(6):777–83.

22 **Brewerton DA, Hart FD, Nicholls A, et al**. Ankylosing spondylitis and HL-A 27. *Lancet* 1973;**1**(7809):904–7.

23 **International Team for the Revision of the International Criteria for Behçet's Disease (ITR-ICBD), Davatchi F, Assaad-Khalil S, et al**. The International Criteria for Behçet's Disease (ICBD): a collaborative study of 27 countries on the sensitivity and specificity of the new criteria. *J Eur Acad Dermatol Venereol* 2014;**28**(3):338–47.

24 **Rudwaleit M, van der Heijde D, Landewe R, et al**. The Assessment of SpondyloArthritis International Society classification criteria for peripheral spondyloarthritis and for spondyloarthritis in general. *Ann Rheum Diseases* 2011;**70**(1):25–31.

25 **Garrett S, Jenkinson T, Kennedy LG, et al**. A new approach to defining disease status in ankylosing spondylitis: the Bath Ankylosing Spondylitis Disease Activity Index. *J Rheumatol* 1994;**21**(12):2286–91.

26 **Lukas C, Landewe R, Sieper J, et al**. Development of an ASAS-endorsed disease activity score (ASDAS) in patients with ankylosing spondylitis. Ann Rheum Dis 2009;**68**(1):18–24.

27 **Anderson JJ, Baron G, van der Heijde D, et al**. Ankylosing spondylitis assessment group preliminary definition of short-term improvement in ankylosing spondylitis. Arthritis Rheum 2001;**44**(8):1876–86.

Paper 3.3: The discovery of the association between ankylosing spondylitis and *HLA-B27*

Reference

Brewerton D, Hart F, Nicholls A et al. (1973). Ankylosing spondylitis and HL-A27. *Lancet* 1973;301(7809):904–7.

Purpose

To search for an association between a form of arthritis with clear clinical evidence of a major genetic component and a newly described set of polymorphic alleles in humans.

Patients

The authors reported data from 75 patients with ankylosing spondylitis; all had Grade 3 or 4 bilateral sacroiliitis, and patients with evidence of other forms of spondyloarthritis (e.g. reactive arthritis) were excluded. Disease duration was ~17 years. Seventy-five blood donors were tested as controls.

Study design

Serological typing for previously defined *HLA* alleles by lymphocytotoxicity; that is, testing the ability of sera from multiparous or multitransfused individuals to kill lymphocytes from patients and controls. Note that the sera used in this technique were not specific for a given allele and therefore the typing required observing the effects of several sera, with an allele being defined by the pattern of cytotoxicity observed using the panel of typing sera—monoclonal antibodies had not yet been invented, so no HLA-B27-specific reagents were available. (Even today, different B27-reactive monoclonal antibodies cross-react with at least one other allele.) At that time, in two series, 26 alleles were recognized, later to be defined as *HLA-A* and *HLA-B* but, at this stage, all simply were termed '*HL-Ax*'—hence the paper's title.

Results

Seventy-two of 75 patients were typed as HL-A27 positive, with a further patient having a 'weak' cytotoxicity result, that is, possibly positive, giving an overall frequency of 96%–97% in ankylosing spondylitis, as compared to 4% in the controls (3/75 positive).

Critique of the paper

The genius in this paper was in selecting ankylosing spondylitis as the rheumatic disease to investigate for an HLA association. Other rheumatic diseases in which patients often have a positive family history could have been chosen—gout is an obvious example and was apparently the disease initially chosen by the US group which also reported the association of ankylosing spondylitis and *HLA-B27* [1]—the AS patients were originally conceived as controls for those with gout! The strength of the association was, and remains, astonishing, with no other disease showing anything like so strong an HLA association. In fact the true frequency of *HLA-B27* in controls in the UK is nearer 8% than 4%, and most larger series of AS patients show frequencies of *HLA-B27* of around 90%. In larger series it is difficult to avoid 'contamination' with patients who have undeclared inflammatory bowel disease or psoriasis with axial spondyloarthritis, conditions where the frequency of *HLA-B27* is only ~50%. Nevertheless, the existence of true AS which is *HLA-B27* negative was clearly pointed out in this paper and has been confirmed many times since. Thus, the clinical phenotype of AS can be achieved without participation of *HLA-B27*. Presumably, in view of what we now know of additional loci which contribute to AS susceptibility, a sufficient 'dose' of additional genetic factors may be able to compensate for the absence of *HLA-B27*, in the same way that psoriasis and inflammatory bowel disease are able to in the 50% B27-negative AS cases which complicate those conditions.

Significance and importance of the paper

In these days of genome-wide association studies and the availability of literally millions of polymorphisms scattered across the genome, it requires some imagination to recall the difficulties of investigating the genetic basis of diseases which do not show clear Mendelian inheritance. Initially, the only polymorphic system available for investigation was the ABO blood group system, and weak associations between several diseases and particular blood groups were demonstrated. The discovery of the HLA system, with vastly greater polymorphism than ABO blood groups, represented an enormous advance in the tools available to geneticists—although the extreme polymorphism of HLA—thousands of alleles are now described at each locus [2]—was not evident at this stage.

When the observation was made, the physiologic function of HLA antigens was quite unknown. It was conceded that they were most unlikely to have evolved simply to frustrate transplant surgeons but demonstration of function was not achieved until the following year when Zinkernagel and Doherty, in a landmark and Nobel prize-winning investigation, showed that viral antigens were recognized in the context of class I MHC antigens—the phenomenon of MHC-restriction [3]. The initial studies in mice MHC antigens (H-2) were soon extended to the human system (HLA). The full meaning of 'recognized in the context of HLA' became clear with the demonstration that HLA antigens were capable of binding a wide range of peptides derived from pathogens or even self-proteins, and that T-cell receptors recognize the combination [4].

Once the physiologic function of HLA molecules was known, an immediate and attractive hypothesis to explain the association between AS and HLA-B27 presented itself: HLA-B27 would be able to bind and present a peptide derived from some component of the axial skeleton to the immune system and generate a pro-inflammatory autoimmune response. Of course this would require the breakage of self-tolerance, since T-cells which recognize self-peptides, whether bound to HLA-B27 or any other HLA protein, should be deleted in the thymus. The main way around this was to postulate 'molecular mimicry' in which a response generated against a B27-binding peptide derived from a pathogen would cross-react with an 'arthritogenic' self-peptide. This still requires breakage of tolerance, and we now know that molecular mimicry is nearly ubiquitous, that is, most foreign peptides will have similar counterparts among self-peptides, or at least ones similar enough to allow T-cell recognition, so mechanisms to prevent this kind of induction of autoimmunity must be fairly robust. Nevertheless, the 'arthritogenic peptide' theory remains conceptually attractive. Sadly, after 40 years of research it has not been shown to be true—despite many attempts—but nor has it been clearly refuted. Perhaps the very exceptional strength of the association between AS and HLA-B27 suggests that some unique property of the molecule is involved rather than its normal physiologic function which it shares with all other HLA molecules. Unique or unusual properties of HLA-B27 which have attracted attention in recent years include its ability to form heavy-chain dimers which are immunologically active [5], and its tendency to mis-fold during synthesis in the endoplasmic reticulum [6], with consequences for HLA-B27-positive antigen-presenting cells, particularly their secretion of cytokines (especially IL-23) which influence T-cell differentiation [7]. All of these theories continue to be tested actively.

There may be some disappointment that such a major discovery, and such a strong association between a disease and a single molecule, should still be unexplained after four decades. In defence, almost all of immunology had to be discovered during this time, and new aspects of the properties of HLA antigens and their role in antigenic peptide presentation continue to be discovered. Since 99% of HLA-B27-positive individuals are healthy, something relatively subtle must occur in those who develop AS, and elucidating what this might be and how it interacts with the other genes which influence AS susceptibility continues to keep many investigators busy.

References

1 **Schlosstein L, Terasaki PI, Bluestone R, et al**. High association of an HL-A antigen, W27, with ankylosing spondylitis. *N Engl J Med* 1973;**288**(14):704–6.

2 **Robinson J, Halliwell JA, McWilliam H, et al**. The IMGT/HLA database. *Nucleic Acids Res* 2013;**41**(D1):D1222–7.

3 **Zinkernagel RM, Doherty PC**. Restriction of in vitro T cell-mediated cytotoxicity in lymphocytic choriomeningitis within a syngeneic or semiallogeneic system. *Nature* 1974;**248**(450):701–2.

4 **Townsend A, Bodmer H**. Antigen recognition by class I-restricted T lymphocytes. *Annu Rev Immunol* 1989;**7**(1):601–24.

5 **Kollnberger S, Bird L, Sun MY, et al**. Cell-surface expression and immune receptor recognition of HLA-B27 homodimers. *Arthritis Rheum* 2002;**46**(11):2972–82.

6 **Colbert RA**. HLA-B27 misfolding: a solution to the spondyloarthropathy conundrum? *Mol Med Today* 2000;**6**(6):224–30.

7 **Goodall JC, Wu C, Zhang Y, et al**. Endoplasmic reticulum stress-induced transcription factor, CHOP, is crucial for dendritic cell IL-23 expression. *Proc Natl Acad Sci U S A* 2010;**107**:17698–703.

Paper 3.4: A syndrome of seronegative enthesopathy and arthropathy in children

Reference

Rosenberg AM, Petty RE. A syndrome of seronegative enthesopathy and arthropathy in children. *Arthritis Rheum* 1982;25(9):1041–7.

Purpose

The study evaluated 39 children with a syndrome of seronegative enthesopathy and arthropathy (SEA). The features demonstrated by these children made it possible to distinguish the syndrome of SEA from other childhood rheumatic conditions such as juvenile rheumatoid arthritis.

Patients

The subjects were 39 children with SEA syndrome as defined by fulfilling four criteria: (1) the onset of musculoskeletal symptoms prior to the age of 16 years; (2) the absence of both classical IgM rheumatoid-factor and antinuclear antibodies (ANA); (3) the presence of enthesopathic signs; and (4) the presence of arthralgia with or without objective signs of arthritis. These patients presented to the paediatric rheumatic disease clinics of the Children's Hospital, Winnipeg, Canada, and the Arthritis Centre, Vancouver, Canada, during a four-year period. The comparator comprised 100 children who conformed to the American Rheumatism Association criteria for juvenile rheumatoid arthritis (JRA) [1].

Results

Of the 39 children with SEA syndrome, 8 children fulfilled diagnostic criteria for ankylosing spondylitis (AS), 2/39 had concurrent inflammatory bowel disease, and 3/39 demonstrated SEA with reactive arthritis; therefore, the remaining 26 children had idiopathic SEA syndrome. Thirty-five of the 39 children (90%) were males; in contrast, 21% of the JRA population were males ($P < 0.0005$). The mean age of onset of musculoskeletal symptoms was older in the SEA group (9.8 years; range, 2–16 years) than in the JRA group (5.1 years; range, 1–15 years; $P < 0.0005$). Family history was more evident in the SEA group than in the JRA group ($P < 0.0025$), with a history of arthritis in first-degree relatives present in 32% of SEA patients but only 4% of JRA patients ($P < 0.0005$).

Peripheral arthritis was apparent in 29/39 patients with SEA syndrome, with the remaining reporting arthralgia. The mean number of affected joints was 4.7 in the SEA group and was 9.2 in the JRA group ($P < 0.01$). Twenty-eight of the 29 patients with SEA syndrome and arthritis had lower limb involvement, with the knee most commonly affected joint. By definition, all the patients demonstrated enthesopathic signs: the calcaneal insertion of the plantar aponeurosis was the most affected site, followed by the tibial tuberosity. Tenderness of one or more metatarsophalangeal joints was present in 18 patients and was mostly localized to the plantar aspect of the metatarsal head. Lower back signs were also significantly more frequent in the SEA group ($P < 0.0005$).

Twenty-six of the 39 patients with SEA syndrome had radiographic studies of the sacro-iliac joints, with bilateral sclerosis and erosions observed in 8 patients with AS and 1 patient with reactive arthritis; 15 of the 26 evaluated had normal sacroiliac joints. Twenty-three patients had radiological studies of the calcanei: 5/23 showed erosions of the Achilles tendon insertion, and 7/23 demonstrated spur formation at either the Achilles tendon or plantar aponeurosis. Radiological studies of the thoracolumbar spine in 6/7 patients studied showed abnormalities. Twenty-three of the 32 SEA syndrome patients (72%) who were HLA typed were HLA-B27 positive, as compared to 13% of patients with JRA (P < 0.0005).

Critique of the paper

This manuscript described epidemiological and clinical characteristics in a group of 39 children with features distinguishing them from those with JRA, as defined by ACR criteria in 1977 [1]. These included lack of autoantibodies, and enthesopathy in the presence of articular involvement. Seronegativity is not uncommon in children, as most patients with JRA have neither rheumatoid factor nor ANA [2]. Enthesopathy has been well documented in seronegative spondylarthropathy (SpA) in adults [3], but the significance and characterization of this phenomenon in children had been less well documented. All 39 children had enthesopathy, compared to 3 females with seropositive polyarticular JRA in the control group. The authors postulated that the entheses of the growing child may be more metabolically active than in adults and that lesions at calcaneal entheses are more frequent in children with AS than in adults with AS [4].

The authors evaluated a relatively small group of individuals over a four-year period, comparing this to a similarly aged group with differentiating clinical symptoms and signs. Despite the size of the group, the study was sufficient to identify unique features. These included male preponderance, later age of onset, positive family history, predominant involvement of large joints of the lower limbs, and increased prevalence of HLA-B27. Long-term follow-up may enable the elucidation of a primary diagnosis in addition to providing prognostic information with respect to this unique category of paediatric rheumatic disease.

Significance and importance of the paper

There have been a number of classification systems proposed for rheumatic conditions in the paediatric population. The 1977 classification considered three broad categories where symptoms were evident in ≥1 joint for ≥6 weeks: (i) systemic-onset JRA (two subtypes); (ii) pauciarticular (four subtypes); or (iii) polyarticular (two subtypes) [1]. This ACR classification did not incorporate juvenile psoriatic arthritis or juvenile AS, which may have been placed within the pauciarticular group. Furthermore, no distinction was made between rheumatoid-factor-positive and rheumatoid-factor-negative polyarticular subtypes. A further evaluation was undertaken in 1986, when it was proposed that the course of disease after the onset period of six months should be incorporated [5]. The European League against Rheumatism (EULAR) meanwhile utilized the term juvenile chronic arthritis (JCA) to include systemic, polyarticular (rheumatoid-factor negative), pauciarticular, and JRA (polyarticular, rheumatoid-factor positive) forms of disease. JCA included, but did not differentiate, juvenile psoriatic arthritis and juvenile AS.

The clinical features of SpA in children differ from those observed in adults, with enthesitis and peripheral arthritis more common than inflammatory back pain [6]. Rosenberg and Petty recognized SEA as an undifferentiated juvenile SpA with minimal axial involvement [7]. The latest (2001) International League of Associations for Rheumatology (ILAR) criteria define seven subtypes of juvenile idiopathic arthritis (JIA) [8]. Enthesis-related arthritis (ERA), psoriatic arthritis, and undifferentiated JIA likely incorporate all patients formerly categorized with SEA syndrome. The disadvantage of the ILAR criteria is that children meeting diagnostic criteria for AS and those with reactive arthritis or co-existing inflammatory bowel disease are not considered independently [9, 10]. The ILAR classification system has been adopted worldwide, thus harmonizing diagnostic and treatment strategies.

The original 39 children with SEA syndrome were followed for a mean of 11 years; half of the group developed definite or possible SpA. They also tended to have arthritis rather than arthralgia, and onset after five years of age influenced progression to SpA [11]. Juvenile SpA and ERA have also been shown to predict worse health outcomes relative to JRA and JIA, respectively [12, 13]. A second important aspect is when considering treatment strategies, and transitioning between paediatric and adult services. Juvenile axial SpA prior to fulfilling criteria for AS may provide a treatment window whereby the early use of TNF inhibitors could influence the progress of axial disease. Importantly, for the purpose of treatment strategies, ILAR has defined five treatment groups (as opposed to the seven diagnostic groups), whereby ERA and PsA may be incorporated into different categories [14].

References

1 **Brewer EJ Jr, Bass J, Baum J, et al**. Current proposed revision of JRA Criteria. JRA Criteria Subcommittee of the Diagnostic and Therapeutic Criteria Committee of the American Rheumatism Section of The Arthritis Foundation. *Arthritis Rheum* 1977;**20**(2 Suppl):195–9.

2 **Petty RE, Cassidy JT, Sullivan DB**. Serologic studies in juvenile rheumatoid arthritis: a review. *Arthritis Rheum* 1977;**20**(2 Suppl):260–7.

3 **Ball J**. Enthesopathy of rheumatoid and ankylosing spondylitis. *Ann Rheum Dis* 1971;**30**(3):213–23.

4 **Riley MJ, Ansell BM, Bywaters EG**. Radiological manifestations of ankylosing spondylitis according to age at onset. *Ann Rheum Dis* 1971;**30**(2):138–48.

5 **Cassidy JT, Levinson JE, Bass JC, et al**. A study of classification criteria for a diagnosis of juvenile rheumatoid arthritis. *Arthritis Rheum* 1986;**29**(2):274–81.

6 **Hofer M**. Spondylarthropathies in children—are they different from those in adults? *Best Pract Res Clin Rheumatol* 2006;**20**(2):315–28.

7 **Rosenberg AM, Petty RE**. A syndrome of seronegative enthesopathy and arthropathy in children. *Arthritis Rheum* 1982;**25**(9):1041–7.

8 **Petty RE, Southwood TR, Manners P, et al**. International League of Associations for Rheumatology classification of juvenile idiopathic arthritis: second revision, Edmonton, 2001. *J Rheumatol* 2004;**31**(2):390–2.

9 Gomez KS, Raza K, Jones SD, Kennedy LG, Calin A. Juvenile onset ankylosing spondylitis—more girls than we thought? *J Rheumatol* 1997;**24**(4):735–7.

10 Tse SM, Laxer RM. Juvenile spondyloarthropathy. *Curr Opin Rheumatol* 2003;**15**(4):374–9.

11 Cabral DA, Oen KG, Petty RE. SEA syndrome revisited: a longterm followup of children with a syndrome of seronegative enthesopathy and arthropathy. *J Rheumatol* 1992;**19**(8):1282–5.

12 Selvaag AM, Lien G, Sorskaar D, et al. Early disease course and predictors of disability in juvenile rheumatoid arthritis and juvenile spondyloarthropathy: a 3 year prospective study. *J Rheumatol* 2005;**32**(6):1122–30.

13 Flato B, Hoffmann-Vold AM, Reiff A, et al. Long-term outcome and prognostic factors in enthesitis-related arthritis: a case-control study. *Arthritis Rheum* 2006;**54**(11):3573–82.

14 Beukelman T, Patkar NM, Saag KG, et al. 2011 American College of Rheumatology recommendations for the treatment of juvenile idiopathic arthritis: initiation and safety monitoring of therapeutic agents for the treatment of arthritis and systemic features. *Arthritis Care Res* 2011;**63**(4):465–82.

Paper 3.5: Yersinia antigens in synovial-fluid cells from patients with reactive arthritis

Reference

Granfors K, Jalkanen S, von Essen R, et al. Yersinia antigens in synovial-fluid cells from patients with reactive arthritis. *N Engl J Med* 1989;320(4):216–21.

Purpose

To demonstrate the presence of yersinia antigens in synovial-fluid cells obtained from patients with reactive arthritis. The patients had a recent history of yersinia infection (1 week to 5 months).

Patients

Fifty-six adults with inflammatory joint disease were studied, with samples collected between 1983 and 1988. The three study groups were as follows: (1) 13 patients with reactive arthritis triggered by *Yersinia enterocolitica* O:3 or *Y. pseudotuberculosis* IA, as identified by an antibody response to the causative organism which was four standard deviations above the mean titre in healthy donors; all patients experienced typical clinical signs of acute yersinia infection followed by acute reactive arthritis; (2) 2 patients with reactive arthritis triggered by *Y. enterocolitica* O:3, who had low antibody titres of IgG or IgA subtype and were stool culture negative; and (3) 20 patients with rheumatoid arthritis plus 21 patients with other inflammatory joint diseases.

Study design

An experimental study used to investigate whether yersinia bacterial antigens could be detected in synovial fluid isolated from patients with reactive arthritis after yersinia infection (15 patients; Groups 1 and 2). Three methodologies were utilized: (i) bacterial culture of synovial fluid on different agar preparations; (ii) demonstration of bacterial antigens in purified mononuclear and polymorphonuclear cells using indirect immunofluorescence of fixed cells; or (iii) demonstration of bacterial antigens in purified mononuclear and polymorphonuclear cells via solubilization of synovial-fluid cells for electrophoresis and western blotting. A rabbit antiserum against *Y. enterocolitica* O:3 or a mouse monoclonal antibody specific for the O-polysaccharide of *Y. enterocolitica* O:3 were used. Subjects were typed for HLA-B27.

Results

Synovial fluid cultured from 13 of 15 patients, using a variety of bacteriological culture conditions, failed to recover viable organisms. This was despite positive stool cultures from 7 of 15 patients, and positive serum antibodies to *Y. enterocolitica* O:3 in all 15 patients with reactive arthritis. Yersinia antigens were detected in synovial-fluid cells by immunofluorescence from 10 of 15 patients with reactive arthritis but not within synovial cells obtained from 41 controls. The majority of positively stained cells were polymorphonuclear phagocytes, but yersinia antigens were also detected in mononuclear phagocytes. Of nine patient synovial cells subjected to western blot analysis, six were positive for an antigen that was 29 KDa in size. Cells from ten patients with rheumatoid arthritis and who were studied as controls were negative.

Critique of the paper

Reactive arthritis (ReA) was first described in 1969 as a joint disease developing after infection elsewhere in the body [1]. This original definition assumed that neither viable microorganisms nor microbial products could be detected in joints. Granfors et al. used a number of different bacteriological culture methodologies to try to isolate viable bacteria from synovial fluid. These included direct culture and the use of enrichment media. A cultivation-independent method for the identification of bacterial DNA using broad-range PCR targeting the 16S rRNA sequence provides a sensitive alternative to conventional culture techniques [2]. While the use of universal primers can produce a positive result due to the presence of commensals in synovial fluid, as demonstrated by Cox et al. [3], species-specific primers can be used to amplify the product obtained with the 'universal' primers. There has been a subsequent report of detection of *Y. pseudotuberculosis* in ReA synovial fluid using this technique [4].

Prior to the publication of this paper, chlamydia antigens had been detected in synovium and synovial fluid by several investigators [5–7]. The authors had also previously demonstrated immune complexes containing yersinia antigens in the synovial fluid of 3/12 patients with ReA [8]. In this study, yersinia antigens were detectable within polymorphonuclear leucocytes and mononuclear phagocytes in 67% of patients with ReA. However, following the paper's publication, a letter to the editor postulated the existence of a synovial antigen which might have a conformation identical to the yersinia antigen and thus cross-react with the anti-yersinia antibodies [9]. The authors contested this hypothesis since the antigenic material was found within an intracellular compartment, most probably the phagolysosome. In addition, a single 29 kDa entity was identified in synovial-fluid cells via western blotting but this moiety was not observed with extracellular yersinia or when peripheral blood mononuclear cells infected ex vivo were tested. It was suggested that this entity might represent a final degradation product of yersinia lipopolysaccharide.

Significance and importance of the paper

This paper was the first to show clear evidence that components of a ReA-triggering organism reach the affected joints and are particularly located in phagocytes. Following on from these observations, a crucial factor in considering the pathophysiology of ReA is whether joints at some time contain metabolically viable bacteria or whether phagocytes from a distant infectious site simply transport non-viable organisms/degradation products to the joint. A later study which amplified *Chlamydia trachomatis* rRNA implied that ongoing multiplication of these organisms occurs in synovial tissue, since rRNA has a short half-life [10]. However, with the exception of the report noted, there has been much less evidence of this kind for enterobacteria [11]. Thus, it seems that, in general, enteric pathogens survive at an extra-articular site (possibly gut-associated lymphoid tissue) and that their antigens are then carried to joints by phagocytic cells.

In conclusion, the authors elegantly demonstrated the presence of yersinia antigens, but not viable bacteria, within the joints of patients with a diagnosis of yersinia-induced ReA. The same authors later published similar findings for salmonella- and shigella-induced ReA [12, 13]. These findings concur with the original definition of reactive arthritis as a non-purulent joint disease developing after infection elsewhere in the body. While the presence of bacterial antigens in the joint does not alter the classification of ReA (it does not thereby become 'septic' arthritis), this finding has important implications for the pathogenesis of the disease, since local bacterial protein antigens could be stimuli for the T-cell-mediated inflammatory responses which are easily identified within the ReA joint, while bacterial cell wall components and nucleic acids also have pro-inflammatory effects acting through Toll-like receptors and other sensors of bacterial products.

References

1 Ahvonen P, Sievers K, Aho K. Arthritis associated with *Yersinia enterocolitica* infection. *Acta Rheumatol Scand* 1969;**15**(3):232–53.

2 Wilbrink B, van der Heijden IM, Schouls LM, et al. Detection of bacterial DNA in joint samples from patients with undifferentiated arthritis and reactive arthritis, using polymerase chain reaction with universal 16S ribosomal RNA primers. *Arthritis Rheum* 1998;**41**(3):535–43.

3 Cox CJ, Kempsell KE, Gaston JS. Investigation of infectious agents associated with arthritis by reverse transcription PCR of bacterial rRNA. *Arthritis Res Ther* 2003;**5**(1):R1–8.

4 Gaston JSH, Cox C, Granfors K. Clinical and experimental evidence for persistent *Yersinia* infection in reactive arthritis. *Arthritis Rheum* 1999;**42**(10):2239–42.

5 Ishikawa H, Ohno O, Yamasaki K, et al. Arthritis presumably caused by Chlamydia in Reiter syndrome. Case report with electron microscopic studies. *J Bone Joint Surg Am* 1986;**68**(5):777–9.

6 Keat A, Thomas B, Dixey J, et al. *Chlamydia trachomatis* and reactive arthritis: the missing link. *Lancet* 1987;**1**(8524):72–4.

7 Schumacher HR Jr., Magge S, Cherian PV, et al. Light and electron microscopic studies on the synovial membrane in Reiter's syndrome. Immunocytochemical identification of chlamydial antigen in patients with early disease. *Arthritis Rheum* 1988;**31**(8):937–46.

8 Lahesmaa-Rantala R, Granfors K, Isomaki H, et al. Yersinia specific immune complexes in the synovial fluid of patients with yersinia triggered reactive arthritis. *Ann Rheum Dis* 1987;**46**(7):510–4.

9 Kennedy, JR. Letter in response to: Yersinia antigens in reactive arthritis. *N Engl J Med* 1989;**321**(3): 189–90.

10 Hammer M, Nettelnbreker E, Hopf S, et al. Chlamydial rRNA in the joints of patients with Chlamydia-induced arthritis and undifferentiated arthritis. *Clin Exp Rheumatol* 1992;**10**(1):63–6.

11 Sibilia J, Limbach FX. Reactive arthritis or chronic infectious arthritis? *Ann Rheum Dis* 2002;**61**(7):580–7.

12 Granfors K, Jalkanen S, Mäki-Ikola O, et al. Salmonella lipopolysaccharide in synovial cells from patients with reactive arthritis. *Lancet* 1990;**335**(8691):685–8.

13 Granfors K, Jalkanen S, Toivanen P, et al. Bacterial lipopolysaccharide in synovial fluid cells in Shigella triggered reactive arthritis. *J Rheumatol* 1992;**19**(3):500.

Paper 3.6: Transgenic expression of *HLA-B27* in rats induces various inflammatory disorders with clear links to spondyloarthritis

Reference

Hammer RE, Maika SD, Richardson JA, et al. Spontaneous inflammatory disease in transgenic rats expressing HLA-B27 and human β_2m: an animal model of HLA-B27-associated human disorders. *Cell* 1990;63(5):1099–112.

Hypothesis

To determine whether transgenic expression of a single human molecule, HLA-B27, associated with human spondyloarthritis, would cause disease or susceptibility to disease in rats.

Study design

The association between HLA-B27 and spondyloarthritis could have two general explanations: first, HLA-B27 itself might be the molecule which confers susceptibility to disease (e.g. by presenting an 'arthritogenic peptide' or altering the function of antigen-presenting cells). Alternatively, HLA-B27 might simply be a polymorphic marker for another gene that lies within the MHC on Chromosome 6 and is the true susceptibility gene. The MHC is an extremely 'gene-rich' region of the human genome, and many of these genes have important immunologic functions. Thus, due to linkage disequilibrium—the tendency to inherit whole blocks of adjacent genes—the polymorphism represented by the *B27* allele might be a way of identifying those who inherit polymorphic variants in other relevant genes. Nowadays, the ability to fine-map susceptibility genes using the huge number of available single nucleotide polymorphisms (SNPs) has allowed this idea to be addressed directly (and discounted). But 20 years ago, the most elegant way of addressing the same question was to express the candidate gene, *HLA-B27*, transgenically and determine whether any disease phenotype resulted.

This is what these investigators did. Transgenic expression of genes in rats is much more difficult than in mice, and only in the last few years have there been advances which allow this to be achieved more readily, so the successful expression of the two genes required to express human HLA-B27 (the genes encoding B27 heavy chain and human β_2 microglobulin) was a considerable achievement—one of the first examples of establishing transgenic rats. It involved the injection of plasmids encoding both genes, including significant upstream (5′) and downstream (3′) sequences to allow regulation of expression, into no fewer than 677 one-cell fertilized rat eggs in order to produce 6 founders which expressed HLA-B27. Five of these also expressed β_2 microglobulin. This technique does not control the number of copies of each plasmid which are integrated into the rat DNA, and this was variable, ranging from 1 to 150 copies of particular transgenes. However, this variability was itself useful since a disease phenotype was limited to those rats with a high copy number of transgenes. In fact, one founder had integration of transgenes at two separate loci, which segregated independently on subsequent breeding, so that descendants of this founder inherited one or other of these loci, resulting in two new strains, 21-4L and 21-4H, with relatively low and high copy numbers of the genes encoding B27 and β_2 microglobulin, respectively (6 + 6 vs 150 + 90). Interestingly, surface expression of HLA-B27 was not notably different in these two strains despite the very different copy numbers.

Results

The spectacular result of this experiment was seen in rats with a high copy number for *HLA-B27* and which developed a remarkable spontaneously arising disease phenotype. This consisted of inflammatory bowel disease, present in essentially all rats, peripheral and axial arthritis, and psoriasiform skin and nail disease (Figures 3.3 and 3.4). The arthritis was much commoner in male rats—70% versus 10%, with a total of 11 rats affected. Together, these various clinical features mimic those seen in human spondyloarthritis and the diseases associated with them. It is still remarkable to consider that all these things could occur spontaneously, through the expression of a single human protein (albeit one whose two subunits happens to be encoded by different genes), in a very different species,

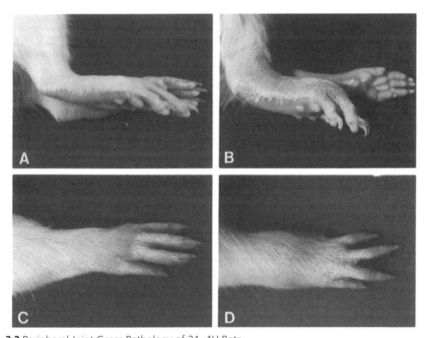

Fig. 3.3 Peripheral Joint Gross Pathology of 21–4H Rats

Normal control specimens are from nontransgenic LEW rats, 3–6 months old.

(A) Normal distal hindlimb.

(B) Distal hindlimb of a 6-month-old 21–4H male showing swelling and erythema.

(C) Normal distal forelimb.

(D) Distal forelimb of a 4-month-old 21–4H male showing swelling and erythema surrounding the carpal joint.

Reprinted from Cell, Vol 63, Robert E. Hammer, Shanna D. Maika, James A. Richardson, Jy-Ping Tang, Joel D. Taurog, Spontaneous inflammatory disease in transgenic rats expressing HLA-B27 and human β2m: An animal model of HLA-B27-associated human disorders, 1099–1112, Copyright 1990, with permission from Elsevier.

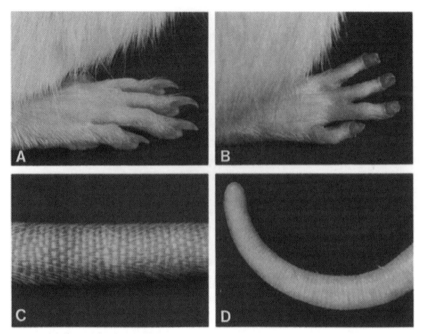

Fig. 3.4 Nail and Skin Gross Pathology of 21–4H Rats
(A) Normal hindlimb digits and nails.
(B) Hindlimb digits and nails of a 3½-month-old 21–4 male, showing hyperkeratosis and dystrophy of the nails and alopecia over the digits.
(C) Normal tail.
(D) Tail of a 3½-month-old 21–4 male (same as in [B]), showing edema, alopecia, flaking, and masking of the normal ridged pattern.
Reprinted from Cell, Vol 63, Robert E. Hammer, Shanna D. Maika, James A. Richardson, Jy-Ping Tang, Joel D. Taurog, Spontaneous inflammatory disease in transgenic rats expressing HLA-B27 and human β2m: An animal model of HLA-B27-associated human disorders, 1099–1112, Copyright 1990, with permission from Elsevier.

although the rat was chosen because of its susceptibility to various kinds of experimental arthritis. The predominance of arthritis in male rats is particularly striking, given the very skewed sex ratio seen in ankylosing spondylitis.

The IBD was reminiscent of Crohn's disease, with involvement of the colon, small intestine, and stomach; there was an inflammatory infiltrate and crypt hyperplasia.

The arthritis histologically resembled the arthritis which can be induced in rats by Freund's adjuvant or streptococcal cell walls, with synovitis, a neutrophilic infiltrate into the joint space, and erosion leading to ankylosis. Tarsal and carpal joints were the commonest to be involved (Figure 3.3). Duration was variable, ranging from a few days at its mildest to a waxing and waning arthritis lasting several weeks. However, as with adjuvant arthritis, it eventually resolved. The axial arthritis was assessed in tail vertebrae, where histology showed features highly suggestive of enthesitis, with inflammation of the outer aspects of the annulus fibrosis and its attachment to the vertebral endplates.

Additional features with relevance to spondyloarthritis were observed, including orchitis/epididymitis and involvement of the heart and large vessels. The former occurred in 'most' male rats and consisted of granulomatous inflammation leading to infertility—and hence an additional difficulty for breeding sufficient stocks of transgenic rats. Heart involvement was assessed histologically and was seen in 4/9 rats examined, with myocarditis, with notable inflammatory changes in the aortic root and even in great vessels in one rat. No consistent uveitis was seen.

These disease features were basically confined to the 21-4H line, which had very high copy numbers for the transgenes (150 B27 heavy chain genes + 90 β_2 microglobulin genes), with some preliminary indications of similar effects in six of seven rats from another founder (33-3, on a Fisher rather than a Lewis background, copy number 55 + 66) developing signs of IBD. The lack of disease of any kind in the 21-4L rats, derived, as noted, from the same founder (which had incorporated different numbers of genes at separate loci), was particularly striking—21-4L rats had a copy number of only six for both transgenes. While surface expression of HLA-B27 was similar in both lines, there were higher levels of *HLA-B27* transcripts in affected tissues of the diseased 21-4H rats, together with marked decrease in transcripts of the endogenous rat Class I MHC gene *RT1*.

Critique of the paper

In view of the dramatic induction of spondyloarthritis-related clinical features as a consequence of transgenic expression of HLA-B27, this paper reported their occurrence relatively soon after the initial observations, almost all from a single diseased transgenic line, 21-4H, with only hints (later confirmed) in another (33-3). The numbers of rats observed were quite small (23 21-4H rats—14 males and 9 females), and for disease features other than IBD, conclusions were inevitably based on limited numbers. Thus, the diagnosis of axial arthritis rested on histological examination of tail vertebrae from only two rats. As noted, the histology was that of enthesitis and interestingly was interpreted as 'extension' of synovitis to involve adjacent ligaments and tendons in rats with peripheral arthritis. Nowadays, one might wonder whether in fact the earliest lesions might have been at peripheral joint entheses, with extension to synovium, but this is speculative. No precise incidence of psoriatic skin and nail disease was given—it occurred in 'several' rats.

Very limited data on the function of the transgenically expressed HLA-B27 were presented—basically, transgenic cells appeared to elicit alloreactive cytotoxic T-cell responses but these were fairly weak, requiring high effector:target ratios to achieve even limited killing, though this was always greater on B27-expressing cells than on non-transgenic cells. Moreover, allorecognition of transgenic cells was similar whether they were derived from diseased (21-4H) or non-diseased (21-4L) rats.

Given the difficulty in producing transgenic rats, the authors could be forgiven for not reporting appropriate controls, such as those expressing an HLA-B antigen other than B27, or β_2 microglobulin alone; all this was done later, with no spondyloarthritis seen when HLA-B7 was expressed or in rats expressing only one of the transgenes needed for HLA-B27 expression [1]. The ubiquitous IBD immediately raised the question of the involvement of an infectious agent. The failure to culture a known pathogen from the gut, and the lack of disease in co-housed non-transgenic rats excluded a conventional 'infectious' diarrhoea but the critical role of commensal flora and our current view of Crohn's disease as some kind of failure of normal tolerance of gut flora nowadays point to a likely role for infectious agents, even if these are commensals rather than pathogens. To their credit the authors recognized this possibility even in this first report and indicated their plan to examine germ-free rats; later, they reported the absence of disease in germ-free rats [2]. How HLA-B27 expression alters the normal relationship between the host and its gut flora remains an open question and one currently being investigated vigorously.

The authors were appropriately conservative in speculating on the mechanism whereby HLA-B27 might bring about the spondyloarthritis, other than emphasizing that it was clearly due to HLA-B27 itself, the primary goal of the experiment. While it is formally possible that expression of B27 could bring about phenotypically similar diseases in rats and humans by completely different mechanisms, this seems rather unlikely, and therefore conclusions drawn from subsequent and ongoing studies of the B27 transgenic rat are almost certainly valid.

Significance and importance of the paper

This paper established two important things; first, it showed that transgenic expression of HLA-B27 was sufficient to induce several features characteristic of human spondyloarthritis, and implicated HLA-B27 itself, and not a linked gene, in the pathogenesis of these diseases. Second, it established a model which, because it mimicked human disease so faithfully, could reasonably be used to address further aspects of spondyloarthritis pathogenesis. Subsequent papers did precisely this, though always limited by the problems in producing further transgenic rat lines which might be informative and which would have been easy to produce in mice. Importantly, subsequent work established the importance of gut flora for the emergence of the disease phenotype, and very surprisingly, the lack of any requirement for CD8+ T-cells in disease pathogenesis [2, 3]. Since CD8+ T-cells interact with Class I MHC proteins such as HLA-B27, it was assumed that these cells must be implicated in disease; instead, CD4+ cells proved critical.

In the most recent elaboration of this work, it has been shown that HLA-B27 transgenic rats with a higher copy number of the gene expressing β_2 microglobulin no longer had inflammatory bowel disease but had a higher incidence of arthritis; these rats also had marked epididymitis [4].

References

1 Taurog JD, Maika SD, Satumtira N, et al. Inflammatory disease in HLA-B27 transgenic rats. *Immunol Rev* 1999;**169**(1):209–23.

2 Taurog JD, Richardson JA, Croft JT, et al. The germfree state prevents development of gut and joint inflammatory disease in HLA-B27 transgenic rats. *J Exp Med* 1994;**180**(6):2359–64.

3 May E, Dorris ML, Satumtira N, et al. CD8αβ T cells are not essential to the pathogenesis of arthritis or colitis in HLA-B27 transgenic rats. *J Immunol* 2003;**170**(2):1099–105.

4 Tran TM, Dorris ML, Satumtira N, et al. Additional human beta-2 microglobulin curbs HLA-B27 heavy chain misfolding and promotes arthritis and spondylitis but not colitis in male B27 transgenic rats. *Arthritis Rheum* 2006;**54**(4):1317–27.

Paper 3.7: The evolution of spondyloarthropathies in relation to gut histology

Reference

Mielants H, Veys EM, Cuvelier C, et al. The evolution of spondyloarthropathies in relation to gut histology. II. Histological aspects. *J Rheumatol* 1995;22(12):2273–78.

Purpose

To examine the clinical evolution of different forms of spondyloarthropathy (SpA) including reactive arthritis (ReA), undifferentiated SpA (uSpA), and ankylosing spondylitis (AS), and to correlate this with gut inflammation shown by ileocolonoscopy and biopsies on recruitment to the study. This paper was the second in a series of three devoted to the same patient cohort, all published back to back. The clinical features were examined in the first paper [1], but the innovative aspects of the study, that is, ileocolonoscopy of a large patient cohort, were described in this paper. The third paper dealt with a subgroup of patients who had follow-up ileocolonoscopy so that evolution of the gut lesions and arthritis could be examined simultaneously [2].

Patients

Using the criteria of the European Spondylarthropathy Study Group (ESSG), 217 patients (149 men and 68 women) were diagnosed with SpA [3]. Four clinical groups were identified, with the following characteristics: (1) a diagnosis of urogenital ReA with proven infection, plus signs of urogenital inflammation at presentation (16 patients); (2) enterogenic ReA with triggering agents identified either by culture from stool or by elevated titres of bacteria-specific antibodies (12 patients); (3) patients with clinical features of SpA that failed to meet the Rome criteria for AS and in whom no triggering agent could be identified (undifferentiated SpA; 97 patients) [4]; and (4) patients who fulfilled the Rome criteria for AS (92 patients) [4]. AS patients were subdivided according to whether patients had only axial involvement (central AS, 27 patients) or also peripheral arthritis (peripheral AS, 65 patients). Importantly, patients with psoriatic arthritis or known inflammatory bowel disease (IBD) were excluded.

Study design

This report describes a prospective observational study of 217 patients; 123/217 patients were regularly monitored and reviewed clinically at 2–9 years post ileocolonoscopy, while 94 patients were followed by telephone consultation only.

Treatment

All patients were treated with low-dosage non-steroidal anti-inflammatory drugs (NSAIDs). Sulphasalazine at 2–3 g/day was added if disease persisted after three months of NSAID treatment. NSAIDs were stopped after one year of clinical remission, and sulphasalazine after two years of remission.

Study end points measured

On enrolment, all 217 patients had (a) clinical evaluation; (b) radiographs of the sacroiliac joints, the axial skeleton, and clinically involved joints; (c) laboratory measurements including erythrocyte sedimentation rate (ESR), C-reactive protein (CRP), IgM rheumatoid factor, antinuclear factor, full blood count, urinalysis, HLA typing, and antibodies to yersinia, campylobacter, salmonella, and chlamydia; and (d) evaluation of terminal ileum and entire colon by ileocolonoscopy, with 10–17 biopsies/patient. Biopsies were categorized as either histologically normal, or showing 'acute' lesions (neutrophil and/or eosinophil infiltration with crypt abscesses but preserved architecture), or 'chronic' lesions (crypt distortion with villous atrophy, with lymphoid aggregates in the lamina propria, and in some cases granulomas indistinguishable from Crohn's disease). Chronic lesions in any biopsy always classified the patient as 'chronic'.

Results

The analysis concentrated on the 123 patients on whom complete clinical evaluation at follow-up was available. Forty patients (32.5%) had normal gut histology, while 28 (22.5%) had acute lesions, and 55 (45%), chronic lesions. In those patients with uSpA, 51/71 (72%) had abnormal gut histology—23 had acute changes, and 28 had chronic changes. A similar proportion of AS patients had abnormal gut histology (32/52 (62%)) but a significantly higher proportion showed chronic changes—27/32. During follow-up, eight patients developed clinical IBD (mostly Crohn's disease—the diagnosis was made by independent clinicians). Seven of these had chronic lesions on initial histology, and one had acute lesions. An additional three patients with chronic lesions reported developing IBD at telephone review. The risk factors for evolution to IBD, other than chronic histological changes, were higher ESR/CRP, lack of HLA-B27, and abnormal sacroiliac joint radiographs.

Patients who were HLA-B27+ were less likely to go into clinical remission but remission occurred in similar proportions of patients with normal, acute, and chronic histology, so chronic inflammatory changes in the gastrointestinal tract per se did not predict the clinical outcome. Having said this, 13 patients evolved to a diagnosis of AS (1 with yersinia-induced ReA and who also developed Crohn's disease, and 12 with uSpA, 3 of whom also developed Crohn's disease), and of these all but one had abnormal gut histology at baseline.

Critique of the paper

An important consideration is the classification criteria used in the study. The authors used the Rome criteria, which requires bilateral sacroiliitis of Grade 2 or above on plain radiographs, to define AS and then classified all those not having ReA as 'undifferentiated SpA'. This group therefore includes patients in the early (pre-radiographic) phase of axial AS, as well as those with predominantly peripheral SpA. These patients are now better defined by the Assessment of Spondylarthritis International Society (ASAS) criteria for axial and peripheral SpA [5–7]. A proportion of those with pre-radiographic AS would be expected to progress to AS and it would be interesting to analyse the gut histology in this subgroup.

This study examined 217 patients defied by ESSG criteria at recruitment but only 123 were regularly monitored and reviewed clinically. The reason for this was not clear but the remission rate was higher in the telephone review group, suggesting disease progression was not the likely cause for non-participation. A further point for consideration is that all patients, regardless of their form of SpA, were treated with NSAIDs, and sulphasalazine was added if symptoms persisted at three months. NSAIDs are known to influence the progression of structural damage in AS [8, 9], and could therefore have had an impact on the proportion progressing to fulfil the Rome criteria for AS. Likewise treatment with sulphasalazine may have limited the number of patients developing symptomatic IBD.

Remission was defined as the absence of peripheral synovitis, peripheral tendinitis, inflammatory axial complaints, and morning stiffness, all for at least six months. Remission of an inflammatory rheumatic disease ideally comprises the absence of its signs and symptoms, along with maximal improvement in physical function, and a halt in structural changes. Alternative ways of defining remission in AS include the Ankylosing Spondylitis Disease Activity Score (ASDAS) [10] or a composite of BASDAI and CRP [10, 11].

Both of the 'evolutionary events'—development of IBD or AS—involved relatively small numbers of patients, despite the investigation of a large cohort of SpA patients. Fourteen of 71 (20%) patients with uSpA developed AS—previous estimates varied between 1.5% and 60%—with predisposing factors in this study being inflammatory axial pain (P < 0.001) and high ESR/CRP (P < 0.05). However, to obtain statistically significant data on other risk factors would require larger numbers of patients evolving to AS.

This study recorded remission rates of 60% in uSpA versus 19% in patients with AS. While the high rate of remission in ReA and uSpA is not unexpected, and others have reported the maintenance of good functional status in AS, [12] long-term remission rates in AS are usually much lower (e.g. 1% [13]). The difference may relate to the treatment regimen used in this study and adopted here from the work of Boersma et al. [14], together with the definition of remission used.

Significance and importance of the paper

The main significance of this paper (and its companions) is a large series of SpA patients investigated by ileocolonoscopy and gut biopsy, in an important advance relating gut pathology to SpA pathogenesis. Previous studies by this group had described a high prevalence of inflammatory gut lesions in patients with SpA [15, 16], and these findings were confirmed by other investigators [17–19]. Leaving aside those with enteropathic ReA, who by definition have 100% incidence of gut inflammation, a high proportion of patients with each of the other forms of SpA had gut lesions in the absence of clinical symptoms of gut involvement—60%–75% of those with uSpA or AS with peripheral joint involvement. These patients would appear to fall into several categories: first, those whose gut inflammation did not lead to sustained arthritis (and whose gut inflammation also remitted [2]), since the rates of remission did not reflect gut histology at baseline; second, those whose IBD would eventually declare itself clinically—these patients were likely to develop AS with peripheral joint involvement and were less likely to be HLA-B27+, in line with observations on those with SpA and overt IBD. However, a third category were those who did not progress to overt IBD but nevertheless had continuing joint disease and evolution to AS. Progression was associated with the presence of chronic histological changes at baseline, and such changes were also prevalent in those with AS at baseline. In line with this, repeat ileocolonoscopy in 49 patients did not show any abnormalities in ReA or uSpA patients who had not developed AS, whereas acute or chronic (mainly chronic) changes persisted in 14/31 of those with continuing AS, especially with peripheral disease (13/19). This suggests that chronic subclinical IBD may be an important factor in development and persistence of AS, particularly in the presence of HLA-B27. Overt IBD appears to be sufficient to drive AS in the absence of HLA-B27 (only ~5% of cases are B27+), whereas ~90% of AS patients without IBD or psoriasis are HLA-B27+. Some patients with subclinical IBD may have mutations in *CARD15/NOD2*, a gene associated with Crohn's disease [20]. The mechanism relating chronic gut inflammation to SpA/AS has not yet been elucidated. One possibility would be altered handling of gut organisms (pathogens or commensals) by macrophages in the gut, perhaps leading to the transport of bacterial antigens to entheseal and/or synovial tissue.

References

1 **Mielants H, Veys EM, De Vos M, et al**. The evolution of spondyloarthropathies in relation to gut histology. I. Clinical aspects. *J Rheumatol* 1995;**22**(12):2266–72.

2 **Mielants H, Veys EM, Cuvelier C, et al**. The evolution of spondyloarthropathies in relation to gut histology. III. Relation between gut and joint. *J Rheumatol* 1995;**22**(12):2279–84.

3 **Dougados M, van der Linden S, Juhlin R, et al**. The European Spondylarthropathy Study Group preliminary criteria for the classification of spondylarthropathy. *Arthritis Rheum* 1991;**34**(10):1218–27.

4 **Kellgren JH, Jeffrey MR, Ball J, eds**. The epidemiology of chronic rheumatism. Oxford: Blackwell; 1963.

5 **Rudwaleit M, Landewe R, van der Heijde D, et al**. The development of Assessment of SpondyloArthritis international Society classification criteria for axial spondyloarthritis (part I): classification of paper patients by expert opinion including uncertainty appraisal. *Ann Rheum Dis* 2009;**68**(6):770–6.

6 **Rudwaleit M, van der Heijde D, Landewe R, et al**. The Assessment of SpondyloArthritis International Society classification criteria for peripheral spondyloarthritis and for spondyloarthritis in general. *Ann Rheum Dis* 2011;**70**(1):25–31.

7 **Rudwaleit M, van der Heijde D, Landewe R, et al**. The development of Assessment of SpondyloArthritis international Society classification criteria for axial spondyloarthritis (part II): validation and final selection. *Ann Rheum Dis* 2009;**68**(6):777–83.

8 **Poddubnyy D, Rudwaleit M, Haibel H, et al**. Effect of non-steroidal anti-inflammatory drugs on radiographic spinal progression in patients with axial spondyloarthritis: results from the German Spondyloarthritis Inception Cohort. *Ann Rheum Dis* 2012;**71**(10):1616–22.

9 **Wanders A, Heijde D, Landewe R, et al**. Nonsteroidal antiinflammatory drugs reduce radiographic progression in patients with ankylosing spondylitis: a randomized clinical trial. *Arthritis Rheum* 2005;**52**(6):1756–65.

10 **Machado P, Landewe R, Lie E, et al**. Ankylosing Spondylitis Disease Activity Score (ASDAS): defining cut-off values for disease activity states and improvement scores. *Ann Rheum Dis* 2011;**70**(1):47–53.

11 **Lukas C, Landewe R, Sieper J, et al**. Development of an ASAS-endorsed disease activity score (ASDAS) in patients with ankylosing spondylitis. *Ann Rheum Dis* 2009;**68**(1):18–24.

12 **Mau W, Zeidler H, Mau R, et al**. Clinical features and prognosis of patients with possible ankylosing spondylitis. Results of a 10-year followup. *J Rheum* 1988;**15**(7):1109–14.

13 **Kennedy LG, Edmunds L, Calin A**. The natural history of ankylosing spondylitis. Does it burn out? *J Rheum* 1993;**20**(4):688–92.

14 **Boersma JW**. Retardation of ossification of the lumbar vertebral column in ankylosing spondylitis by means of phenylbutazone. *Scand J Rheumatol* 1976;**5**(1):60–4.

15 **Mielants H, Veys EM, Cuvelier C, et al**. Ileocolonoscopic findings in seronegative spondylarthropathies. *Br J Rheumatol* 1988;**27**(Suppl 2):95–105.

16 **Mielants H, Veys EM, Cuvelier C, et al**. HLA- B27 related arthritis and bowel inflammation. Part 2. Ileocolonoscopy and bowel histology in patients with HLA-B27 related arthritis. *J Rheum* 1985;**12**(2): 294–8.

17 **Dougados M, Alemanni M, Tulliez M, et al**. [Systematic ileocolonoscopy in seronegative spondylarthropathies]. *Rev Rhum Mal Osteoartic* 1987;**54**(3):279–83.

18 **Leirisalo-Repo M, Turunen U, Stenman S, et al**. High frequency of silent inflammatory bowel disease in spondylarthropathy. *Arthritis Rheum* 1994;**37**(1):23–31.

19 **Simenon G, Van Gossum A, Adler M, et al**. Macroscopic and microscopic gut lesions in seronegative spondyloarthropathies. *J Rheum* 1990;**17**(11):1491–4.

20 **Laukens D, Peeters H, Marichal D, et al**. CARD15 gene polymorphisms in patients with spondyloarthropathies identify a specific phenotype previously related to Crohn's disease. *Ann Rheum Dis* 2005;**64**(6):930–5.

Paper 3.8: A hypothesis that enthesitis is the primary pathological process occurring in spondylarthropathy

Reference

McGonagle D, Gibbon W, Emery P. Classification of inflammatory arthritis by enthesitis. *Lancet* 1998;352(9134):1137–40.

Purpose

This manuscript proposed the hypothesis that enthesitis is the primary pathological process occurring in spondylarthropathy (SpA), whereas synovitis is a secondary event. In contrast, synovitis is the primary manifestation of rheumatoid arthritis (RA) (Figure 3.5).

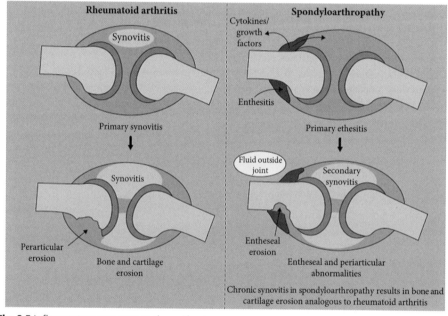

Fig. 3.5 Inflammatory response at the enthesis.
Reprinted from The Lancet, Vol. 352, Dennis McGonagle, Wayne Gibbon, Paul Emery, Classification of inflammatory arthritis by enthesitis, 1137–1140, Copyright 1998, with permission from Elsevier.

Hypothesis

The authors began by stating that synovitis accounts for all signs of disease in the joints in RA. In contrast, the clinical features of the spondyloarthropathies (reactive arthritis, psoriatic arthritis, ankylosing spondylitis, enteropathic arthritis, and undifferentiated spondylarthropathy), and related non-RA conditions, include enthesitis and other features not readily explained by synovitis. While the synovitis of SpA is histologically similar to that of RA [1], it has generally been regarded as something which occurs independently of enthesitis [2]. Instead, this paper suggested that enthesitis is the *primary* lesion in SpA; they further argued that this idea provides a unifying concept for considering the clinical features of diseases within the SpA spectrum. Synovitis which occurs in SpA would then be seen to be driven by the primary, and adjacent, enthesitis. An important implication of this hypothesis is to distinguish primary synovitis (classically RA) from primary entheseal-associated inflammation, since the former has a poorer prognosis and may therefore merit different treatment approaches.

Evidence to support the hypothesis

1. Experimental studies suggest that the synovium is particularly sensitive to pro-inflammatory cytokines (e.g. direct injection of TNF or IL-1) and therefore might react to these cytokines if they are made in adjacent entheses (though interestingly enthesitis is prominent in TNF-overexpressing mice [3]). Likewise, while bacterial components and bacteria-specific T-cells have been detected in SpA joints (mainly in reactive arthritis) [4–6], these may primarily be deposited or recruited to entheses and merely be 'bystanders' in the synovium, causing synovitis through their production of cytokines in the enthesis.

2. Sacroiliitis cannot be a primary synovitis, since bone erosion may occur in the upper third of the joint which lacks synovium.

3. The use of fat-suppressed MRI in early knee SpA demonstrates enthesopathy (Figure 3.6) [7].

4. Other features of SpA, such as dactylitis, may be due to inflammation of several entheseal insertions resulting in synovitis and tenosynovitis, in addition to soft tissue swelling; (dactylitis is not seen in RA, despite prominent tenosynovitis, hence the need to invoke alternative mechanisms). Likewise, the pencil-in-cup deformity associated with hand SpA can be seen as a consequence of distal capsular calcification with erosion at the insertions of the central flexor or extensor tendons.

5. In the SpA-related condition SAPHO, osteolysis adjacent to entheseal insertions predates new bone formation [8].

6. Aortic valve disease is associated with SpA, and the aortic valve insertion has anatomical similarities to an enthesis.

Critique of the paper

This paper was crucial is drawing attention to the enthesis as a distinct anatomical structure which might participate in inflammatory responses and thereby explain many of the features of SpA. In fact, the authors were more ambitious in also suggesting that enthesitis might underlie many other forms of arthritis with a good prognosis, including post-viral arthritis, but this was perhaps stretching the hypothesis further than the evidence would take it. In addition, even if enthesitis is critical to SpA, this does not necessarily imply good prognosis—psoriatic arthritis can be chronic, destructive, and disabling. The prognosis relates more to the intensity

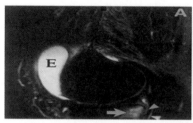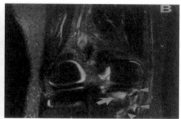

Fig. 3.6 Magnetic resonance images of the right knee of a patient with reactive arthritis, showing entheseal bone oedema at one site. A, Sagittal section through the medial knee compartment shows tibial plateau bone marrow oedema (arrow) and oedema of the adjacent capsular insertion (arrowheads). A joint effusion is present (E). B, Coronal section through the posterior knee also shows bone marrow oedema (arrow) and peri-entheseal oedema of the adjacent semimembranosus insertion (arrowheads; adapted from [7]).

Reproduced from McGonagle D, Gibbon W, O'Connor P, Green M, Pease C, Emery P. Characteristic magnetic resonance imaging entheseal changes of knee synovitis in spondylarthropathy. Arthritis and rheumatism. 1998 Apr;41(4):694–700 with permission from Wiley.

and duration of the inflammation, rather than whether it involves synovitis versus enthesitis. For instance, 20% of individuals with HLA-B27-positive reactive arthritis and 50%–60% of HLA-B27-positive patients with inflammatory bowel disease progress to ankylosing spondylitis [9], again a chronic disease with significant disease burden. There is a suggestion that the chronicity of these conditions may be due to persistent bacterial triggers localized to the bowel or skin in psoriasis, driving entheseal inflammation.

Some of the claims in the paper were disputed: Francois contested the notion that enthesitis accounts for all of the rheumatological findings of SpA [10]. In particular, he argued that the principal lesion of sacroiliitis in patients with ankylosing spondylitis is localized to a region devoid of entheses deep to the synovial joint, with additional changes in the ligamentous area, and also that bony fusion occurs in the absence of sacroiliac ligament ossification. At a histological level, subchondral bone marrow changes could account for the widespread joint destruction in sacroiliitis [11]. Braun and Sieper also questioned the role of enthesitis in sacroiliitis [12]. However, McGonagle et al. responded that enthesitis is observed as bone marrow oedema when using fat-suppressed MRI, as shown in Figure 3.6 [7], arguing that the sacroiliac joint has strong intra-articular ligament and circumferential capsular insertions. Additionally, the hypothesis sheds no light on the mechanisms which might account for the association between HLA-B27 and sacroiliitis and enthesitis.

Significance and importance of the paper

While earlier studies may have proposed the enthesis as a primary site for disease pathology in SpA [13], this paper and subsequent studies by McGonagle et al. clearly demonstrated the importance of the enthesis in accounting for SpA pathology [7, 14, 15]. More recently, the term synovio-entheseal complex (SEC) has been coined to identify the relationship between entheses and adjacent synovium [16].

An interesting experimental validation of the enthesis concept was recently provided by Sherlock et al. [17]. They showed that the arthritis which developed in mice overexpressing IL-23 was driven by IL-23-receptor-expressing T-cells resident in the enthesis (with an unusual phenotype—CD3+ CD4– CD8– RORγt+). These then secrete pro-inflammatory cytokines such as IL-6, IL-17, and IL-22 in response to IL-23. Furthermore, the in vivo expression of excessive IL-23 was sufficient to promote enthesitis and entheseal new bone formation in the initial complete absence of synovitis. This study confirms that resident entheseal cells are sufficient to elicit joint pathology given the appropriate stimulus. Polymorphisms in the IL-23 receptor gene and genes encoding components of IL-23 and its downstream signalling pathway are all associated with susceptibility to SpA. The physiologic function of this entheseal population of lymphocytes remains mysterious.

In contrast with this intriguing animal model, findings in the HLA-B27 transgenic rat, the most faithful mimic of human SpA, have not been thought to support the 'primary enthesitis' hypothesis [18]. However, this study was not able to observe the very earliest lesions in the diseased rats, so enthesitis might still have been an initiating event.

References

1 **Revell PA, Mayston V**. Histopathology of the synovial membrane of peripheral joints in ankylosing spondylitis. *Ann Rheum Dis* 1982;**41**(6):579–86.

2 **Ball J**. Enthesopathy of rheumatoid and ankylosing spondylitis. *Ann Rheum Dis* 1971;**30**(3):213–23.

3 **Armaka M, Apostolaki M, Jacques P, et al**. Mesenchymal cell targeting by TNF as a common pathogenic principle in chronic inflammatory joint and intestinal diseases. *J Exp Med* 2008;**205**(2):331–7.

4 **Schumacher HR Jr, Magge S, Cherian PV, et al**. Light and electron microscopic studies on the synovial membrane in Reiter's syndrome. Immunocytochemical identification of chlamydial antigen in patients with early disease. *Arthritis Rheum* 1988;**31**(8):937–46.

5 **Taylor-Robinson D, Gilroy CB, Thomas BJ, et al**. Detection of *Chlamydia trachomatis* DNA in joints of reactive arthritis patients by polymerase chain reaction. *Lancet* 1992;**340**(8811):81–2.

6 **Viner N, Bailey L, Life P, et al**. Isolation of *Yersinia*-specific T cell clones from the synovial membrane and synovial fluid of a patient with reactive arthritis. *Arthritis Rheum* 1991;**34**(9):1151–7.

7 **McGonagle D, Gibbon W, O'Connor P, et al**. Characteristic magnetic resonance imaging entheseal changes of knee synovitis in spondylarthropathy. *Arthritis Rheum* 1998;**41**(4):694–700.

8 **Maugars Y, Berthelot JM, Ducloux JM, et al**. SAPHO syndrome: a followup study of 19 cases with special emphasis on enthesis involvement. *J Rheumatol* 1995;**22**(11):2135–41.

9 **Lahesmaa-Rantala R, Granfors K, Isomaki H, et al**. Yersinia specific immune complexes in the synovial fluid of patients with yersinia triggered reactive arthritis. *Ann Rheum Dis* 1987;**46**(7):510–4.

10 **Francois RJ**. Classification of inflammatory arthritis. *Lancet* 1998;**352**(9144):1938–9.

11 **Francois RJ, Gardner DL, Degrave EJ, et al**. Histopathologic evidence that sacroiliitis in ankylosing spondylitis is not merely enthesitis. *Arthritis Rheum* 2000;**43**(9):2011–24.

12 **Braun J, Sieper J**. Spondyloarthropathy. *Lancet* 1999;**353**(9163):1526–7.

13 **Paolaggi JB, Struz P, Goutet MC et al**. [Systematic research on enthesopathies in chronic rheumatism. Results and pathological significance. Relation to erosive spondylitis and other tendinous or synovial lesions]. *Rev Rhum Mal Osteoartic* 1984;**51**(9):451–6.

14 **McGonagle D, Gibbon W, Emery P**. Classification of inflammatory arthritis by enthesitis. *Lancet* 1998 Oct 3;**352**(9134):1137–40.

15 **McGonagle D, Khan MA, Marzo-Ortega H, et al**. Enthesitis in spondyloarthropathy. *Curr Opin Rheumatol* 1999 Jul;**11**(4):244–50.

16 **Benjamin M, McGonagle D**. Histopathologic changes at 'synovio-entheseal complexes' suggesting a novel mechanism for synovitis in osteoarthritis and spondylarthritis. *Arthritis Rheum* 2007 Nov;**56**(11):3601–9.

17 **Sherlock JP, Joyce-Shaikh B, Turner SP, et al**. IL-23 induces spondyloarthropathy by acting on ROR-gammat + CD3 + CD4-CD8- entheseal resident T cells. *Nat Med* 2012 Jul;**18**(7):1069–76.

18 **van Duivenvoorde LM, Dorris ML, Satumtira N, et al**. Relationship between inflammation, bone destruction, and osteoproliferation in the HLA-B27/human beta2 -microglobulin-transgenic rat model of spondylarthritis. *Arthritis Rheum* Oct;**64**(10):3210–9.

Paper 3.9: First, and dramatic, indication of the effectiveness of tumour necrosis factor α blockade in ankylosing spondylitis

Reference

Brandt J, Haibel H, Cornely D, et al. Successful treatment of active ankylosing spondylitis with the anti-tumor necrosis factor α monoclonal antibody infliximab. *Arthritis Rheum* 2000;43(6):1346–52.

Hypothesis

The authors, having shown the presence of TNFα mRNA and protein in AS sacroiliac joints through their pioneering biopsies studies [1], concluded that anti-TNF therapy would be worth testing. This was reinforced by its effectiveness in Crohn's disease, which is associated with spondyloarthritis. Efficacy in RA, which was well recognized by this time, did not especially point to a high likelihood that the same strategy would be successful in AS.

Patients

Eleven patients were treated, although one (the only female) had to withdraw after a single infusion due to an adverse reaction (urticaria). All patients had AS by modified New York criteria, and a range of disease durations (0.5 to 13 years), although half had accumulated at least three syndesmophytes and/or fusions. They had active disease for at least three months, as judged by BASDAI >4 and VAS for spinal pain >4.

Study design

This was an open-label pilot study.

Treatment

Infliximab (5 mg/kg) was given as an infusion on weeks 0, 2, and 6. The timing of the initial infusions followed experience in the treatment of RA. The authors chose the dose of 5 mg/kg rather than the 3 mg/kg which has become standard in RA treatment, arguing that higher doses might be required to control axial inflammation.

Study end points measured

Clinical end points were BASDAI, BASFI, BASMI, VAS spinal pain score, and SF36. Laboratory measures included CRP and IL-6 levels; MRI studies were carried out in five patients, with post-treatment scans in only three of these.

Follow-up

Patients were followed through week 12 (i.e. six weeks after the final infusion) with comments on their progress in the subsequent three months and need for additional infusions.

Results

The results are readily summarized in the authors' justified comment that 'all (patients) showed dramatic clinical improvement in all parameters measured.' Improvement was reported by some patients within 24 hours of the first infusion. Details of the responses are summarized in Table 3.3, which is reproduced from the paper. The most striking results were actually at week 2 when nine of ten treated patients showed >50% improvement in BASDAI. By week 12, two had further improvements in BASDAI by >80% of the pretreatment level, and another two by week 14, giving an early indication of excellent clinical efficacy achieved by blockade of a principal pro-inflammatory cytokine, without effect on the underlying pathogenic processes leading to its production. Interestingly the SF36, as a more general measurement of improvement, showed significant changes in six of nine domains and trends in the other three, with changes in vitality and social functioning indicative of the major systemic effects of active AS, quite apart from inflammatory back pain, and their response to TNFα blockade. NSAID doses required for symptom control decreased by >50%—in fact, five patients discontinued them. Peripheral arthritis and arthralgias improved in all the patients with these features prior to treatment (two and four patients, respectively). Only two patients had a history of uveitis and, interestingly, one had a further episode during treatment, described as mild. MRI assessments in this study were minimal, but two of the three patients in whom pre- and post-treatment scans were obtained showed decreased signs of inflammation. Laboratory results showed the expected improvements in ESR, CRP and IL-6 in those (the majority) in whom they were initially elevated.

Infections were actually rather frequent in this short study, with five episodes: four required antibiotics (two tonsillitis, one sinusitis, and one otitis media), and there was one case of herpes labialis.

Table 3.3 Comparison of outcome parameters before treatment, after 2 weeks of treatment with infliximab and after 12 weeks of treatment with infliximab, in patients with severe ankylosing spondylitis*

	Week 0	Week 2	P[†]	Week 12	P[†]
BASDAI	6.5 (5.2–8.5)	1.9 (0.4–4.6)	0.001	2.4 (0.4–6.3)	0.004
BASFI	5.3 (1.3–8.2)	2.3 (0.2–6.4)	0.002	2.4 (0.2–6.5)	0.008
BASMI	3.0 (0.0–6.0)	1.0 (0.0–6.0)	0.031	1.5 (0.0–5.0)	0.100
VAS for inflammatory back pain	7.8 (6.0–9.8)	2.0 (0.3–5.1)	0.002	2.5 (0.7–5.1)	0.004
CRP, mg/litre	15.5 (<6.0–90.8)	<6.0 (<6.0–18.5)	0.005	<6.0 (<6.0–13.6)	0.008
ESR, mm/hour	32.0 (4.0–110.0)	<15.0 (2.0–34.0)	0.005	<15.0 (2.0–40.0)	0.008

* Values are the median (range). BASDAJ = Bath Ankylosing Spondylitis Disease Activity Index; BASFI = Bath AS Functional Index; BASMI = Bath AS Metrology Index; VAS = visual analogue scale; CRP = C-reactive protein; ESR = erythrocyte sedimentation rate.

[†] Week 2 or 12 versus week 0, by Wilcoxon's rank sum test.

Reproduced from Brandt J, Haibel H, Cornely D, Golder W, Gonzalez J, Reddig J, et al. (2000) Successful treatment of active ankylosing spondylitis with the anti-tumor necrosis factor α monoclonal antibody infliximab. *Arthritis Rheum*: 43:1346–52 with permission from Wiley.

Critique of the paper

It is self-evident that this is a tiny, open-label, non-randomized study but that is scarcely the point, since really major therapeutic effects should be evident in these kinds of pilot study (remember penicillin in pneumococcal pneumonia). The authors were surely justified in their understated conclusion—'it is very unlikely that the high percentage of responders (90% of the treated patients) was due to a placebo response'. Indeed the results with infliximab and other anti-TNF biologics were subsequently fully verified in much larger conventional double-blind randomized placebo-controlled trials [2–4].

Significance and importance of the paper

The importance of this paper was its clear demonstration that TNFα blockade had a major therapeutic effect in ankylosing spondylitis in patients whose symptoms were inadequately controlled by NSAIDs. In the absence of any efficacious disease-modifying drug for axial disease in AS, with limited evidence for the usefulness of drugs such as bisphosphonates, thalidomide, and parenteral corticosteroids, and with problems with tolerability, the introduction of anti-TNF therapy has revolutionized the management of this condition for thousands of patients worldwide. Almost all physicians treating AS will recall several incidences where patients spontaneously volunteer that their lives have been completely changed by the introduction of anti-TNF therapy.

Of course, the short-term trial demonstrated symptom relief, albeit substantial, and not disease modification. Whether anti-TNF therapy is truly disease modifying continues to be debated, and the answer to the question is not straightforward. Unlike erosions in RA, bony changes in AS proceed rather slowly, so many years of follow-up may be required to demonstrate a disease-modifying action. No true control group can be followed for similar periods—this would require them to be denied the symptomatic benefits—and therefore historical cohorts with regular radiographic follow-up have been the only alternative. Even if a true control group could be assembled, the symptomatic benefit of anti-TNF therapy permits a much higher level of physical activity and exercise, and this in itself is already known to be 'disease modifying' in the sense of maintaining better mobility, and it could be difficult to disentangle this effect from 'biological' disease modification. Suffice to say that, while analysis at two years failed to show an alteration in bony progression as compared to historical controls for any of the anti-TNF therapies [5], more recent data on patients followed for five to eight years do suggest that they are diverging significantly from the controls [6].

Nevertheless, as was immediately evident in this trial, relapse is inevitable when therapy is withdrawn, indicating that the basic pro-inflammatory predisposition remains unaffected. Would this be the case if treatment were to be introduced in very early (pre-radiographic) disease? This is under investigation. However, given the ability to achieve good symptomatic control in most patients, there is much work to be done to determine what else needs to be done to bring about 'drug-free' remission—for example, what other cytokines might need to be inhibited? The IL-17/IL-23 axis currently attracts most attention in this respect. The trial reminds us that even small pilot studies should be capable of detecting major treatment effects: thus, if >90% of current anti-TNF treated patients relapse on treatment withdrawal in approximately three months, a novel intervention which reduced this by 50%–60% should be detected in a trial with similar numbers to those used in this study. Such work needs to be done urgently.

References

1 Francois RJ, Neure L, Sieper J, et al. Immunohistological examination of open sacroiliac biopsies of patients with ankylosing spondylitis: detection of tumour necrosis factor alpha in two patients with early disease and transforming growth factor beta in three more advanced cases. *Ann Rheum Dis* 2006;**65**(6):713–20.

2 Braun J, Brandt J, Listing J, et al. Treatment of active ankylosing spondylitis with infliximab: a randomised controlled multicentre trial. *Lancet* 2002;**359**(9313):1187–93.

3 van der Heijde D, Kivitz A, Schiff MH, et al. Efficacy and safety of adalimumab in patients with ankylosing spondylitis—Results of a multicenter, randomized, double-blind, placebo-controlled trial. *Arthritis Rheum* 2006;**54**(7):2136–46.

4 Brandt J, Khariouzov A, Listing J, et al. Six-month results of a double-blind, placebo-controlled trial of etanercept treatment in patients with active ankylosing spondylitis. *Arthritis Rheum* 2003;**48**(6):1667–75.

5 van der Heijde D, Landewe R, Baraliakos X, et al. Radiographic findings following two years of infliximab therapy in patients with ankylosing spondylitis. *Arthritis Rheum* 2008;**58**(10):3063–70.

6 Baraliakos X, Haibel H, Listing J, et al. Continuous long-term anti-TNF therapy does not lead to an increase in the rate of new bone formation over 8 years in patients with ankylosing spondylitis. *Ann Rheum Dis* 2005;**73**(4):710–15.

Paper 3.10: Additional genes which influence susceptibility to ankylosing spondylitis, including *ERAP1*, which affects HLA-B27 assembly

Reference

Evans DM, Spencer CC, Pointon JJ, et al. Interaction between *ERAP1* and HLA-B27 in ankylosing spondylitis implicates peptide handling in the mechanism for HLA-B27 in disease susceptibility. *Nat Genet* 2011;43(8):761–7.

Purpose

To detect genes which influence susceptibility to ankylosing spondylitis, using a high density of single nucleotide polymorphisms (SNPs) across the whole genome, together with patient and control cohorts sufficiently large to have the power to detect relatively small effects. To examine the biologic function of any genes identified.

Patients

The patients examined in this study consisted of 1,787 AS patients meeting the modified New York criteria (i.e. they had radiographic sacroiliitis) recruited from UK and Australia, all of European descent. The controls were 4,800 healthy subjects. The data were later combined with subjects used in a previous study of UK, Australian, and US patients to give 3,023 cases and 8,779 controls. This group was termed the 'discovery set', and a further 'replication set' of 2,111 UK, Australian, and Canadian cases with 4,483 controls was used to confirm findings made in the discovery set.

Study design

All cases and controls were genotyped for a large number of SNPs spanning the whole genome—660,000 SNPs for cases and 1.2 million for controls. It is worth pausing to consider the size of the datasets required to detect genes altering susceptibility to disease by 10%–20% (i.e. OR 1.1–1.2)—the discovery set generated ~2 billion data points for AS patients and ~8 billion for the controls. This in turn means that P values of $<5 \times 10^{-8}$ are required for significance.

In addition to the main work of genotyping and analysis, some in vitro analysis of the enzymatic properties of different variants of the exopeptidase ERAP1 was carried out.

Results

This analysis confirmed some loci previously shown to be associated with AS and positively identified three others, while producing strong evidence (i.e. P values which did not quite attain the $<5 \times 10^{-8}$ cut-off) for four additional loci, two of which were novel. Several, such as *RUNX3*, *PTGER4*, and *IL12B*, had apparent relevance to AS pathogenesis: RUNX3 is a transcription factor involved in the differentiation of CD8+ T-cells, the subset which would normally be expected to interact with HLA-B27. Decreased numbers of circulating

CD8+ T-cells were noted in AS patients as compared to controls, and the *RUNX3* variants associated with AS were also associated with CD8+ T-cell numbers. Expression of PTGER4, a receptor for prostaglandins, was found by the investigators to be increased in synovial biopsies from spondyloarthritis patients, and PTGER4 expression is modulated by mechanical stress, of the kind which operates at entheses, the principal sites of pathology in AS. Prostaglandins also influence the differentiation of the Th17 helper T-cell subset which was already implicated in AS pathogenesis by earlier genetic findings and direct measurement of the T-cell subset in AS patients [1, 2]. Indeed, *IL12B* encodes the p40 subunit, which is a component of both IL-23 and IL-12, and IL-23 plays a crucial role in development of IL-17-producing cells of various kinds [3].

This study was large enough, and had sufficient density of SNP coverage, to detect significant and independent effects of more than one SNP in genes previously identified as affecting susceptibility to AS. Thus, for *IL-23R*, two SNPs were identified, one of which conferred susceptibility while the other was protective; in *ERAP1*, two protective SNPs were identified. For *ERAP1*, the combined effect of the two protective SNPs was quite impressive—HLA-B27+ subjects homozygous for both SNPs had a three-to-fourfold lower risk of developing AS as compared to those with risk-conferring alleles. There was dense coverage of class I MHC but no SNP was as strongly associated with AS as HLA-B27 itself. Two SNPs outside *HLA-B* were markers for *HLA-B27* (and therefore may present a new and cheap way of typing large numbers of patients for *HLA-B27* status) but this only applied to *HLA-B2705*—other subtypes known to be associated with AS, particularly in non-European populations, were not identified by these SNPs, and therefore these SNPs outside *HLA-B* have no causal role in disease.

A particularly important finding in this study was the interaction between *ERAP1* polymorphisms and HLA-B27, such that no association between *ERAP1* and AS was seen in HLA-B27-negative subjects with AS (see Figure 3.7; the SNP outside *HLA-B*, which served as a marker for HLA-B27 (rs4349849) was used to identify *B27*-positive subjects). Importantly, this did not apply to any of the other disease-associated genes, for which effects were seen in both HLA-B27-positive and HLA-B27-negative subjects. Since the function of ERAP1 is to trim the short antigenic peptides which are bound by all class I MHC molecules, this finding implies that in HLA-B27-negative subjects, the disease phenotype is achieved without a contribution to pathogenesis from class I MHC molecules. Similar findings have been presented in psoriasis, where *ERAP1* polymorphisms also affect susceptibility to disease but only in those who carry the disease-associated class I HLA allele, *HLA-Cw6* [4], and the same applies to Behçet's disease, associated with *HLA-B51* [5].

The biologic significance of the findings on *ERAP1* polymorphisms was addressed in a brief experimental 'addendum' to the main genetic findings. By producing recombinant ERAP1 molecules with the amino acid changes produced by the polymorphisms, the authors were able to show that protective alleles had a slower ability to trim substrate peptides, and could be regarded by 'defective', in turn implying that optimal loading of HLA-B27 with antigenic peptides predisposes to disease. However these findings have

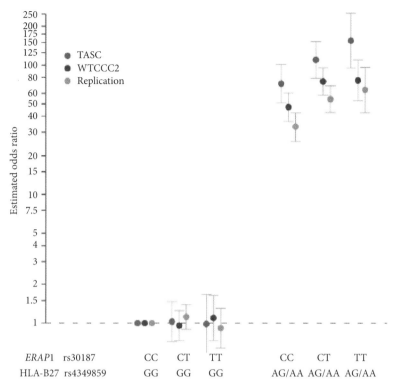

Fig. 3.7 Lack of any effect of *ERAP1* alleles at SNP rs30187 in HLA-B27-negative subjects (tagged by SNP rs4349859, where the *A* allele indicates *B27*).

recently been challenged: whilst individual protective *ERAP1* SNPs may produce amino acid changes which reduce the efficiency of peptide trimming in vitro, the picture is more complicated. It has now been shown that many *ERAP1* genes contain several amino acid changes and the cumulative effects of these need to be considered. When the major forms of *ERAP1* (haplotypes) which are inherited were examined and classified as efficient or inefficient peptide trimmers, AS patients were found to have a combination of haplotypes (i.e. their maternally and paternally inherited forms of *ERAP1*) which resulted in inefficient trimming whereas healthy subjects had efficient forms [6, 7]. Further studies will be required to settle this controversy.

Critique of the paper

The paper represents a very substantial achievement but also perhaps begins to point out the limits of this kind of approach—Will it be possible to recruit even larger patient cohorts with careful control of the quality of clinical data? Will such studies be fundable? Encouragements on this front come from the rapidly decreasing costs of genotyping. There remain substantial statistical challenges to the analysis of the huge datasets which result from studies of this kind but again this is a very active field in bioinformatics.

The studies on the function of different ERAP1 molecules incorporating amino acid changes resulting from significant polymorphisms were essentially illustrative of the approach which needs to be taken in following up a GWAS but are not the last word on the subject. Enzymes may display very different properties when tested in vitro as compared to their intracellular activity when acting in conjunction with the rest of the antigen processing machinery. Further studies of variant ERAP1 molecules are required, and indeed some were published subsequent to this paper [6, 7].

Significance and importance of the paper

This paper succeeded in bringing together the major factors needed for genetic studies of this kind—sufficiently large populations of clinically well-defined patients/controls (with both discovery and replication cohorts), and a sufficient density of SNPs to cover the whole genome with multiple SNPs in many of the regions of interest. This allowed it to have the power to confirm previous findings made in affecting susceptibility. Additional important features of the study were the ability to demonstrate interaction between susceptibility genes, notably *ERAP1* and *HLA-B27*—an interaction which has obvious physiologic relevance but could be demonstrated without any a priori assumption that such an interaction should be evident. Lastly, fine-mapping allowed the effects of different polymorphisms in the same gene, most impressive when these were in opposite directions, that is, increasing or decreasing susceptibility. Such findings lead naturally to experiments of the kind which the authors began to perform looking directly at the effect of single amino acid changes on the function of the molecule concerned. This is the ultimate aim of all genetic studies of disease susceptibility—genetics ideally leads to functional genomics—but this has rarely been achieved in complex multigenic disorders.

References

1 Reveille JD, Sims AM, Danoy P, et al. Genome-wide association study of ankylosing spondylitis identifies non-MHC susceptibility loci. *Nat Genet* 2010;**42**(2):123–7.

2 Shen H, Goodall JC, Hill Gaston JS. Frequency and phenotype of peripheral blood Th17 cells in ankylosing spondylitis and rheumatoid arthritis. *Arthritis Rheum* 2009;**60**(6):1647–56.

3 McKenzie BS, Kastelein RA, Cua DJ. Understanding the IL-23-IL-17 immune pathway. *Trends Immunol* 2006;**27**(1):17–23.

4 Strange A, Capon F, Spencer CC, et al. A genome-wide association study identifies new psoriasis susceptibility loci and an interaction between *HLA-C* and *ERAP1*. *Nat Genet* 2010;**42**(11):985–90.

5 Kirino Y, Bertsias G, Ishigatsubo Y, et al. Genome-wide association analysis identifies new susceptibility loci for Behçet's disease and epistasis between *HLA-B*51* and *ERAP1*. *Nat Genet* **45**(2):202–7.

6 Reeves E, Edwards CJ, Elliott T, et al. Naturally occurring ERAP1 haplotypes encode functionally distinct alleles with fine substrate specificity. *J Immunol* 2013;**191**(1):35–43.

7 Reeves E, Colebatch-Bourn A, Elliott T, et al. Functionally distinct ERAP1 allotype combinations distinguish individuals with Ankylosing Spondylitis. Proc Natl Acad Sci USA 2014; **111**:17594–9.

Chapter 4

Systemic lupus erythematosus

Benjamin Parker and Ian N. Bruce

Introduction

Major advances in our understanding of systemic lupus erythematosus and its related disorders have taken place over the past 50 years. Our understanding has increased as we have gained insights in to the key pathological processes that underlie these conditions. It is now clear that systemic lupus erythematosus fits within the family of systemic autoimmune rheumatic diseases (AIRDs); however, this started as a hypothesis as recently as the 1940s (Paper 4.1). The inflammatory and autoimmune nature of the condition has also taken time to be confirmed and several landmark papers have been chosen that describe key discoveries that lead us to a better understanding of systemic lupus erythematosus pathogenesis and how this understanding translates to better diagnostic tests and systems to classify patients with systemic lupus erythematosus (Papers 4.2, 4.3, 4.6, and 4.7). While survival has increased over the past 50 years, the number of successful clinical trials in systemic lupus erythematosus has been limited. We have also chosen three landmark papers that illustrate successful trials that have advanced the field. These trials confirmed efficacy of a particular agent (Papers 4.8 and 4.9), and the National Institutes of Health (NIH) lupus nephritis trials taught us how long-term follow-up is needed to truly show efficacy in this organ manifestation (Paper 4.5). Finally, two major complications that can complicate the clinical presentation, anti-phospholipid syndrome and premature atherosclerosis (Papers 4.4 and 4.10), were chosen to show how the clinical pattern of disease is not always driven by overt inflammatory processes. These features require a different management approach and need to be considered in the differential diagnosis of key manifestations such as chest pain and cerebral involvement.

Paper 4.1: Common overlapping pathological features of systemic autoimmune rheumatic diseases

Reference

Klemperer P. The concept of collagen diseases. *Amer J Pathol* 1950;26(4):505–19.

Background

Techniques and approaches to the diagnosis of disease have evolved dramatically over the last 150 years. The initial description of the disease usually began with a clinical description of a group of patients with common clinical features and, in the nineteenth century, this became correlated with the gross and microscopic pathological changes seen at post-mortem. The general historical teaching of Morgagni was that a key organ drove the pathological and clinical features of a particular disease entity [1]. Over the years, however, a number of clinical entities evolved and were described that seemed to defy the 'single organ' theory, and these conditions were originally described separately and include conditions such as systemic lupus erythematosus, scleroderma, dermatomyositis, and polyarteritis nodosa. Each condition was considered separately and described in detail as within its own discreet pathological entity. In 1941 Banks published a case report of a 51-year-old secretary who first presented in 1937 and developed a condition which rapidly evolved over two years and from which she eventually died in 1939 [2]. The condition initially presented as a case of scleroderma with facial skin tightness and hyperpigmentation associated with Raynaud's phenomenon and pulmonary fibrosis. She had also developed intermittent fevers without evidence of infection, nephrotic syndrome, and renal failure. She also had polyarthritis noted during her disease course. Her post-mortem examination included extensive myocardial and pulmonary fibrosis as well as a glomerulonephritis and 'arteriolitis' in the kidney. This case report also contained a review of the literature to date on the pathological features on several conditions of relevance, including scleroderma, dermatomyositis, and systemic lupus erythematosus. A number of common features were highlighted, including the 'vascular' involvement seen across a number of conditions. Banks pointed out that, while these conditions may exist as discrete entities, significant overlaps could be observed within individual cases but that 'a widespread vascular involvement' may be a common thread within these conditions.

Paper summary

Klemperer in this paper gives an historical perspective on our understanding of collagen and 'connective tissue' up until the time of publication in 1950 [3]. Once again, the starting point for this idea was based on the anatomical pathology teachings of Morgagni. By thinking of 'connective tissue' as an organ system, then one could begin to think about diffuse multi-organ diseases as sharing this 'organ system' as the primary seat of pathology. It had been noted in a number of earlier pathological descriptions that a number of these conditions had expansion of connective tissue as well as fibrinoid changes within the extracellular matrix and also around vascular structures. Klemperer also reviewed the role of the fibroblast and how certain nutrients such as vitamin C were important in the development of collagen. He also noted the important negative effects of cortisone on experimental wound healing as well as the influence of cortisone and adrenocorticotropic hormone on reducing hexosamines in patients with systemic lupus erythematosus. His group had also noted that steroids improved serum albumin and reduced gamma globulins in systemic lupus erythematosus patients. All of this confirmed the dynamic nature of production and alterations in connective tissue.

By 1950, a lot was known about common features across these conditions but a lot more needed to be understood about the nature of collagen and how and when fibronoid reactions occurred. Klemperer was aware of additional upcoming techniques and approaches which might help clarify this situation further, such as improved tissue culture techniques and electron microscopy. He was also aware that, while there did seem to be a broad concept at work, there were limitations of the science to date, and therefore was careful not to conflate common morphological observations with a single pathogenic process or pathway. The intention was also not for the phrase 'collagen diseases' to become a 'catchall term for maladies with puzzling clinical and anatomical features'. He argued that this was not a diagnosis in its own right but, nevertheless, that developing this concept would stimulate further research and understanding of these diseases. As such, he described the concept as 'not an idle speculation' and actually pointed forwards to a day when this concept may have 'served its purpose'.

Significance of the paper

The phrase 'collagen disease and collagen vascular diseases' has remained in use for many years subsequent to this publication, later being changed to 'connective tissue diseases', which reflects the same root concept at work. Latterly, the phrase 'systemic autoimmune rheumatic diseases' has replaced these older names as the preferred overarching term for these conditions. Nevertheless, a number of the same conditions remain within this family. While significant research efforts remain focused on particular disease entities such as systemic lupus erythematosus, dermatomyositis, systemic sclerosis, and others, there remains a broad acceptance that many patients present with overlapping features across a number of these conditions. In addition, entities have been described that also reflect the evolving nature of these conditions and that early in their disease course it can be difficult to distinguish one from another. Therefore, concepts such as undifferentiated connective tissue disease and mixed connective tissue disease have both been described [5, 6]. Patients may remain with an indistinct phenotype throughout their disease course, or over time may evolve towards a more distinct diagnostic category.

At the serological level, antinuclear antibodies, rheumatoid factor and extractable nuclear antigen subsets show overlap between a number of these syndromes. For example, SSA (Ro) and SSB (La) antibodies are associated with Sjögren's syndrome but are not confined to this condition. They are also seen in photosensitive patients with systemic and cutaneous lupus. Also, follow-up of mothers of babies born with congenital heart block (also associated with Ro and La antibodies) shows that many of these women do not express any clinical phenotype themselves [4]. At a more fundamental level, pathological processes such as that reflected by the so called 'interferon signature' have also been found to be common across a number of these conditions, an observation suggesting significant overlap in their immunopathogenesis [7]. More recently, a number of the genetic markers described also show overlap between a number of these entities [8].

Klemperer's observations and proposed concept of 'collagen diseases' still remain useful today. In clinical practice, it serves as a reminder to clinicians to remain alert to the evolving and changing nature of the clinical features patients may present with over time. It is also useful from a research point of view as it enables investigators to address common pathogenic mechanisms that may be shared across related disease entities while also enabling us to consider novel therapies that may have usefulness in similar and related conditions.

References

1 **Klemperer P, Pollack AD, Baehr G**. Diffuse collagen disease: acute disseminated lupus erythematosus and diffuse scleroderma. JAMA 1942;**119**(4):331–2.

2 **Banks BM**. Is there a common denominator in scleroderma, dermatomyositis, disseminated lupus erythematosus, the Libman–Sachs syndrome and polyarteritis nodosa? *New Engl J Med* 1941;**225**(12):433–44.

3 **Klemperer P**. The concept of collagen diseases. *Amer J Pathol* 1950;**26**(4):505–19.

4 **Waltuck J, Buyon JP**. Autoantibody-associated congenital heart block: outcome in mothers and children. *Ann Intern Med* 1994;**120**(7):544–51.

5 **Mosca M, Tani C, Talarico R, et al**. Undifferentiated connective tissue diseases (UCTD): simplified systemic autoimmune diseases. *Autoimmun Rev* 2011;**10**(5):256–8.

6 **Sharp GC, Anderson PC**. Current concepts in the classification of connective tissue diseases. Overlap syndromes and mixed connective tissue disease (MCTD). *J Am Acad Dermatol* 1980;**2**(4):269–79.

7 **Higgs BW, Liu Z, White B, et al**. Patients with systemic lupus erythematosus, myositis, rheumatoid arthritis and scleroderma share activation of a common type I interferon pathway. *Ann Rheum Dis* 2011;**70**(11):2029–36.

8 **Martin JE, Assassi S, Diaz-Gallo LM, et al**. A systemic sclerosis and systemic lupus erythematosus pan-meta-GWAS reveals new shared susceptibility loci. *Hum Mol Genet* 2013;**22**(19):4021–9.

Paper 4.2: The LE cell phenomenon

Reference

Hargraves MM, Richmond H, Morton R. Presentation of two bone marrow elements: the 'Tart' cell and the L.E. cell. *Proc Staff Meet, Mayo Clin* 1948;23(2):25–8.

Background

The diagnosis of systemic lupus erythematosus has presented physicians with major challenges throughout the years. Identifying specific tests to support the diagnosis has been aided in the last 30–40 years by the description of autoantibodies. Prior to such testing becoming mainstream, the diagnosis of lupus in the first half of the twentieth century was on the basis of the presence of a combination of clinical presentation and suggestive changes in routine testing. The earliest test primarily associated with lupus was the LE cell phenomenon.

Purpose

To describe the LE cell phenomenon.

Paper summary

Hargraves et al. first reported their observation of the LE cell phenomenon in 1948. In the original description, they outlined two distinct phenomena from bone marrow preparations [1].

The LE cell got its name from the fact that it was seen in patients with acute systemic lupus erythematosus. The phenomenon describes the presence of nuclear material that has been phagocytosed into a mature neutrophil or macrophage. The nuclear origins of the ingested material were demonstrated using Feulgen stain. Within these preparations and aspirates, neutrophils appeared to be attracted towards the debris and two to three neutrophils could be observed around such nuclear material. After the material had been completely ingested into one of the cells, the other neutrophils were observed to move away, thus suggesting a chemotactic process was being observed. In the original report, the authors stated that they had not seen this phenomenon in peripheral blood but that it was confined to the bone marrow and that 25 cases of systemic lupus erythematosus had been observed to have this phenomenon, although they did point out that 'the diagnosis of acute disseminated lupus erythematosus might be questioned clinically in some of the more than 25 cases observed'. They therefore concluded that further observations were required to understand the significance and specificity of this test.

In addition to the LE cell phenomenon, the group had also identified a similar but distinct phenomenon known as the 'tart cell'. This phenomenon appeared to be general to many bone marrow preparations from a wide range of conditions, although occurring in greater quantities in bone marrow preparations from diseases such as lymphoblastoma, respiratory infections, and metastatic cancer. This phenomenon consisted of a histiocyte containing a second nucleus. The second nucleus usually stained reddish/purple with

Wright's stain rather than the dark purple seen in the original histiocyte nucleus. The authors were, however, clear that this was a more generalized phenomenon and was distinct from the LE cell phenomenon.

Subsequent work from the same group did however show that, when peripheral blood was prepared in a standardized fashion, a small number of LE cells could be identified within peripheral blood as well as within the bone marrow [2]. Again, this was associated with systemic lupus erythematosus. The observation of the LE cell phenomenon raised the possibility of a circulating factor associated with lupus that could induce LE cell production.

Haserick and Bortz noted that plasma from systemic lupus erythematosus patients when added to bone marrow from patients with other conditions and incubated at body temperature could induce the development of LE cells [3]. The LE cell phenomenon has subsequently been confirmed to relate to the presence of histone-binding autoantibodies and it was noted that the LE cell phenomenon was completely inhibited by mixing positive serum with core mononucleosomes, the basic histone–DNA subunit of chromatin [4]. This reactivity of histones was also noted in NZB/NZW mice in which LE cell formation is a feature [5].

Significance of the paper

Following on from the LE cell phenomenon description and discovery, further novel tests to contribute to the diagnosis of autoimmune diseases such as systemic lupus erythematosus included the description of antinuclear antibodies (ANAs) and specific staining of ANA subsets using immunofluorescence. Both the LE cell phenomenon and ANA production were shown not to be specific for lupus but were found in other contexts such as autoimmune liver disease, systemic sclerosis, dermatomyositis, etc.

Later discovery of antibodies to double-stranded DNA and, in particular, refinement of the technique using the Farr assay improved the specificity for lupus [6]. Indeed, DNA antibody titres in some patients reflected levels of disease activity, and therefore double-stranded DNA antibodies were seen to have both a diagnostic and a monitoring role in patients with lupus. Other discoveries included the Sm antibody and its high specificity for lupus [7]. The LE cell phenomenon, as well as specific autoantibodies such as anti-dsDNA and Sm, was among the tests included within the American College of Rheumatology 1982 criteria for systemic lupus erythematosus [8]. Hargraves's original description of the LE cell phenomenon did however point out early that none of these tests are actually specific for a particular diagnosis and therefore cannot be seen as definitive diagnostic tests. In later years, the widespread availability of ANA testing and similar associated tests have now lead to the wider problem of patients being found to have a positive antibody but without a direct clinical correlate to support the diagnosis of lupus or other autoimmune rheumatic diseases. The widespread 'false positivity' means that, like all such testing, clear guidelines are still required to ensure that the right test is done at the right time. This means that such tests should only be performed in clinical situations where the diagnosis is suggested. In such cases, positive tests do increase the post-test probability that the patient has the diagnosis of interest. In contrast, widespread use of such testing in the context of a low prior probability of disease can lead to over-diagnosis, over-treatment, and great anxiety for the patient.

The LE cell phenomenon stands as a landmark in the diagnosis and management of systemic lupus erythematosus, as it was the first test clearly and primarily associated with systemic lupus erythematosus. Subsequent understanding of the mechanism of the LE cell phenomenon has improved our understanding of the autoimmune nature of the disease. Nevertheless, it was never absolutely diagnostic; yet, it proved extremely useful in the diagnosis and management of patients who had highly suggestive clinical and other laboratory features. Also, in contrast to autoantibody testing, which can sometimes take several days to be reported, the LE cell phenomenon remains a test which can be performed in a short period and could help support a rapid diagnosis.

References

1 **Hargraves MM, Richmond H, Morton R**. Presentation of two bone marrow elements: the 'Tart' cell and the 'L.E.' cell. *Proc Staff Meet, Mayo Clin* 1948;**23**(2):25–8.

2 **Hargraves MM**. Production in vitro of the L.E. cell phenomenon; use of normal bone marrow elements and blood plasma from patients with acute disseminated lupus erythematosus. *Proc Staff Meet Mayo Clin* 1949;**24**(9):234–7.

3 **Haserick JR, Bortz DW**. Normal bone marrow inclusion phenomena induced by lupus erythematosus plasma. *J Invest Dermatol* 1949;**13**(2):47–9.

4 **Rekvig OP, Hannestad K**. Lupus erythematosus (LE) factors recognize both nucleosomes and viable human leucocytes. *Scand J Immunol* 1981;**13**(6):597–604.

5 **Miller MM, Goto R, Phillips ML, et al**. Monoclonal autoantibody directed toward histone and capable of inducing LE cell formation. *Hybridoma* 1983;**2**(2):201–9.

6 **Aarden LA, Lakmaker F, Feltkamp TE**. Immunology of DNA. I. The influence of reaction conditions on the Farr assay as used for the detection of anti-ds DNA. *J Immunol Methods* 1976;**10**(1):27–37.

7 **Notman DD, Kurata N, Tan EM**. Profiles of antinuclear antibodies in systemic rheumatic diseases. *Ann Intern Med* 1975;**83**(4):464–9.

8 **Tan EM, Cohen AS, Fries JF, et al**. The 1982 revised criteria for the classification of systemic lupus erythematosus. *Arthritis Rheum* 1982;**25**(11):1271–7.

Paper 4.3: Complement deposition demonstrated in systemic lupus erythematosus tissue

Reference

Lachmann PJ, Muller-Eberhard HJ, Kunkel HG, et al. The localization of in vivo bound complement in tissue sections. *J Exp Med* 1962;115(1):63–82.

Background

Autoimmunity as a concept was first mooted in the early 1900s, with observations in paroxysmal cold haemoglobinuria that suggested autoantibodies against the patient's own erythrocytes were central to the pathogenesis of this disease [1]. This concept did, however, take a long time to be accepted. In the 1950s a number of studies began to demonstrate the presence of immunoglobulins in the lesions of certain human conditions, including systemic lupus erythematosus. Such deposition was also demonstrated in experimental models such as serum sickness. It was, however, argued that the simple demonstration of immunoglobulin deposition in lesions did not necessarily mean they were playing a pathogenic role. In order to demonstrate a cytotoxic effect of such deposits, other mediators of an inflammatory response were argued to be necessary. A key potential candidate for this was complement, as studies had begun to show a cytotoxic effect of complement in experimental systems. Demonstrating complement deposition at the site of lesions in human disease had proven a major challenge.

Purpose

The purpose of this paper was to demonstrate whether the authors could identify bound complement in tissue samples from patients with conditions which might be due to autoimmunity.

Study design

The authors set out to demonstrate whether they could identify bound complement in tissue samples from patients with a number of conditions some of which may have an autoimmune aetiology [2]. They had identified an antigenic moiety on the third: complement (β_{1c}). A purified form of this antigen had been used to raise anti-β_{1c} serum in rabbits, and this antiserum had been conjugated to fluorescein. The authors obtained tissue blocks from biopsies or post-mortem samples from patients with a range of conditions, including systemic lupus erythematosus. The tissues examined included kidney, liver, lymph nodes, spleen, and heart. The range of conditions studied included other types of glomerulonephritis as well as hypertension, polyarteritis nodosa, and generalized atherosclerosis. The experiments also included anti-7S gamma globulin to demonstrate immunoglobulin deposition in parallel.

Results

In the samples from patients with systemic lupus erythematosus, strong staining was noted, particularly in lesions from patients with lupus nephritis, and this staining co-localized with immunoglobulin deposition. The staining was predominantly focused around the glomeruli. Samples from patients with more severe and advanced lesions including fibrosis showed much less staining. In lupus patients, there was also complement deposition co-localized with immunoglobulin in the vessel walls of kidneys and splenic vessels. Samples from other conditions such as hypertension, atherosclerosis, and polyarteritis nodosa all showed much less intense complement deposition, although some cases of 'subacute glomerulonephritis' did show significant complement deposition. This was also true in patients with amyloid disease. Interestingly, cardiac lesions from patients with acute rheumatic fever, renal and splenic tissue from Waldenström's macroglobulinaemia, and splenic tissue from patients with idiopathic thrombocytopaenic purpura also demonstrated complement deposition.

Significance of the paper

This paper demonstrated the technical feasibility of identifying complement deposition in vivo in tissue samples from patients with systemic lupus erythematosus. From these early observations, the authors concluded that complement binding localized with immunoglobulin binding, especially in glomeruli and in vascular lesions from patients with systemic lupus erythematosus. This suggested that immune complex deposition was an important feature of the disease and that complement binding may mediate cytotoxic effects in vivo. They also postulated that complement binding explained the hypocomplementaemia noted in these patients.

Complement is now widely accepted as being a major factor in the pathogenesis of systemic lupus erythematosus. Indeed, several deficiencies in the complement pathway, particularly in early factors such as C1q, are among only a few proven monogenic causes of systemic lupus erythematosus [3]. In these individuals, systemic lupus erythematosus begins at an early age and has a more severe clinical phenotype. Two distinct features of the complement pathway are now believed to be important in lupus pathogenesis. As suggested by Lachmann et al., activation of the complement cascade results in pro-inflammatory responses in part mediated by the membrane attack complex (MAC) assembled by later complement components [2]. This MAC is directly damaging to cells and drives the cytotoxic effects of complement activation.

Second, complement deficiencies, particularly C1q deficiency, have been shown in model systems to be associated with impaired clearance of apoptotic cells. The failure to clear apoptotic cells in an efficient manner may render cell components more antigenic, thus provoking immune complex formation and stimulating a pro-inflammatory response [4]. There is also some evidence that immune complex formation in the absence of C1q is more likely to provoke interferon production from plasmacytoid dendritic cells [5].

It is also been observed over the past decade or so that C1q antibodies are strongly associated with lupus nephritis in systemic lupus erythematosus cohorts. C1q antibodies have been noted to bind particularly to C1q located within immune complexes and in so doing may further amplify the activation of the complement pathway and thus enhance further inflammation at sites of immune complex deposition. Similarly, others have found that C1q antibodies may also bind more avidly to C1q already bound to apoptotic cells [6]. Both of these mechanisms may therefore enhance further the pro-inflammatory effects of complement binding in tissue sites such as the kidney.

References

1 **Silverstein AM**. Autoimmunity versus horror autotoxicus: the struggle for recognition. *Nat Immunol* 2001;**2**(4):279–81.

2 **Lachmann PJ, Muller-Eberhard HJ, Kunkel HG, et al**. The localization of in vivo bound complement in tissue section. *J Exp Med* 1962;**115**(1):63–82.

3 **Thompson RA, Haeney M, Reid KB, et al**. A genetic defect of the C1q subcomponent of complement associated with childhood (immune complex) nephritis. *N Engl J Med* 1980;**303**(1):22–4.

4 **Taylor PR, Carugati A, Fadok VA, et al**. A hierarchical role for classical pathway complement proteins in the clearance of apoptotic cells in vivo. *J Exp Med* 2000;**192**(3):359–66.

5 **Santer DM, Hall BE, George TC, et al**. C1q deficiency leads to the defective suppression of IFN-alpha in response to nucleoprotein containing immune complexes. *J Immunol* 2010;**185**(8):4738–49.

6 **Pickering MC, Botto M**. Are anti-C1q antibodies different from other SLE autoantibodies? *Nat Rev Rheumatol* 2010;**6**(8):490–3.

Paper 4.4: Premature cardiovascular disease in systemic lupus erythematosus patients

Reference

Urowitz MB, Bookman AA, Koehler BE, et al. The bimodal mortality pattern of systemic lupus erythematosus. *Am J Med* 1976;60(2):221–5.

Background

For many years systemic lupus erythematosus was recognized as an illness with an extremely poor prognosis. Prior to the advent of modern therapy, mortality rates of 50% at five years were described [1]. With the advent of steroid therapy and improved diagnostic awareness, longer-term survival became a realistic expectation. There was, however, a feeling in the mid-1960s and early 1970s that survival rates had effectively plateaued. A number of large clinical cohorts had also begun to emerge following patients with lupus prospectively over time to study the disease in more detail. One of the earliest of these cohorts was established in 1970 in Toronto, where patients were followed according a standard clinical and laboratory assessment protocol. One of the earlier papers from the Toronto cohort examined mortality in the initial group of patients recruited.

Purpose

The aim of this paper was to examine mortality in a well-described cohort of patients with systemic lupus erythematosus.

Patients

Patients were recruited to the Toronto Lupus Cohort from 1970, and this paper describes deaths in the first 81 patients who were followed [2]. The average disease duration at the time of study was six years. The majority of patients (73%–90%) were taking corticosteroids, with an average daily prednisone dose of 18.1 mg per day. Forty patients (49%) had clinical evidence of renal involvement.

Study design

This report comprised an observational study.

Results

Between 1970 and 1974, 11 deaths (three men and eight women) occurred in the cohort. The mean age and disease duration at death were 44 years and 4.2 years, respectively. The investigators divided patients into two groups based on the time of death related to their diagnosis. In Group 1, six patients died within one year of diagnosis and, in Group 2, five patients died at a mean (range) of 8.6 (2.5–19.5) years after their lupus was diagnosed. The early deaths (Group 1) were characterized by patients having active lupus, with four of the six having active lupus nephritis. In addition, four of the Group 1 patients had a major infective episode at the time of their death. The mean prednisone dose at time of death in this first group was 53.3 mg per day.

In Group 2, the five patients (four women and one man) died after a mean disease duration of 8.6 years. At the time of death, the average prednisone dose was 10.1 mg per day. Only one of these five patients had evidence of active lupus at time of death, with no evidence of active nephritis on biopsy report or post-mortem. Strikingly, every patient in Group 2 had a fresh myocardial infarction (MI) at the time of death and this MI was the key cause of death in four of the five patients. Post-mortem examination in these patients revealed established atherosclerotic coronary heart disease. Three of the four women were premenopausal at the time of death in Group 2.

Subsequent analysis of the entire cohort of 81 patients found six MIs in this population (7.4%). Increased blood pressure and increased triglyceride levels were noted in those patients with coronary heart disease. The average age at time of first event was 39.6 years.

Significance of the paper

Accelerated atherosclerosis and premature coronary heart disease are now recognized as major long-term complications of lupus and indeed other inflammatory rheumatic diseases such as rheumatoid arthritis [3]. This paper was the first to highlight the phenomenon of clinical coronary heart disease as a major cause of late morbidity and mortality in systemic lupus erythematosus. Around the same time, Bulkley et al. had reported a post-mortem series of patients with systemic lupus erythematosus who died in the era since steroid therapy came into use [4]. In this study, 36 such patients' post-mortems were compared to a historical group of patients who died prior to steroid therapy being used in systemic lupus erythematosus. Pathological evidence of hypertension was seen in 25 (69%), left ventricular hypertrophy in 23 (64%), and congestive cardiac failure in 15 (43%). Atherosclerotic narrowing (>50%) of at least one major coronary artery was observed in 42% of patients who had taken steroids for more than one year but in none of the 17 patients in the series treated for less than one year (Figure 4.1) [4]. A number of subsequent studies have confirmed the early and excess mortality from coronary heart disease in systemic lupus erythematosus. Manzi et al. estimated that women with lupus age 35–44 have a >50-fold relative risk of MI compared to women in the general population and, in a UK study, Haque et al. noted that the first clinical event in a nationwide lupus study occurred under the age of 55 years old and in over half of the patients [5, 6]. Subclinical atherosclerosis has also been noted to underpin these clinical observations by a number of investigators using a range of techniques including myocardial perfusion imaging, coronary calcification, and carotid Doppler ultrasound [7]. Subsequent work has noted that, while classic risk factors play an important role in accelerated atherosclerosis, the chronic inflammatory state also plays an important role [7].

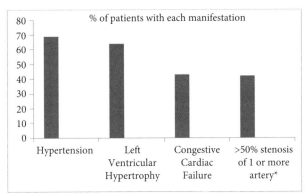

Fig. 4.1 Percentage of patients with evidence of cardiac pathology on post-mortem in a series of 36 systemic lupus erythematosus patients treated since the introduction of glucocorticoids for management; * denotes the percentage of patients with this feature who had received steroids for >1 year [4].
Source data from Bulkley BH, Roberts WC. The heart in systemic lupus erythematosus and the changes induced in it by corticosteroid therapy. A study of 36 necropsy patients. Am J Med. 1975;58:243–64.

Recent studies have also focused on the contribution of therapies used in lupus to atherosclerosis. There is strong evidence from a number of studies of both clinical and subclinical cardiovascular disease that corticosteroid exposure increases the risk of future clinical events. A recent study by Magder et al. suggested that higher doses of prednisone were a particularly important risk factor [8]. At the same time, there is evidence that antimalarial drugs may have a modulating role on cardiovascular risk factors, with a potential to improve lipid profiles and reduce the tendency towards insulin resistance and metabolic syndrome, as well as having potential antithrombotic effects [7].

Cardiovascular risk is now accepted as an important co-morbidity to consider in the long-term management of patients with systemic lupus erythematosus, and heightened awareness of the early age at which this complication may emerge, particularly its ability to present in premenopausal women, has important clinical implications when considering the differential diagnosis of, for example, chest pain or breathlessness in younger patients with systemic lupus erythematosus.

The study by Urowitz et al. also highlights the significant contribution that long-term observational cohorts make to our knowledge of less common rheumatic diseases such as systemic lupus erythematosus. A number of large clinic cohorts have all contributed significantly to our knowledge of atherosclerosis in lupus and have served as a template for larger multicentre studies that have also been able to address aspects of long-term outcomes in diseases such as systemic lupus erythematosus.

References

1 **Merrill JT**. Cortisone in disseminated lupus erythematosus during pregnancy; report of a case and review of the literature. *Obstet Gynaecol* 1955;**6**(6):637–43.

2 Urowitz MB, Bookman AA, Koehler BE, et al. The bimodal mortality pattern of systemic lupus erythematosus. *Am J Med* 1976;**60**(2):221–5.

3 Aviña-Zubieta JA, Choi HK, Sadatsafavi M, et al. Risk of cardiovascular mortality in patients with rheumatoid arthritis: a meta-analysis of observational studies. *Arthritis Rheum* 2008;**59**(12):1690–7.

4 Bulkley BH, Roberts WC. The heart in systemic lupus erythematosus and the changes induced in it by corticosteroid therapy. A study of 36 necropsy patients. *Am J Med* 1975;**58**(2):243–64.

5 Manzi S, Meilahn EN, Rairie JE, et al. Age-specific incidence rates of myocardial infarction and angina in women with systemic lupus erythematosus: comparison with the Framingham Study. *Am J Epidemiol* 1997;**145**(5):408–15.

6 Haque S, Gordon C, Isenberg D, et al. Risk factors for clinical coronary heart disease in systemic lupus erythematosus: the lupus and atherosclerosis evaluation of risk (LASER) study. *J Rheumatol* 2010;**37**(2):322–9.

7 Bruce IN. 'Not only . . . but also': factors that contribute to accelerated atherosclerosis and premature coronary heart disease in systemic lupus erythematosus. *Rheumatology* 2005;**44**(12):1492–502.

8 Magder LS, Petri M. Incidence of and risk factors for adverse cardiovascular events among patients with systemic lupus erythematosus. *Am J Epidemiol* 2012;**176**(8):708–19.

Paper 4.5: Long-term trials demonstrate the efficacy of immunosuppression for lupus nephritis

Reference

Austin HA 3rd, Klippel JH, Balow JE, et al. Therapy of lupus nephritis. Controlled trial of prednisone and cytotoxic drugs. *N Engl J Med* 1986;314(10):614–9.

Background

Lupus nephritis represents one of the more serious complications of systemic lupus erythematosus. Prior to the advent of steroids and immunosuppressive agents, proliferative glomerulonephritis had a high mortality within two years of onset [1]. Modification of this outcome was only in part affected by high-dose glucocorticoids, and better therapies were needed. In the late 1960s and 1970s, additional immunosuppressive agents were being investigated in the treatment of lupus nephritis, including azathioprine, nitrogen mustard, and oral cyclophosphamide. Such agents did show early promise in controlling lupus nephritis [2], and early data did not appear to show any excess of adverse events, probably in part due to their steroid-sparing capabilities. Whether use of these agents fundamentally altered the long-term prognosis in systemic lupus erythematosus and in particular renal outcomes, remained uncertain although early reports did suggest a trend towards more patients remaining dialysis free following such therapies.

Purpose

To describe the outcomes of a series of trials using immunosuppressive agents in lupus nephritis.

Patients

Patients were enrolled between 1969 and 1981. All patients had systemic lupus erythematosus as confirmed by standard criteria, and all patients had biopsy-proven lupus nephritis.

Study design

The NIH established a clinical trials programme to investigate newer therapies for lupus nephritis [3]; this programme consisted of a series of open-label randomized control trials.

Treatment

The trials randomized patients to one of five treatment arms, one of which was the use of oral steroids only (prednisone 1 mg/kg daily for 4–8 weeks and then tapered; Group 1; $n = 30$). The four other groups received oral prednisone (0.5 mg/kg daily) and also received one of the following treatments: oral azathioprine (up to 4 mg/kg daily; Group 2; $n = 20$), oral cyclophosphamide (up to 4 mg/kg daily; Group 3; $n = 18$), combined oral cyclophosphamide and azathioprine (1 mg/kg daily of both; Group 4; $n = 23$), or IV cyclophosphamide (0.5–1.0 g/m^2 monthly; Group 5; $n = 20$). Patients continued immunosuppressives for up to 18 months after remission, or for at least four years. As such, the median duration of immunosuppressive use was between four and seven years, with the azathioprine group having a median of seven years of therapy. Patients also remained on alternate day maintenance steroids. The groups were not all recruited contemporaneously. Group 1 was recruited over the whole period, Groups 2–3 were recruited from 1969 to 1973, and Groups 4–5 were recruited from 1976 onwards.

Follow-up

Of the patients recruited, 107 had at least three months follow-up and were included in the analysis (four were excluded due to early infection or a non-renal death).

Study end points measured

Clinical end points were mortality, serum creatinine, and end-stage renal failure.

Results

The cohort for analysis included 92 (86%) women and had a median age of onset and duration of nephritis of 27 years and 9 months, respectively. Six patients did not have a biopsy and seven had WHO Class II lesions. The rest had WHO Class III–V lupus nephritis.

There was no difference in mortality between the groups. Numerically, more patients taking oral prednisone alone experienced a doubling of their serum creatinine or went on to develop end-stage renal failure. Survival analyses showed that these differences began to be apparent after five years of follow-up. Formal statistical analysis showed that this difference was significant when Group 1 (oral prednisone alone) was compared to Group 5, which was the IV cyclophosphamide group ($P = 0.027$; Figure 4.2). This significant difference between Groups 1 and 5 were also observed in a subset analysis of patients with evidence of chronicity on biopsy ($P = 0.014$). Adverse events noted included a higher risk of amenorrhoea and herpes zoster with cyclophosphamide-based regimes, and haemorrhagic cystitis, which occurred in the oral cyclophosphamide groups.

Significance of the paper

This paper represented analysis of a 'trials programme' in which the protocol varied over a long period of time but in which the primary comparator (oral steroids alone) remained constant. Such trials were pivotal in moving us into the modern era of lupus nephritis trials. A number of previous studies had suggested that immunosuppressive regimes were well tolerated and may have some advantages when compared to steroid-only regimes for lupus nephritis, and there was some evidence that cyclophosphamide in particular helped modify the rate of developing chronic lesions on serial biopsies [2]. There was, however, very limited evidence of a long-term effect of such regimes on clinically important end points such as doubling of serum creatinine or end-stage renal failure. By extending the observation period out to more than five years, this trial for the first time demonstrated a long-term benefit to immunosuppression added to steroids in lupus nephritis. It also

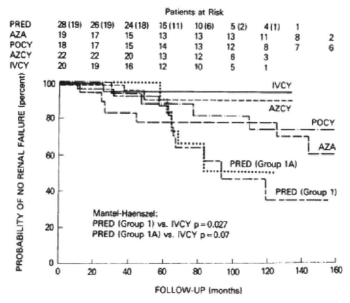

Fig. 4.2 Probability of being free of renal failure according to treatment assignment in early NIH trials of lupus nephritis; AZA, azathioprine; AZACY, azathioprine and cyclophosphamide; IVCY, intravenous cyclophosphamide; POCY, oral cyclophosphamide; PRED, methylprednisolone only [3]. From New England Journal of Medicine, Austin H.A. et al, Therapy of lupus nephritis. Controlled trial of prednisone and cytotoxic drugs, 314, 614–9, Copyright © 1986 Massachusetts Medical Society. Reprinted with permission from Massachusetts Medical Society.

emphasized the need for long-term end points in lupus nephritis trials. Lupus nephritis is a life-long condition and needs a long-term management plan. Early improvements in proteinuria and urinary sediment are surrogates of the really important 'hard' clinical end points and need to be recognized as such. This trial was the first to also show that, while still associated with significant toxicity, IV cyclophosphamide allowed a reduction in the risk of haemorrhagic cystitis, a risk factor for future bladder malignancy [3].

Subsequent research and lupus nephritis trials have also included longer-term follow-up. The Euro-Lupus Group have also shown that low-dose cyclophosphamide regimes are equally effective in maintaining long-term renal function compared to the higher-dose NIH regimes [4, 5]. The Euro-Lupus regime also reduces total cyclophosphamide exposure and risk of amenorrhoea [4, 5]. A further major development has been the advent of mycophenolate mofetil (MMF) for use in induction and maintenance of lupus nephritis. While overall toxicity in the trials of MMF was comparable to 'NIH' cyclophosphamide, amenorrhoea is not seen with this agent [6, 7]. Long-term maintenance regimes with MMF have also been shown to be superior to azathioprine in maintaining relapse-free disease and maintaining renal function [7]. We are also learning more about subgroups of lupus nephritis. A key observation recently has been the poorer response to cyclophosphamide-based regimes in patients of African origin, and better overall outcomes in African and Hispanic origin patients in the MMF trials [6]. Although newer agents such as rituximab have been disappointing in clinical trials [8], it is hoped that targeted biological therapies may help to further improve clinical outcomes in patients with lupus nephritis and allow long-term preservation of renal function with less toxicity than current therapeutic regimes produce.

References

1 **Pollak VE, Pirani CL, Kark RM**. Effect of large doses of prednisone on the renal lesions and life span of patients with lupus glomerulonephritis. *J Lab Clin Med* 1961;**57**:495–511.

2 **Dillard MG, Dujovne I, Pollak VE, et al**. The effect of treatment with prednisone and nitrogen mustard on the renal lesions and life span of patients with lupus glomerulonephritis. *Nephron* 1973;**10**(5):273–91.

3 **Austin HA 3rd, Klippel JH, Balow JE, et al**. Therapy of lupus nephritis. Controlled trial of prednisone and cytotoxic drugs. *N Engl J Med* 1986;**314**(10):614–9.

4 **Houssiau FA, Vasconcelos C, D'Cruz D, et al**. Immunosuppressive therapy in lupus nephritis: the Euro-Lupus Nephritis Trial, a randomized trial of low-dose versus high-dose intravenous cyclophosphamide. *Arthritis Rheum* 2002;**46**(8):2121–31.

5 **Houssiau FA, Vasconcelos C, D'Cruz D, et al**. The 10-year follow-up data of the Euro-Lupus Nephritis Trial comparing low-dose and high-dose intravenous cyclophosphamide. *Ann Rheum Dis* 2010;**69**(1):61–4.

6 **Appel GB, Contreras G, Dooley MA, et al**. Mycophenolate mofetil versus cyclophosphamide for induction treatment of lupus nephritis. *J Am Soc Nephrol* 2009;**20**(5):1103–12.

7 **Dooley MA, Jayne D, Ginzler EM, et al**. Mycophenolate versus azathioprine as maintenance therapy for lupus nephritis. *N Engl J Med* 2011;**365**(20):1886–95.

8 **Rovin BH, Furie R, Latinis K, et al**. Efficacy and safety of rituximab in patients with active proliferative lupus nephritis: the Lupus Nephritis Assessment with Rituximab study. *Arthritis Rheum* 2012;**64**(4):1215–26.

Paper 4.6: Development of classification criteria for systemic lupus erythematosus

Reference

Tan EM, Cohen AS, Fries JF, et al. The 1982 revised criteria for the classification of systemic lupus erythematosus. *Arthritis Rheum* 1982;25(11):1271–7.

Background

Systemic lupus erythematosus is a heterogeneous disease that can manifest a wide variety of clinical and laboratory features. Although the cutaneous manifestations of systemic lupus erythematosus have been recognized since the mid-nineteenth century, it was not until 1971 that the first preliminary criteria for the classification of the disease were agreed by the American College of Rheumatology (ACR) [1]. However, the initial classification criteria in 1971 did not have access to many important immunological disease markers such as autoantibodies and serum complement; markers that became more widely available over the subsequent decade. Of equal importance was the development of sophisticated epidemiological methodology that could be utilized in the development of classification criteria. Therefore, in 1979 a subcommittee of the American Rheumatism Association was established and tasked with updating and revising the preliminary 1971 classification criteria for systemic lupus erythematosus.

Purpose

To describe the revised classification criteria for systemic lupus erythematosus.

Methods

The authors describe in detail the methodological steps involved with developing an updated classification criteria, and the assessment of sensitivity and specificity in various clinical cohorts. Initially, 30 potential criteria variables (including the original criteria set) were agreed by the subcommittee and were then tested in two cohorts of 177 systemic lupus erythematosus patients and 162 control patients with a range of rheumatic conditions. Variables were eliminated that were not commonly performed, such as biopsies, or that did not achieve statistical significance, such as Raynaud's phenomenon. Interestingly, the LE cell test was infrequently performed within the cohort (just 45% of the lupus cohort underwent the investigation) despite being highly specific for systemic lupus erythematosus. The sensitivity and specificity of individual criteria were then assessed and selections of potential criteria sets were developed. The final potential combinations of variables were tested in a dataset of 172 patients with systemic lupus erythematosus and more than 400 patients with either scleroderma or dermatomyositis.

Results

Overall, at least 12 final criteria sets were analysed, and the addition of the fluorescence ANA (FANA) test proved the strongest addition to the classification criteria. In total,

174/175 systemic lupus erythematosus patients had been positive for FANA over the course of their disease, and the test was almost universally used in clinical practice. It was noted, however, that, although the FANA was very sensitive, it was relatively non-specific, as it was positive in 51% of controls. The committee suggested that the FANA could potentially operate as an entry point into the final criteria, as it would immediately exclude approximately half the non-lupus patients, although they did not eventually pursue this recommendation. An organ system approach was utilized to aid simplification of the criteria set, which did not appear to lose accuracy, apart from the cutaneous manifestations which were kept separate (Table 4.1).

Table 4.1 1982 American College of Rheumatology Classification Criteria for systemic lupus erythematosus*

Malar rash	Haematological disorder
Oral ulceration	- Leucopaenia
Discoid rash	- Lymphopaenia
Photosensitivity	- Haemolytic anaemia
Arthritis	- Thrombocytopaenia
Serositis	Immunological disorder
Neurological disorder	- Anti-ds DNA antibodies
(seizures or psychosis)	- Anti Sm antibodies
Renal disorder	- †Anticardiolipin antibodies or lupus Anticoagulant
(proteinuria >0.5 g/day or cellular casts)	ANA positive

* Patient are required to have four or more criteria to be classified as systemic lupus erythematosus; ANA, antinuclear antibody.

Source data from 1982 American College of Rheumatology Classification Criteria for SLE.

† Revised in 1997 by Hochberg et al. (Tan EM, Cohen AS, Fries JF et al. The 1982 revised criteria for the classification of systemic lupus erythematosus. *Arthritis Rheum* 1982;25:1271–7, Hochberg MC. Updating the American College of Rheumatology revised criteria for the classification of systemic lupus erythematosus. *Arthritis Rheum* 1997;40:1725).

Compared to the 1971 criteria, the final 1982 criteria excluded Raynaud's phenomenon and alopecia and included FANA and anti-dsDNA and anti-Sm antibodies. Overall, the new criteria were 96% sensitive and 96% specific when tested in the systemic lupus erythematosus and control groups collected by the subcommittee. The sensitivity of the 1982 criteria for systemic lupus erythematosus was 83%, and the specificity was 89%, versus 78% and 87%, respectively, for the 1971 criteria.

Significance of the paper

The development of classification criteria to standardize research cohorts is an essential first step when attempting to study any disease. This is especially true in a complex and heterogeneous disease such as lupus. However classification criteria also have to keep up to date with advances in our understanding of disease processes to ensure they remain relevant, while also being applicable to large groups of patients drawn from daily clinical practice. This updated criteria set was the first to include the ANA, which was noted to be highly sensitive in systemic lupus erythematosus.

Of course, the 1982 classification criteria set was itself updated in 1997 to include the presence of anti-phospholipid antibodies [2]. In this update, the positive LE cell preparation criterion was also deleted. More recently the Systemic Lupus International Collaborating Clinics group developed classification criteria in an attempt to incorporate new knowledge into clinically relevant criteria, using updated methodology [3]. This new criteria set includes 17 criteria, and a patient must satisfy at least one clinical criteria and one immunological criteria (as initially proposed in the 1982 criteria), or have biopsy-proven lupus nephritis in the presence of positive immunology (ANA or anti-dsDNA).

The development of such systemic lupus erythematosus criteria sets, that utilize essential immunological criteria, mirrors the recent progress of drug development in systemic lupus erythematosus. For example, recent clinical trials have noted that systemic lupus erythematosus patients with positive antibodies and/or immunological abnormalities at entry appear to respond better than those without, leading to many patients with antibody-negative lupus being excluded from such studies [4, 5]. As always, we must also be aware that classification criteria such as these are meant primarily for clinical research to standardize research cohorts and are not diagnostic criteria for use in patients in daily clinical practice.

References

1 **Cohen AS, Reynolds W, Franklin EC**. Preliminary criteria for the classification of SLE. *Bull Rheum Dis* 1971;**21**:643–5.

2 **Hochberg MC**. Updating the American College of Rheumatology revised criteria for the classification of systemic lupus erythematosus. *Arthritis Rheum* 1997;**40**(9):1725.

3 **Petri M, Orbai AM, Alarcon GS, et al**. Derivation and validation of the Systemic Lupus International Collaborating Clinics classification criteria for systemic lupus erythematosus. *Arthritis Rheum* 2012;**64**(8):2677–86.

4 **Navarra SV, Guzmán RM, Gallacher AE, et al**. Efficacy and safety of belimumab in patients with active systemic lupus erythematosus: a randomised, placebo-controlled, phase 3 trial. *Lancet* 2011;**377**(9767):721–31.

5 **Rovin BH, Furie R, Latinis K, et al**. Efficacy and safety of rituximab in patients with active proliferative lupus nephritis: the Lupus Nephritis Assessment with Rituximab study. *Arthritis Rheum* 2012;**64**(4):1215–26.

Paper 4.7: Interferon implicated in immunopathogenesis of systemic lupus erythematosus

Reference

Hooks JJ, Moutsopoulos HA, Geis SA, et al. Immune interferon in the circulation of patients with autoimmune disease. *N Engl J Med* 1979;301(1):5–8.

Background

Our understanding of the immunopathogenesis of systemic lupus erythematosus has improved greatly over recent decades, and the role of interferon has become increasingly acknowledged. Type 1 interferons (including interferon-α and interferon-β) are produced by all cells in response to infection, particularly viruses, and are involved in the development of autoimmunity. The mechanisms behind this remain unclear; however, the therapeutic use of Type I interferon has been associated with the development of autoimmunity, including systemic lupus erythematosus [1]. Several cytokine and cellular pathways appear to be associated with systemic lupus erythematosus, and clinical studies now frequently test for interferon activity, such as by assaying the 'interferon gene signature', as a surrogate marker for inflammatory disease activity. Novel therapeutics targeting the interferon pathway are also in advanced clinical trial development, and this study by Hooks et al., published in 1979, was the first to describe elevated interferon levels in patients with systemic lupus erythematosus and other connective tissue diseases.

Purpose

To investigate whether interferon might be produced in patients with diseases involving an immune response.

Patients

This study involved 28 patients with systemic lupus erythematosus, 10 patients with rheumatoid arthritis, 10 patients with scleroderma, 15 patients with Sjögren's syndrome, and 47 controls.

Study design

This study investigated the relationship between interferon levels and clinical and serological disease activity (C3 and anti-dsDNA) in patients with lupus.

Results

Overall, interferon levels were higher in autoimmune disease patients than in controls, although elevated levels were not universal. For example, only 46% of systemic lupus erythematosus patients and 60% of scleroderma patients had detectable interferon levels, as compared to just 3% of controls. Interferon was present in 71% of patients with active lupus compared to 21% with inactive lupus, and interferon titres correlated positively with anti-dsDNA titres and negatively with C3 levels. Nine lupus patients were also assessed serially over time but the relationship between interferon levels and clinical and serological disease activity was less clear. No relationship was found between drug treatments and interferon titres.

Commentary

This was the first description of elevated interferon levels in systemic lupus erythematosus cohort and intriguingly this study also described a potential relationship between disease activity and interferon titres. Similar findings were subsequently reported by Ytterberg et al [2]. Measurement of interferon by traditional ELISA is challenging and, more recently, investigations have focused on the genetic signature induced in both peripheral blood mononuclear cells and leucocytes by higher circulating levels of Type I interferon. For example, Bennett et al. demonstrated an upregulation of interferon-induced genes in patients with active systemic lupus erythematosus, and this 'interferon signature' also appears to correlate with disease activity [3]. Interestingly, the interferon signature is abrogated following treatment with high-dose steroids doses in vivo, and subsequent cell culture experiments have shown that anti-interferon-α antibody inhibits the interferon signature in blood cells treated with interferon-α [4].

Abnormalities in both the innate and adaptive immune response are seen in systemic lupus erythematosus, and the immunopathology of the disease remains incompletely understood. However, our increased understanding of the cytokine and signalling pathways, such as those involving interferon-α, in patients with systemic lupus erythematosus has led to the development of targeted biological therapies for active and resistant disease [5].

References

1 **Rönnblom LE, Alm GV, Öberg KE**. Autoimmunity after alpha-interferon therapy for malignant carcinoid tumors. *Ann Intern Med* 1991;**115**(3):178–83.

2 **Ytterberg SR, Schnitzer TJ**. Serum interferon levels in patients with systemic lupus erythematosus. *Arthritis Rheum* 1982;**25**(4):401–6.

3 **Bennett L, Palucka AK, Arce E, et al**. Interferon and granulopoiesis signatures in systemic lupus erythematosus blood. *J Exp Med* 2003;**197**(6):711–23.

4 **Yang WS, Chuang LM**. Human genetics of adiponectin in the metabolic syndrome. *J Mol Med* 2006;**84**(2):112–21.

5 **Petri M, Wallace DJ, Spindler A, et al**. Sifalimumab, a human anti-interferon-alpha monoclonal antibody, in systemic lupus erythematosus: a phase I randomized, controlled, dose-escalation study. *Arthritis Rheum* 2013;**65**(4):1011–21.

Paper 4.8: Successful clinical trials of belimumab in systemic lupus erythematosus

Reference

Navarra SV, Guzmán RM, Gallacher AE, et al. Efficacy and safety of belimumab in patients with active systemic lupus erythematosus: a randomised, placebo-controlled, phase 3 trial. *Lancet* 2011;377(9767):721–31.

Background

The advent of the biological area in rheumatoid arthritis transformed the care and management of this disease and has led to a proliferation of targeted biological therapies. For decades, systemic lupus erythematosus was managed with an unlicensed and narrow therapeutic armamentarium, despite advances in our knowledge of the underlying pathogenic mechanisms involved in the disease. Shortly before this landmark study describing the efficacy of belimumab in systemic lupus erythematosus was published, rituximab had (to many rheumatologists) surprisingly failed its clinical trial programme in lupus and lupus nephritis, despite promising open-label studies. The BLISS clinical trial programme therefore changed the landscape of clinical trials and treatment of systemic lupus erythematosus and became the first drug to be approved and licensed for use in systemic lupus erythematosus in more than half a century.

Purpose

To describe the effectiveness of belimumab in systemic lupus erythematosus.

Patients

The BLISS-52 study was performed in Latin America, Asia, and Eastern Europe and recruited 867 patients with active systemic lupus erythematosus into a randomized clinical trial of belimumab and standard care versus placebo and standard care. A similar clinical trial (BLISS-76) was run concurrently in Europe and North America and published later the same year [1]. Only patients with serologically and clinically active disease were included in the clinical trial.

Study design

This study involved a randomized, double-blind, placebo-controlled Phase 3 trial.

Treatment

Patients were randomized in a 1:1:1 ratio to belimumab 1 mg/kg, belimumab 10 mg/kg, or placebo; treatment was administered by intravenous infusion over 1 h given on days 0, 14, and 28, and then every 28 days until 48 weeks, with standard of care.

Study end points measured

Response to treatment was assessed using the Systemic Lupus Erythematosus Responder Index (SRI), a combination of SELENA-SLEDAI, BILAG, and physician global assessment score. The SRI was the primary outcome assessed at week 52.

Follow-up

Follow-up was at 52 weeks.

Results

Overall, significantly higher response rates were seen in patients receiving belimumab at week 52 (at both 1 mg/kg and 10 mg/kg) than in those receiving the placebo (51%, 58%, and 44%, respectively), and more patients receiving belimumab had no new severe disease flare (BILAG A) than those in placebo group (78%, 81%, and 73%, respectively). A number of other secondary outcomes were also met, including improvement in complement levels, reduction in anti-dsDNA titres, and lower steroid doses in the belimumab treatment arms compared to placebo. Similar response rates were observed in the BLISS-76 trial programme [1].

Significance of the paper

B-lymphocyte stimulator (BLyS), also known as BAFF (B-cell activating factor), is a transmembrane protein expressed on monocytes, macrophages, and dendritic cells and its levels are regulated by cytokines, in particular interferon [2]. Activation of the BLyS receptors leads to B-cell and plasma cell proliferation, differentiation, and survival and to IgG class switching [3]. The importance of BLyS in the immunopathogenesis of systemic lupus erythematosus was demonstrated initially in animal studies [4]. Human clinical studies reveal that 20%–40% of patients have significantly elevated levels of circulating BLyS, and plasma BLyS protein levels appear to correlate with disease activity [5, 6]. However, belimumab does not deplete peripheral B-cells (unlike rituximab) but instead appears to reduce their ability to proliferate and differentiate into mature B-cells, although the exact mode of action is incompletely understood.

The BLISS clinical trials programme successfully achieved its primary outcome in 2 pivotal phase 3 trials involving almost 1,700 patients from across the globe. Unlike previous studies, these trials required patients to have both moderate–severe active systemic lupus erythematosus (SLEDAI >6) and positive serology at study entry and restricted the use of concurrent therapies (including steroids) after 16 weeks. The trials also used an innovative composite response index (SRI) based on secondary analyses of earlier Phase 2 clinical trials [7]. Secondary analyses of the study programme also confirmed that patients with higher disease activity, serologically active disease, or those using steroids responded better to belimumab [8].

The changes in clinical trial design, combined with the large study population from multiple centres across the globe, led to a successful clinical trials programme in systemic lupus erythematosus and have set the standard for how future clinical trials in lupus are conducted.

References

1 **Furie R, Petri M, Zamani O, et al**. A phase III, randomized, placebo-controlled study of belimumab, a monoclonal antibody that inhibits B lymphocyte stimulator, in patients with systemic lupus erythematosus. *Arthritis Rheum* 2011;**63**(12):3918–30.

2 Nardelli B, Belvedere O, Roschke V, et al. Synthesis and release of B-lymphocyte stimulator from myeloid cells. *Blood* 2001;**97**(1):198–204.

3 Moore PA, Belvedere O, Orr A, et al. BLyS: member of the tumor necrosis factor family and B lymphocyte stimulator. *Science* 1999;**285**(5425):260–3.

4 Jacob CO, Pricop L, Putterman C, et al. Paucity of clinical disease despite serological autoimmunity and kidney pathology in lupus-prone New Zealand mixed 2328 mice deficient in BAFF. *J Immunol* 2006;**177**(4):2671–80.

5 Cheema GS, Roschke V, Hilbert DM, et al. Elevated serum B lymphocyte stimulator levels in patients with systemic immune-based rheumatic diseases. *Arthritis Rheum* 2001;**44**(6):1313–9.

6 Petri M, Stohl W, Chatham W, et al. Association of plasma B lymphocyte stimulator levels and disease activity in systemic lupus erythematosus. *Arthritis Rheum* 2008;**58**(8):2453–9.

7 Wallace DJ, Stohl W, Furie RA, et al. A phase II, randomized, double-blind, placebo-controlled, dose-ranging study of belimumab in patients with active systemic lupus erythematosus. *Arthritis Rheum* 2009;**61**(9):1168–78.

8 Van Vollenhoven RF, Petri MA, Cervera R, et al. Belimumab in the treatment of systemic lupus erythematosus: high disease activity predictors of response. *Ann Rheum Dis* 2012;**71**(8):1343–9.

Paper 4.9: The first description of the association between the lupus anticoagulant and thrombosis in systemic lupus erythematosus

Reference

Boey ML, Colaco CB, Gharavi AE, et al. Thrombosis in systemic lupus erythematosus: striking association with the presence of circulating lupus anticoagulant. *Br Med J* 1983;287(6398):1021–3.

Background

The association between a biological false test for syphilis with the lupus anticoagulant (LAC) had been known since the 1950s and reports of an association with a hypercoagulable state had been made in 1980 [1, 2]. The authors of this study, reported the association between the LAC and clinical and serological features of patients with systemic lupus erythematosus and related connective tissue diseases. The research group also published shortly afterwards a study describing the development of a radioimmunoassay for the detection of anti-cardiolipin antibodies, and their correlation with clinical thrombotic events in a cohort of patients with systemic lupus erythematosus [3].

Purpose

To describe the association between thrombosis and systemic lupus erythematosus.

Patients

The authors assembled a cohort of 49 patients with systemic lupus erythematosus, and 11 patients with related disorders (such as vasculitis and systemic sclerosis); the patients had a mean age of 32.7 years and a mean symptom duration of 5.4 years. Each patient provided a clinical history of their connective tissue disease and any thrombotic events they had suffered.

Methods

The LAC was tested using a modified mixing partial thromboplastin time with kaolin.

Results

Overall, 31/60 patients had a positive LAC; of these, 25 had systemic lupus erythematosus, although no significant association was noted between the presence of LAC and autoantibodies. However, thrombotic episodes (venous and arterial thromboses) were significantly more numerous in those patients with a positive LAC compared to those without in all patients (18/31 vs 3/29, P < 0.01). Similarly, thrombocytopenia was more frequent in LAC positive patients (9/31 vs 1/29). Although previous miscarriages were more numerous in women with the LAC than those without, this relationship was not statistically different (9/26 vs 5/27). The authors discuss that thrombosis is a common complication of systemic lupus erythematosus and that the LAC could be a useful marker for a subset of patients at risk for thromboembolic complications.

Significance of the paper

Together with the study by the same group describing the detection of anti-cardiolipin antibodies in systemic lupus erythematosus and their association with systemic lupus erythematosus [3], this landmark paper confirmed the association between systemic lupus erythematosus and thrombosis and introduced the entity that became recognised as the anti-phospholipid syndrome (APS). Although the relationship was not clear in this study, the link between systemic lupus erythematosus and pregnancy morbidity was also increasingly recognized and rapidly became part of the developing syndrome. Additionally, it became apparent that the phenomenon was also observed in patients without other autoimmune disease and this was termed 'primary APS' [4].

The subsequent discovery that anti-cardiolipin antibodies are directed against a phospholipid-binding protein rather than against a phospholipid led to the discovery that some autoantibodies bind directly to β_2-glycoprotein I in the absence of phospholipids and the development of assays to detect anti- β_2-glycoprotein I [5]. The first international consensus definition of the APS was reached in 1999 [6], and was updated in 2006 (Table 4.2) [7]. APS is now recognized as a major clinical problem in patients with the full

Table 4.2 Revised Sapporo criteria for anti-phospholipid syndrome

Clinical	Laboratory
Vascular thrombosis: one or more episodes of venous, arterial, or small vessel thrombosis, with unequivocal imaging or histologic evidence of thrombosis in any tissue or organ. Pregnancy morbidity: otherwise unexplained foetal death at ≥10 weeks gestation of a morphologically normal foetus, OR one or more premature births before 34 weeks of gestation due to eclampsia, preeclampsia, or placental insufficiency, OR three or more embryonic (<10 weeks gestation) unexplained pregnancy losses.	The presence of antiphospholipid antibodies on two or more occasions at least 12 weeks apart and no more than five years prior to clinical manifestations: i.e. IgG and/or IgM anti-cardiolipin antibodies in moderate/high titre, OR antibodies to β2-glycoprotein I (IgG or IgM) at >99th percentile for the testing laboratory, OR lupus anticoagulant.

Definite anti-phospholipid syndrome occurs if at least one clinical criteria *and* at least one laboratory criterion are satisfied.

Source data from Miyakis S, Lockshin MD, Atsumi T, et al. International consensus statement on an update of the classification criteria for definite antiphospholipid syndrome (APS). *J Thromb Haemost* 2006;4:295–306.

spectrum of autoimmune rheumatic diseases including systemic lupus erythematosus. Its recognition is of course of pivotal importance in patient management as it points to manifestations that require anti-thrombotic medications rather than more immunosuppression. Beyond rheumatology and haematology, APS is also of relevance to all branches of medicine including obstetrics, neurology, respiratory medicine, and dermatology, to name but a few. There is no doubt that recognition of this syndrome has markedly improved patient outcomes over the past 30 years.

References

1 **Laurell AB, Nilsson IM**. Hypergammaglobulinemia, circulating anticoagulant, and biologic false positive Wassermann reaction; a study in two cases. *J Lab Clin Med* 1957;**49**(5):694–707.

2 **Mueh JR, Herbst KD, Rapaport SI**. Thrombosis in patients with the lupus anticoagulant. *Ann Intern Med* 1980;**92**(2):156–9.

3 **Harris EN, Gharavi AE, Boey ML, et al**. Anticardiolipin antibodies: detection by radioimmunoassay and association with thrombosis in systemic lupus erythematosus. *Lancet* 1983;**2**(8361):1211–14.

4 **Asherson RA, Khamashta MA, Ordi-Ros J, et al**. The 'primary' antiphospholipid syndrome: major clinical and serological features. *Medicine (Baltimore)* 1989;**68**(6):366–74.

5 **Galli M, Comfurius P, Maassen C, et al**. Anticardiolipin antibodies (ACA) directed not to cardiolipin but to a plasma protein cofactor. *Lancet* 1990;**335**(8705):1544–7.

6 **Wilson WA, Gharavi AE, Koike T, et al**. International consensus statement on preliminary classification criteria for definite antiphospholipid syndrome: report of an international workshop. *Arthritis Rheum* 1999;**42**(7):1309–11.

7 **Miyakis S, Lockshin MD, Atsumi T, et al**. International consensus statement on an update of the classification criteria for definite antiphospholipid syndrome (APS). *J Thromb Haemost* 2006;**4**(2):295–306.

Paper 4.10: The impact of withdrawal of hydroxychloroquine in stable systemic lupus erythematosus

Reference

The Canadian Hydroxychloroquine Study Group. A randomised study of the effect of withdrawing hydroxychloroquine in systemic lupus erythematosus. *N Engl J Med* 1991;324(3):150–4.

Background

Antimalarial therapies such as hydroxychloroquine and chloroquine are commonly recommended for patients with mild–moderate systemic lupus erythematosus, especially those with cutaneous and musculoskeletal features. Antimalarial therapies may also be steroid sparing and thereby permit the use of lower doses of corticosteroids over time, as well as having a multitude of additional benefits in the lupus patient. These therapies are generally considered to be safe and well tolerated by patients but the small risk of retinal toxicity can lead to a reluctance to prescribe these medicines in the longer term. The lack of experimental clinical trial evidence to inform prescribing of antimalarial therapies, a cornerstone of many patients' treatment regimens, had meant that physicians were unsure whether or not it was safe to withdraw these drugs. The Canadian Hydroxychloroquine Study Group therefore developed an innovative approach to inform the clinician's decision to withdraw hydroxychloroquine in patients with stable systemic lupus erythematosus.

Purpose

To determine the effectiveness of hydroxychloroquine in systemic lupus erythematosus.

Patients

The study examined patients with stable systemic lupus erythematosus.

Study design

This report describes a randomized, placebo-controlled, double-blind, multicentre study of the effect of withdrawing hydroxychloroquine therapy in patients with stable systemic lupus erythematosus.

Treatment

Hydroxychloroquine therapy was withdrawn in a randomized fashion.

Study end points

The primary outcome measure was time to develop a clinical flare of systemic lupus erythematosus, with secondary outcomes including changing prednisolone dose and frequency of severe exacerbations. Assessments were performed at monthly intervals for six months.

Follow-up

Follow-up was performed at 24 weeks.

Results

Overall, 25 patients were assigned to continue hydroxychloroquine, and 22 were assigned to receive placebo. The cohorts were well matched for age (mean age, 45 years vs 44 years) and disease duration (mean 94 months vs 83 months), and no significant differences between the groups in terms of steroid dose hydroxychloroquine dose or disease activity were noted.

A clinical flair of symptoms occurred in 16/22 (73%) patients assigned placebo and 9/25 (36%) assigned hydroxychloroquine, with a relative risk of flare after withdrawing hydroxychloroquine of 2.5 (CI 1.08, 5.58) as compared to continuing treatment. Severe exacerbations of lupus were also numerically more common in the withdrawal arm than in the ongoing treatment arm (5/22 vs 1/25) with a non-significant relative risk of 6.1% (95% CI, 0.72–52.4). No significant differences in steroid dose were noted between the study groups; however, the small sample size may have limited the ability of the study to detect significant differences in the secondary outcomes. Overall, the authors concluded that patients with quiescent lupus were less likely to flare if they continued their hydroxychloroquine.

Significance of the paper

Hydroxychloroquine is commonly prescribed in many patients with systemic lupus erythematosus, particularly in those with cutaneous and musculoskeletal disease but also in combination with other immunosuppressive agents in more severe disease. In addition to its anti-inflammatory properties, hydroxychloroquine has been to shown to have a multitude of other potential benefits in lupus that have led to its central role in therapeutic regimens in systemic lupus erythematosus [1]. For example, studies have shown a beneficial effect of antimalarial therapy on lipid profiles, and the use of antimalarials has been associated with reduced damage accrual overall in systemic lupus erythematosus [2–4]. Hydroxychloroquine also has apparent anti-thrombotic properties and beneficial metabolic effects and is therefore considered by many to confer a protective effect against the development of atherosclerosis in systemic lupus erythematosus [5, 6]. For these reasons, many clinicians are reluctant to withdraw hydroxychloroquine, even in long-term stable patients, an approach supported by the results of this study. However, many of the additional benefits of antimalarial therapies have not been tested in randomized clinical trials and there remains a need to better understand the role of longer-term antimalarial therapy in patients with systemic lupus erythematosus.

References

1 **Ruiz-Irastorza G1, Ramos-Casals M, Brito-Zeron P, et al**. Clinical efficacy and side effects of antimalarials in systemic lupus erythematosus: a systematic review. *Ann Rheum Dis* 2010;**69**(1):20–8.

2 **Petri M, Lakatta C, Magder L, et al**. Effect of prednisone and hydroxychloroquine on coronary artery disease risk factors in systemic lupus erythematosus: a longitudinal data analysis. *Am J Med* 1994;**96**(3):254–9.

3 **Cairoli E, Rebella M, Danese N, et al**. Hydroxychloroquine reduces low-density lipoprotein cholesterol levels in systemic lupus erythematosus: a longitudinal evaluation of the lipid-lowering effect. *Lupus* 2012;**21**(11):1178–82.

4 **Fessler BJ, Alarcon GS, McGwin G Jr, et al**. Systemic lupus erythematosus in three ethnic groups: XVI. Association of hydroxychloroquine use with reduced risk of damage accrual. *Arthritis Rheum* 2005;**52**(5):1473–80.

5 **Ho KT, Ahn CW, Alarcon GS, et al**. Systemic lupus erythematosus in a multiethnic cohort (LUMINA): XXVIII. Factors predictive of thrombotic events. *Rheumatology* 2005;**44**(10):1303–7.

6 **Parker, B, Urowitz MB, Gladman DD, et al**. Impact of early disease factors on metabolic syndrome in systemic lupus erythematosus: data from an international inception cohort. *Ann Rheum Dis* 2014 Apr 1. doi: 10.1136/annrheumdis-2013-203933. [Epub ahead of print].

Chapter 5

Vasculitis

Haroon Khan, David G. I. Scott, and Richard A. Watts

Introduction

The initial description of one of the conditions that we now recognize as the systemic vasculitides was by Heberden in the eighteenth century followed by Schönlein, Henoch, and Kussmaul, and Meier in the nineteenth century [1]. William Heberden described two children with IgA vasculitis (Henoch Schönlein purpura). The first generally recognized case of systemic vasculitis was described by Kussmaul and Meier in 1866 and was called periarteritis nodosa [2]. They described a patient with a systemic illness characterized by numerous palpable nodules along the course of small muscular arteries. During the twentieth century, a number of other entities were described, including granulomatosis with polyangiitis (Wegener's granulomatosis) (7), eosinophilic granulomatosis with poly-angiitis (Churg–Strauss syndrome) (8), and microscopic polyangiitis. Initially, these were descriptions without much idea of aetiopathogenesis and therefore the definition and classification was the matter of much debate. Most classification systems are based on a division by vessel size—large, medium, and small, a notion introduced by Zeek [3]. The two major developments were the elaboration of the American College of Rheumatology criteria for the classification of the seven types of vasculitis in 1990 and the Chapel Hill Consensus Conference in 1994, which provided clear definitions for each condition [4, 5]. The latter have been recently updated [6].

The pathogenesis of certain types of vasculitis has also advanced significantly with the recognition of the relationship between hepatitis B infection and polyarteritis nodosa, the role of IgA in Henoch–Schönlein purpura (now known as IgA vasculitis), and the presence of anti-neutrophil cytoplasmic antibodies in granulomatosis with polyangiitis, microscopic polyangiitis, and eosinophilic granulomatosis with polyangiitis (Churg–Strauss syndrome). The latter has led to these conditions being recognized as a specific group—anti-neutrophil cytoplasmic antibodies-associated vasculitis (AAV)—within the revised Chapel Hill Consensus Conference nomenclature.

The treatment of the vasculitides has evolved rapidly, initially following the discovery of the potent anti-inflammatory effects of glucocorticoids by Hench and colleagues at the Mayo Clinic during the 1940s [9]. Oral prednisolone significantly reduces the risk of blindness in giant cell arteritis and was responsible for the first improvements in mortality in other vasculitides [10, 11]. Mortality was subsequently further improved by Fauci with introduction of the alkylating agent cyclophosphamide [12], which laid the basis for the European series of randomized controlled trials in AAV and the modern approach to treatment of AAV. During the last decade, targeted therapies using rituximab to deplete B-cells have been introduced to treat AAV, following the results of two large trials, and are used on an empirical basis in many other types of vasculitis.

We have selected ten papers which illustrate these seminal developments in the field of vasculitis and present them within their context.

References

1 **Matteson EL**. Notes on the history of eponymic idiopathic vasculitis: the diseases of Henoch and Schönlein, Wegener, Churg and Strauss, Horton, Takayasu, Behçet, and Kawasaki. *Arthritis Care Res* 2000;**13**(4):237–45.

2 **Kussmaul A, Meier R**. Über eine nicht bisher beschriebene eigenthümliche Arterienerkrankung (Periarteritis nodosa), die mit Morbus Brightii und rapid fortschreitender allgemeiner Muskelahmung einhergeht. *Dtsch Arch Klin Med* 1866;**1**:484–518.

3 **Zeek PM**. Periarteritis nodosa; a critical review. *Am J Clin Pathol* 1952;**22**(8):777–90.

4 **Hunder GG, Arend WP, Bloch DA, et al**. The American College of Rheumatology 1990 criteria for the classification of vasculitis. Introduction. *Arthritis Rheum* 1990;**33**(8):1065–7.

5 **Jennette JC, Falk RJ, Andrassy K, et al**. Nomenclature of systemic vasculitides. Proposal of an international consensus conference. *Arthritis Rheum* 1994;**37**(2):187–92.

6 **Jennette J, Falk R, Bacon P, et al**. 2012 Revised International Chapel Hill Consensus Conference Nomenclature of Vasculitides. *Arthritis Rheum* 2013;**65**(1):1–11.

7 **Wegener F**. Über generalisierte, septische Gefässer- krankungen. *Verh Dtsch Ges Pathol* 1936;**29**:202–10.

8 **Churg J, Strauss L**. Allergic granulomatosis, allergic angiitis, and periarteritis nodosa. *Am J Pathol* 1951;**27**(2):277–301.

9 **Hench PS, Slocumb CH**. The effects of the adrenal cortical hormone 17-hydroxy-11-dehydrocorticosterone (Compound E) on the acute phase of rheumatic fever; preliminary report. *Proc Staff Meet Mayo Clin* 1949;**24**(11):277–97.

10 **Bennett G**. Cortisone therapy of visual loss in temporal arteritis. *Brit J Ophthalmol* 1956;**40**(7):430–3.

11 **Frohnert PP, Sheps SG**. Long-term follow-up study of periarteritis nodosa. *Am J Med* 1967;**43**(1):8–14.

12 **Fauci A, Wolff S**. Wegeners granulomatosis: studies in 18 patients and a review of the literature. *Medicine* 1973;**52**:535–61.

Paper 5.1: Earliest description of systemic vasculitis

Reference

Kussmaul A, Meier R. Über eine nicht bisher beschriebene eigenthümliche Arterienerkrankung (Periarteritis nodosa), die mit Morbus Brightii und rapid fortschreitender allgemeiner Muskelahmung einhergeht. *Dtsch Arch Klin Med* 1866;1:484–518.

Translation: Matteson EL. Polyarteritis nodosa: commemorative translation on the 130-year anniversary of the original article by Adolf Kussmaul and Rudolf Meier. Rochester, MN: Mayo Press; 1996.

Purpose

To describe a new form of arterial disease.

Study design

This work comprises a single case report.

Follow-up

The study covers the five weeks prior to the patient's death.

Results

This report comprises a detailed description of the case of Carl Seufarth, a 27-year-old tailor's journeyman who presented with severe malaise, muscle wasting, and nephritis, together with a description of his course in hospital over the five-week period prior to his death. At the post-mortem examination, there was nodular thickening of arteries smaller than the hepatic artery, including the coronary artery, the mesenteric artery, the bronchial artery, and the phrenic artery (Figure 5.1). Kussmaul termed this syndrome 'periarteritis nodosa'.

Significance and importance

This case is generally accepted to be the first detailed clinical description of a systemic vasculitis. Kussmaul termed the case periarteritis nodosa on the basis of the pathological appearance of the arteries.

  Conditions that we now recognize as vasculitis had been previously described, for example, by William Heberden in 1802, and by Eduard Henoch and Johann Schönlein in the mid-nineteenth century [1]. This was the first detailed clinico-pathological description of a medium-vessel vasculitis. The condition subsequently became known as polyarteritis nodosa, a term which by the mid-twentieth century was used to encompass most types of systemic vasculitis. In 1948, Davson et al. described a variant which they called microscopic polyarteritis, which was subsequently called MPA, recognizing that vasculitis could involve smaller vessels and was only observable using microscopy [2]. Other forms of systemic vasculitis were gradually recognized, including Wegener's granulomatosis, which

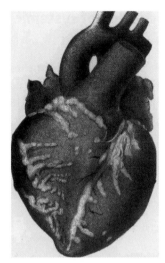

Fig. 5.1 Macroscopic appearance of the heart showing nodular aneurysms on the coronary arteries. From Matteson EL. Polyarteritis nodosa: Commemorative translation on the 130-year anniversary of the original article by Adolf Kussmaul and Rudolf Meier. Mayo Press 1996. Rochester, MN, USA.

was first described in the 1930s, and Churg–Strauss syndrome, which was first described in the 1950s [3, 4]. These two conditions gradually became more clearly delineated from polyarteritis nodosa. Following the first Chapel Hill Consensus Conference in 1994 (vide infra) [5], it was recognized that polyarteritis nodosa was a very uncommon form of vasculitis and was defined as a distinct type of vasculitis. Classification criteria were produced by the American College of Rheumatology in 1990 [6], and more recently by Henegar [6]; the later also noted that polyarteritis nodosa was not associated with the presence of antineutrophil cytoplasmic antibodies. Polyarteritis nodosa was also the first type of vasculitis for which a specific cause was identified, namely, infection with hepatitis B.

References

1 **Matteson EL**. Notes on the history of eponymic idiopathic vasculitis: the diseases of Henoch and Schönlein, Wegener, Churg and Strauss, Horton, Takayasu, Behçet, and Kawasaki. *Arthritis Care Res* 2000;**13**(4):237–45.

2 **Davson J, Ball J, Platt R**. The kidney in periarteritis nodosa. *QJM* 1948;**17**(3):175–202.

3 **Wegener F**. Über generalisierte, septische Gefässerkrankungen. *Verh Dtsch Ges Pathol* 1936;**29**:202–10.

4 **Churg J, Strauss L**. Allergic granulomatosis, allergic angiitis, and periarteritis nodosa. *Am J Pathol* 1951;**27**(2):277–301.

5 **Jennette JC, Falk RJ, Andrassy K, et al**. Nomenclature of systemic vasculitides. *Arthritis Rheum* 1994;**37**(2):187–92.

6 **Henegar C, Pagnoux C, Puéchal X, et al**. A paradigm of diagnostic criteria for polyarteritis nodosa: analysis of a series of 949 patients with vasculitides. *Arthritis Rheum* 2008;**58**(5):1528–38.

Paper 5.2: Pathology of giant cell arteritis

Reference

Horton BT, Magath TB, Brown GE. Undescribed form of arteritis of temporal vessels. *Proc Staff Meet Mayo Clin* 1932;7:700–1.

Purpose

Description of patients with a previously undescribed type of arteritis affecting the temporal vessels.

Patients

Seven patients presenting with tender areas over the scalp and temporal arteries, headaches, malaise, fevers, and weight loss were described.

Study design

This article reports a case series describing the clinical and pathological features of temporal arteritis.

Results

The cases of seven patients, presenting to the Mayo Clinic between 1931 and 1937 with classical symptoms of giant cell arteritis (temporal arteritis) were described. All patients shared the common symptoms of temporal headaches, malaise, fevers, and weight loss and had tender areas over the scalp and temporal arteries; these areas later on became nodular (Figure 5.2). The average duration of these symptoms was 4–6 weeks; four of the patients

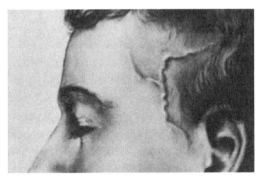

Fig. 5.2 Artist's sketch of the enlarged temporal artery of Horton's first patient with temporal arteritis. From Horton BT. Temporal arteritis: a focal localization of a systemic disease. AMA Scientific Exhibits 1955. Boes CJ. Bayard Horton's clinicopathological description of giant cell (temporal) arteritis. *Cephalalgia* 2007;27:68–75 London. ISSN 0333-©-1024. CJ Boes, Bayard Horton's Clinicopathological Description of Giant Cell (Temporal) Arteritis, Cephalalgia (Vol 27, No 1), copyright © 2007
Reprinted by Permission of SAGE.

were female, the mean age was 67.5 years, and all the patients were white. Five of the seven had temporal artery biopsies performed which showed identical pathologic changes. The course of the disease ran from 4 to 6 months, with patients often confined to bed. However, the illness was not fatal; although some of the patients relapsed, they all eventually made a complete recovery. Interestingly there was no mention of ophthalmic complications of the condition. The treatment was largely symptomatic.

On biopsy, it was noted that the temporal artery was thrombosed. There was necrosis and destruction of the media, together with granulomatous lesions with giant cells and intimal thickening. Nodular areas were present but aneurysms such those seen in polyarteritis nodosa were specifically noted to be absent.

Critique of the paper

This paper is a careful pathological study of a previously unknown condition in which the key clinical and pathological features of giant cell arteritis are well described in a series of seven patients.

Significance and importance

This paper was the first description of giant cell arteritis and distinguished it from other types of vasculitis such as poly- (peri-)arteritis nodosa. The original term temporal arteritis has gradually been replaced by the term giant cell arteritis to reflect the presence of giant cells within inflamed artery as well as occurrence of the disease in large vessels other than the temporal arteries. The ease with which the temporal artery could be biopsied (and this was noted in the paper) led to this rapidly becoming a widely used diagnostic procedure and the recognition that giant cell arteritis is one of the more common forms of systemic vasculitis [1]. Epidemiological studies from the same hospital have noted the marked age tropism, with a peak age of incidence in those aged >70 years; the original seven patients had a mean age of 67.5 years [2].

Subsequent pathology studies confirmed the appearance and also demonstrated at post-mortem that there was widespread involvement of large arteries often clinically undetectable [3]. However, the development of modern imaging techniques, including ^{18}FDG-PET/CT, has clearly demonstrated the widespread nature of arterial inflammation in this condition [4], and the technique is now being used for diagnosis.

The authors, however, believed that a positive diagnosis could always be made on temporal artery biopsy. It is now widely recognized that the arterial lesions in giant cell arteritis are not continuous and therefore inflamed segments of artery may not be observed if the biopsy taken is too short or an insufficient number of sections are examined.

The common occurrence of visual loss in giant cell arteritis was rapidly realized, although not noted by Horton in this paper. In 1938, Jennings recognized blindness as a complication of giant cell arteritis [5], and in 1941 Gilmour recognized the possible systemic onset [6]. Paulley and Hughes in 1960 finally made the clear link between giant cell arteritis and polymyalgia rheumatica as well as describing the various patterns of disease onset [7].

References

1 **MacDonald JA, Moser RH**. Periarteritis and arteritis of the temporal vessels; a case report. *Ann Int Med* 1937;**10**(11);1721–6.

2 **Salvarani C, Crowson CS, O'Fallon WM, et al**. Reappraisal of the epidemiology of giant cell arteritis in Olmsted County, Minnesota, over a 50 year period. *Arthritis Rheum* 2004;**51**(2):264–8.

3 **Cooke WT, Cloake PC**. Temporal arteritis; a generalized vascular disease. *QJM* 1946;**15**(57):47–75.

4 **Prieto-González S, Depetris M, García-Martínez A, et al**. Positron emission tomography assessment of large vessel inflammation in patients with newly diagnosed, biopsy-proven giant cell arteritis: a prospective, case-control study. *Ann Rheum Dis* 2014;**73**(7):1388–92.

5 **Jennings GH**. Arteritis of temporal vessels. *Lancet* 1938;**1**(5973):424–8.

6 **Gilmour JR**. Giant-cell chronic arteritis. *J Pathol Bacteriol* 1941;**53**(2):263–77.

7 **Paulley JW, Hughes JP**. Giant-cell arteritis, or arteritis of the aged. *BMJ* 1960;**2**(5212):1562–7.

Paper 5.3: Original description of Kawasaki disease

Reference

Kawasaki T, Kosaki F, Okawa S, et al. A new infantile acute febrile mucocutaneous lymph node syndrome (MLNS) prevailing in Japan. *Pediatrics* 1974;54(3):271–6.

Purpose

To describe a new acute febrile mucocutaneous lymph node syndrome occurring in Japan.

Patients

This report describes cases of mucocutaneous lymph node syndrome seen at a single centre in Japan between 1961 and 1972 and contains the results of a nationwide questionnaire survey of all paediatric units in Japan conducted in 1971.

Study

This report describes an observational and a questionnaire study.

Results

The single-centre observational study reported on 168 cases; four of these died during the acute illness, and post-mortem examination showed a 'periarteritis nodosa-like' arteritis located in the coronary artery and accompanied by thrombosis and aneurysm formation. The principal symptoms were noted to be fever lasting 1–2 weeks, bilateral conjunctival congestion, erythema of the mucous membranes and mouth, swelling of the tongue, and cervical lymphadenopathy (Figure 5.3) During the third to the fifth days of the illness, a macular eruption developed in the palms and soles and desquamated during the second week (Table 5.1).

In the observational study the authors noted that most patients were aged <5 years and approximately half were aged <2 years. The prognosis was usually good, but 1%–2% died suddenly due to coronary thrombosis.

Questionnaire survey

Two national surveys were conducted in 1971 and 1973, with response rates of 43% and 57%, respectively. A total of 3,265 cases were identified, with a mortality rate of 1.7%.

Thirteen post-mortems were conducted which showed coronary artery thrombosis and aneurysm formation.

Critique of the paper

This is an observational single-centre description of a large number of cases of KD, combined with a nationwide survey of paediatric units in Japan. The clinical features are well described, including the important cardiac outcomes. The frequency of coronary artery involvement is underestimated, primarily because echocardiography was in its infancy at the time and not widely practised. Relatively little long-term outcome data are presented.

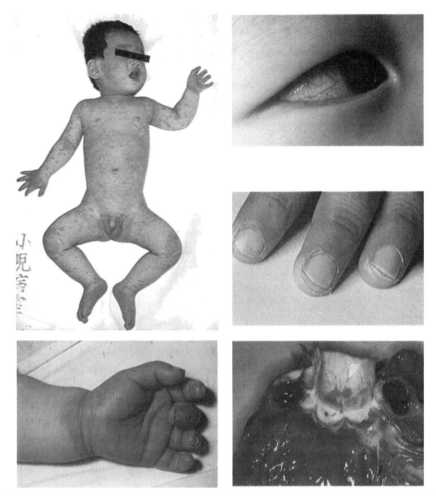

Fig. 5.3 A. Typical exanthema of mucocutaneous lymph node syndrome in a 10-month-old male infant on the fourth day of illness. B. Congestion of ocular conjunctiva in an 8-month-old female infant on the fifth day of illness. C. Desquamation at fingertips in an 18-month-old infant on the fourteenth day of illness. D. Erythema and indurative oedema of the palm in an 11-month-old infant on the fourth day of illness. E. Thrombosis and aneurysm of bilateral coronary arteries at autopsy in a 9-month-old male infant who suddenly died from mucocutaneous lymph node syndrome on the fifty-ninth day.

Investigations as to causation were not performed in a systematic fashion and the suggestion of rickettsia infection has not been subsequently borne out.

Significance and importance

Although the features of KD had been reported by Kawasaki in 1967, this paper was not widely known, as it was not translated from Japanese [1]. This paper was the first in English to describe a large series of patients with mucocutaneous lymph node syndrome, now

Table 5.1 Features of Kawasaki disease

Feature	%
Fever	95
Congestion of conjunctivae	88
Dryness, redness of lips	90
Protuberance of tongue papillae	77
Redness of oral mucosa	90
Reddening palms and soles	88
Indurative oedema	76
Desquamation form finger tips	94
Polymorphous exanthema of body trunk	92
Swelling of cervical lymph nodes	75

Source data from Kawasaki T, Kosaki F, Okawa S, Shigematsu I, Yanagawa H. A new infantile acute febrile mucocutaneous lymph node syndrome (MLNS) prevailing in Japan. *Pediatrics*. 1974;54:271–6.

commonly known by its eponym Kawasaki disease, and its significance was immediately recognized [2]. Mucocutaneous lymph node syndrome has now been recognized in most populations across the world but with pronounced geographical variations in the incidence of KD [3]. KD is most common in the far East, especially in Japan, Korea, and China, and is relatively uncommon in white Caucasian populations in the United States and Europe. The highest incidence rates come from Japan. The key observation, that it is a disease of infancy with most cases occurring in children aged <5 years, was noted in this paper and has been seen in all populations.

This early paper clearly recognizes the importance of coronary involvement. In 1973, Kato performed coronary angiography on 20 children after resolution of symptoms, demonstrating that multiple aneurysms were present in both the right and left coronary arteries, and showed for the first time that aneurysms were present in survivors as well as fatal cases [4]. The development of coronary aneurysms has been extensively investigated subsequently using echocardiography, and two-dimensional echocardiography is now routine in the assessment of KD.

The inefficacy of antibiotics was noted by Kawasaki, together with the possible beneficial effects of glucocorticoids. Intravenous immunoglobulin combined with aspirin has been shown to be effective in reducing the rate of coronary artery aneurysms from 25% to 5% and is now the main therapeutic approach [5].

References

1 **Kawasaki T.** [Acute febrile mucocutaneous syndrome with lymphoid involvement with specific desquamation of the fingers and toes in children]. *Arerugi* 1967;**16**(3):178–222.

2 **Fetterman GH, Hashida Y.** Mucocutaneous lymph node syndrome (MLNS): a disease widespread in Japan, which demands our attention. *Pediatrics* 1974;**54**(3):268–70.

3 **Uehara R, Belay R**. Epidemiology of Kawasaki disease in Asia, Europe, and the United States. *J Epidemiol* 2012;**22**(2):79–85.

4 **Kato H, Kpoike S, Yamamoto M, et al**. Coronary aneurysms in infants and young children with acute febrile mucocutaneous lymph node syndrome. *J Pediatr* 1975;**86**(6);892–8.

5 **Newburger JW, Takahashi M, Gerber MA, et al**. Diagnosis treatment, and long term management of Kawasaki disease: a statement from health professionals from the committee on rheumatic fever, endocarditis and Kawasaki disease, Council on Cardiovascular Disease in the Young, American Heart Association. *Circulation* 2004;**110**(17):2747–71.

Paper 5.4: Relationship between infection with hepatitis B virus and polyarteritis nodosa

Reference

Two groups simultaneously reported the occurrence of hepatitis-associated antigen in patients with polyarteritis nodosa:

Trepo C, Thivolet J. Hepatitis associated antigen and periarteritis nodosa (PAN). *Vox Sang* 1970;19(3):410–11.

Gocke D, Hsu K, Councilman, M, et al. Association between polyarteritis and Australia antigen. *Lancet* 1970;296(7684):1149–53.

Purpose

The purpose of both papers was to describe the occurrence of hepatitis-associated antigen in patients with polyarteritis nodosa.

Patients

The paper by Trepo and Thivolet described 7 patients with histologically proven polyarteritis nodosa, and Gocke et al. described 11 patients.

Study

Both papers simply report the occurrence of hepatitis antigen in patients with biopsy-proven polyarteritis nodosa. The antigen was detected by Trepo via an immunodiffusion assay. Circulating immune complexes were detected by Gocke et al. by using serological, ultracentrifugal, and electron microscopic studies.

Follow-up

No details of follow-up were provided by either group.

Results

Trepo and Thivolet reported hepatitis-associated antigen in six of seven biopsy-confirmed cases of polyarteritis nodosa. Not all cases had evidence of hepatitis: only two presented with an initial icteric hepatitis. In four cases there was no history of blood transfusion. In one case the antigen persisted for 30 months.

Gocke et al. reported that 4 of 11 patients with biopsy-proven polyarteritis nodosa were positive for hepatitis-associated antigen. The four patients positive for the hepatitis antigen had a typical polyarteritis syndrome, with mild hepatic damage. Circulating immune complexes were demonstrated in sera from three of the four antigen-positive patients.

Critique

The numbers of patients in both studies was small, and no follow-up, of either the clinical status of the patients or the persistence of the hepatitis-associated antigen was provided.

Significance and importance

These two papers demonstrated for the first time that a form of systemic vasculitis could be caused by a viral infection. Despite intensive searches in other types of vasculitis for evidence of an infectious aetiology, the association between hepatitis B virus and polyarteritis nodosa remains the best established. Hepatitis C virus infection has been associated with essential cryoglobulinaemia.

The formation of immune complexes in patients with polyarteritis nodosa and infected with hepatitis B virus was subsequently confirmed in a number of other studies [1, 2]. Most cases of hepatitis B virus-associated polyarteritis nodosa are caused by infection with wild-type hepatitis B virus and are associated with HBe antigenaemia and high hepatitis B virus replication; this observation which supports the notion that vasculitic lesions can result from the deposition of soluble viral antigen–antibody immune complexes in conditions of antigen excess. These immune complexes then activate the complement cascade.

Epidemiological data support this association. In an Alaskan native population endemic for hepatitis B virus, 13 of 14 patients with polyarteritis nodosa showed serological evidence of hepatitis B virus infection [3]. None of the survivors of the initial hepatitis B virus infection and polyarteritis nodosa subsequently relapsed over a 55-month follow-up. These results lead to the suggestion that polyarteritis nodosa occurs early in the course of hepatitis B virus infection and is unlikely to recur, an observation confirmed in a large-series study conducted in France and in which only 10% of patients relapsed [4]. Hepatitis B virus polyarteritis nodosa has become a much rarer condition over the last two decades since the introduction of vaccination of high-risk groups and reliable screening of blood products. In France, as hepatitis B virus infection rates have fallen due to vaccination, the prevalence of polyarteritis nodosa has also decreased [5, 6].

The discovery of the association between hepatitis B virus and polyarteritis nodosa also led to the development of treatment strategies based on elimination of the underlying infection rather than just intensive immunosuppression. Use of conventional corticosteroids and cyclophosphamide permits the virus to replicate, thereby enabling development of chronic hepatitis and cirrhosis. The current preferred therapy is plasma exchange and an antiviral drug combined with corticosteroids to control the most severe manifestations, followed by rapid withdrawal of corticosteroids to enhance clearance of infection and seroconversion from HBeAg positive to anti-HBeAb positive. Use of antiviral agents as such lamivudine increases the seroconversion rate to 60% [4].

References

1 **Prince A, Trepo C.** Role of immune complexes involving SH antigen in pathogenesis of chronic active hepatitis and polyarteritis nodosa. *Lancet* 1971;**1**(7713):1309–12.

2 **Guillevin L, Lhote F, Cohen P, et al.** Polyarteritis nodosa related to hepatitis B virus. A prospective study with long term observation of 41 patients. *Medicine (Baltimore)* 1995;**74**(5):238–53.

3 **McMahon BJ, Heyward W L, Templin DW, et al.** (1989). Hepatitis B associated polyarteritis nodosa in Alaskan eskimos: clinical and epidemiological features and long term follow up. *Hepatology* **9**(1);97–101.

4 **Guillevin L, Mahr A, Callard P, et al.** Hepatitis B virus associated polyarteritis nodosa: clinical characteristics, outcome, and impact of treatment in 115 patients. Medicine (Baltimore) 2005;**84**(5):313–22.

5 **Mahr A, Guillevin L, Poissonnet M, et al.** Prevalences of Polyarteritis nodosa, microscopic polyangiitis, Wegener's granulomatosis, and Churg-Strauss syndrome in a French urban multiethnic population in 2000: a capture-recapture estimate. *Arthritis Rheum* 2004;**51**(1):92–9.

6 **Pagnoux C, Seror R, Heneger C, et al.** Clinical features and outcomes in 348 patients with polyarteritis nodosa. *Arthritis Rheum* 2010;**62**(2):616–6.

Paper 5.5: The discovery of anti-neutrophil cytoplasmic antibodies as a marker of Wegener's granulomatosis

Reference

Van der Woude FJ, Rasmussen N, Lobatto S, et al. Autoantibodies against neutrophils and monocytes: tool for diagnosis and marker of disease activity in Wegener's granulomatosis. *Lancet* 1985:1(8426):425–9.

Purpose

To describe the use of antibodies against the cytoplasm of ethanol-fixed neutrophils and monocytes (anti-neutrophil cytoplasmic antibodies) in the diagnosis and assessment of patients with Wegener's granulomatosis (now known as granulomatosis with polyangiitis (GPA)).

Patients

Forty-one patients (22 females; mean age 55.1 years) with active GPA were studied. Fifty-nine serum samples were available from the 41 patients. Serial samples were available from the 19 patients who were followed up.

The control group consisted of 500 sera from healthy blood donors and patients with other types of granulomatous disease, vasculitis, or connective tissue disease.

Study design

This report describes the development and characterization of an indirect immunofluorescence assay to detect anti-neutrophil cytoplasmic antibodies on ethanol-fixed human neutrophils. The assay was characterized using 500 normal and disease controls. Its utility was investigated in a retrospective study of patients with active vasculitis.

Trial end points

Retrospective scoring for disease activity was performed; patients with activity in one or more systems were considered to have active disease.

Follow-up

One-year follow-up was carried out for 19 patients.

Results

Anti-neutrophil cytoplasmic antibodies were detectable in 25/27 patients with active disease, as compared with 4/32 samples from patients with inactive disease. During follow-up, the disease remained inactive in 10/19 patients. Overall IgG anti-neutrophil cytoplasmic antibodies correlated with active disease (P < 0.01). Anti-neutrophil cytoplasmic antibodies were not detectable in the sera from the controls.

Critique

The development and characterization of the anti-neutrophil cytoplasmic antibodies test is well described. However, the number of patients included, particularly in the follow-up study, was small. Disease assessment was relatively crude but, at the time of the study, objective validated scoring tools had not yet been developed.

Significance and importance

The relationship of autoantibodies against cytoplasmic components of granulocytes was initially reported by Davies in a few patients with glomerulonephritis [1]. The study by van der Woude and colleagues was the first demonstration of an antibody specific for GPA, and their results supported the view that GPA should be considered as a distinct disease from polyarteritis nodosa. This discovery directly stimulated a flourishing of research activity in the field of systemic vasculitis, and the establishment of a European-wide network of clinicians, resulting in the successful conduct of multinational trials in systemic vasculitis. The first study of the European group was a multinational collaboration to standardize anti-neutrophil cytoplasmic antibody assays [2]. The discovery of anti-neutrophil cytoplasmic antibodies also heightened awareness of systemic vasculitis, and several studies have shown an increase in the occurrence of GPA in the decade following this paper [3, 4].

The nature of the antigen responsible for the cytoplasmic staining was not identified by van der Woude and colleagues but was subsequently identified as proteinase 3 (PR3), a 29 kDa serine protease located in azurophilic granules [5].

Subsequent studies showed that there were several patterns of immunofluorescence detectable in patients with vasculitis, including the classical cytoplasmic pattern described by van der Woude and a perinuclear pattern recognized in patients with MPA (Figure 5.4) [6]. Myeloperoxidase was shown to be the antigen most commonly responsible for the anti-neutrophil cytoplasmic antibody pattern seen in systemic vasculitis [6, 7].

The long-term follow-up of patients in a number of clinical trials has led to the recognition that anti-neutrophil cytoplasmic antibody specificity is a determinant of outcome; the presence of PR3 antibodies is associated with lower mortality but an increased risk of relapse compared with myeloperoxidase (MPO)-positive patients [8]. Recent genetic data

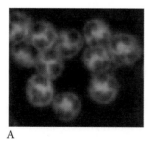
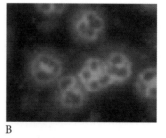

A   B

Fig. 5.4 Indirect immunofluorescence of human neutrophils showing the typical staining pattern for anti-neutrophil cytoplasmic antibodies. A. Cytoplasmic staining. B. Perinuclear staining.

suggest that PR3 plays a central role in the pathogenesis of some types of vasculitis and has led to the suggestion that AAV should be classified by anti-neutrophil cytoplasmic antibody subtype rather than the clinical phenotype [9–11].

References

1 **Davies DJ, Moran JE, Niall JF, et al**. Segmental necrotizing glomerulonephritis with antineutrophil antibody: possible arbovirus aetiology? *BMJ (Clin Res Ed)* 1982;**285**(6342):606.

2 **Hagen EC, Andrassy K, Csernok E, et al**. Development and standardization of solid phase assays for the detection of anti-neutrophil cytoplasmic antibodies (ANCA). A report on the second phase of an international cooperative study on the standardization of ANCA assays. *J Immunol Methods* 1996;**196**(1):1–15.

3 **Andrews M, Edmunds M, Campbell A, et al**. (1990). Systemic vasculitis in the 1980's—is there an increasing incidence of Wegener's granulomatosis and microscopic polyarteritis? *J R Coll Physicians Lond* 1990;**24**(4):284–8.

4 **Watts RA, Scott DGI**. 'Epidemiology of vasculitis' in Oxford textbook of vasculitis, 3rd edn (Ball GV, Fessler BJ, Bridges SL Jr, eds); Oxford: Oxford University Press; 2014; pp. 7–25.

5 **Niles JL, McCluskey RT, Ahmad MF, et al**. Wegener's granulomatosis autoantigen is a novel neutrophil serine proteinase. *Blood* 1989;**74**(6):1888–93.

6 **Cohen Tervaert JW, Huitema M, van der Geissen M, et al**. Wegener's granulomatosis and anti-cytoplasmic antibodies: the Groningen experience. *Acta Pathol Microbiol Immunol Scand* 1989;**97**(6):36.

7 **Falk RJ, Jennette JC**. Anti-neutrophil cytoplasmic autoantibodies with specificity for myeloperoxidase in patients with systemic vasculitis and idiopathic necrotizing and crescentic glomerulonephritis. *N Engl J Med* 1988;**318**(25):1651–7.

8 **Walsh M, Flossmann O, Berden A, et al**. Risk factors for relapse of antineutrophil cytoplasmic antibody-associated vasculitis. *Arthritis Rheum* 2012;**64**(2):542–8.

9 **Lyons PA, Rayner TF, Trivedi S, et al**. Genetically distinct subsets within ANCA-associated vasculitis. *N Engl J Med* 2012;**367**(3):214–23.

10 **Watts R A, Scott DGI**. ANCA vasculitis: to lump or split? Why we should study MPA and GPA separately. *Rheumatology* 2012;**51**(12):2115–17.

11 **Millet A, Pederzoli-Ribeil M, Guillevin L, et al**. Antineutrophil cytoplasmic antibody-associated vasculitides: is it time to split up the group? *Ann Rheum Dis* 2013;**72**(8):1273–9.

Paper 5.6: Definitions and nomenclature of vasculitis—the Chapel Hill Consensus Conferences, 1994 and 2012

Reference

Jennette JC, Falk RJ, Andrassy K, et al. Nomenclature of systemic vasculitides. Proposal of an international consensus conference. *Arthritis Rheum* 1994;37(2):187–92.

Jennette J, Falk R, Bacon P, et al. Revised International Chapel Hill Consensus Conference Nomenclature of Vasculitides. *Arthritis Rheum* 2013;65(1):1–11.

Purpose

The goal of both conferences was to reach a consensus on the names for most types of systemic vasculitis and to construct root definitions for the vasculitides so named.

Study design

Two consensus conferences (1994 and 2012) were held to develop a nomenclature system and definitions for the systemic vasculitides.

The 1994 conference was composed of an ad hoc group of 16 internists, rheumatologists, nephrologists, immunologists, and pathologists from six countries; a modified nominal group process was used to achieve unanimous consensus by the end of the conference. The 1994 conference focused on the seven most common types of non-infectious vasculitis.

The 2012 conference included 28 participants from 12 different countries and from the fields of internal medicine, nephrology, pulmonology, paediatrics, otolaryngology, pathology, and rheumatology. A modified nominal group technique was also used, with one of the lead authors as the moderator. Each name and definition was voted on at least once by every member of the group. More than 80% consensus was needed to make a change in a Chapel Hill Consensus Conference 1994 name or definition or to add a new name or definition. Vote was by show of hand, and all definitions that were adopted received >80% agreement (23 or more votes). Discussions for which consensus that had not been achieved during the round table meeting were continued by email with the same voting system and level of consensus.

Results

The 1994 Chapel Hill Consensus Conference produced a classification and nomenclature system for the systemic vasculitides. The vasculitides were classified according to vessel size—large, medium, and small, and formal definitions for ten types of vasculitis were produced (Table 5.2).

In 2011, in recognition of the progress in the understanding of systemic vasculitides since 1994, including the role of anti-neutrophil cytoplasmic antibodies, a second conference was held. A new tree hierarchy was developed which recognized that some conditions cannot be simply classified by vessel size. AAV was recognized as a specific type of small-vessel vasculitis, along with immune-complex-mediated vasculitis (Table 5.3).

Table 5.2 1994 Chapel Hill Consensus Conference definitions for vasculitis

CHCC 1994 Name	CHCC 1994 Definition
Large vessel vasculitis	
Giant cell (temporal) arteritis	Granulomatous arteritis of the aorta and its major branches, with a predilection for the extra cranial branches of the carotid artery. Often involves the temporal artery. Usually occurs in patients older than 50 and often is associated with polymyalgia rheumatica.
Takayasu's arteritis	Granulomatous inflammation of the aorta and its major branches. Usually occurs in patients younger than 50
Medium sized vessel vasculitis	
Polyarteritis nodosa† (classic polyarteritis nodosa)	Necrotizing inflammation of medium-sized or small arteries without glomerulonephritis or vasculitis in arterioles, capillaries, or venules.
Kawasaki disease	Arteritis involving large, medium sized, small arteries, and associated with mucocutaneous lymph node syndrome. Coronary arteries are often involved. Aorta and veins may be involved. Usually occurs in children.
Small vessel vasculitis	
Wegener's granulomatosis‡	Granulomatous inflammation involving the respiratory tract, and necrotizing vasculitis affecting small to medium-sized vessels (e.g., capillaries, venules, arterioles, and arteries). Necrotizing glomerulonephritis is common.
Churg Strauss syndrome‡	Eosinophil-rich and granulomatous inflammation involving the respiratory tract, necrotizing vasculitis affecting small to medium-sized vessels, and associated with asthma and eosinophilia.
Microscopic polyangiitis† (microscopic polyarteritis)‡	Necrotizing vasculitis, with few or no immune deposits, affecting small vessels (i.e., capillaries, venules, or arterioles). Necrotising arteritis involving small and medium sized arteries may be present. Necrotizing glomerulonephritis is very common. Pulmonary capillaritis often occurs
Henoch Schönlein Purpura	Vasculitis, with IgA-dominant immune deposits, affecting small vessels (i.e., capillaries, venules, or arterioles). Typically involves skin, gut, and glomeruli, and is associated arthralgia or arthritis.
Essential cryoglobulinaemic vasculitis	Vasculitis, with cryoglobulin immune deposits, affecting small vessels (i.e., capillaries, venules, or arterioles), and associated with cryoglobulins in serum. Skin and glomeruli are often involved.
Cutaneous leucocytoclastic angiitis	Isolated cutaneous leucocytoclastic angiitis without systemic vasculitis glomerulonephritis.

* Large vessel refers to the aorta and the largest branches directed towards the major body regions (e.g., to the extremities and the head and neck); medium sized vessel refers to the main visceral arteries (e.g., renal, hepatic, coronary, and mesenteric arteries); small vessel refers to venules, capillaries, arterioles, and the intraparenchymal distal arterial radicals that connect with arterioles. Some small and large vessel vasculitides may involve medium-sized arteries, but large and medium sized vessel vasculitides do not involve smaller than arteries. Essential components are represented by normal type; italicised type represents usual, but not essential, components; CHCC, Chapel Hill Consensus Conference.

† Preferred term.

‡ Strongly associated with antineutrophil cytoplasmic antibodies.

Reproduced from Jennette JC, Falk RJ, Andrassy K, Bacon PA, Churg J, Gross WL, et al. Nomenclature of systemic vasculitides. Proposal of an international consensus conference. *Arthritis Rheum* 1994;37:187–92 with permission from Wiley.

Table 5.3 2012 Chapel Hill Consensus Conference definitions for vasculitis*

CHCC 2012 Name	CHCC 2012 Definition
Large Vessel Vasculitis	Vasculitis affecting large arteries more often than other vasculitides. Large arteries are the aorta and its major branches. Any size artery may be affected.
Takayasu Arteritis	Arteritis, often granulomatous, predominantly affecting the aorta and/or its major branches. Onset usually in patients younger than 50.
Giant Cell Arteritis	Arteritis, often granulomatous, usually affecting the aorta and/or its major branches, with a predilection for the branches of the carotid artery. Often involves the temporal artery. Onset usually in patients older than 50 and often associated with polymyalgia rheumatica.
Medium Vessel Vasculitis	Vasculitis predominantly affecting medium-sized arteries defined as the main visceral arteries and their branches. Any size artery may be affected. Inflammatory aneurysms and stenoses are common.
Polyarteritis Nodosa	Necrotizing arteritis of medium-sized or small arteries without glomerulonephritis or vasculitis in arterioles, capillaries, or venules; and not associated with ANCA.
Kawasaki Disease	Arteritis associated with the mucocutaneous lymph node syndrome and predominantly affecting medium-sized and small arteries. Coronary arteries are often involved. Aorta and large arteries may be involved. Usually occurs in infants and young children.
Small Vessel Vasculitis	Vasculitis predominantly affecting small vessels, defined as small intraparenchymal arteries, arterioles, capillaries and venules. Medium sized arteries and veins may be affected.
ANCA Associated Vasculitis	Necrotizing vasculitis, with few or no immune deposits, predominantly affecting small vessels (i.e., capillaries, venules, arterioles and small arteries), associated with MPO-ANCA or PR3-ANCA. Not all patients have ANCA. Add a prefix indicating ANCA reactivity (e.g., PR3-ANCA, MPO-ANCA, ANCA-negative).
Microscopic Polyangiitis	Necrotizing vasculitis, with few or no immune deposits, predominantly affecting small vessels (i.e., capillaries, venules, or arterioles). Necrotizing arteritis involving small and medium sized arteries may be present. Necrotizing glomerulonephritis is very common. Pulmonary capillaritis often occurs. Granulomatous inflammation is absent.
Granulomatosis with Polyangiitis (Wegener's)	Necrotizing granulomatous inflammation usually involving the upper and lower respiratory tract, and necrotizing vasculitis affecting predominantly small to medium-sized vessels (e.g., capillaries, venules, arterioles, arteries and veins). Necrotizing glomerulonephritis is common.
Eosinophilic Granulomatosis with Polyangiitis (Churg Strauss)	Eosinophil-rich and necrotizing granulomatous inflammation often involving the respiratory tract, and necrotizing vasculitis predominantly affecting small to medium-sized vessels, and associated with asthma and eosinophilia. ANCA is most frequent when glomerulonephritis is present.
Immune Complex Small Vessel Vasculitis	Vasculitis with moderate to marked vessel wall deposits of immunoglobulin and/or complement components predominantly affecting small vessels (i.e., capillaries, venules, arterioles and small arteries). Glomerulonephritis is frequent.
Anti-GBM Disease	Vasculitis affecting glomerular capillaries, pulmonary capillaries, or both, with basement membrane deposition of anti-basement membrane autoantibodies. Lung involvement causes pulmonary hemorrhage, and renal involvement causes glomerulonephritis with necrosis and crescents.

Table 5.3 (continued) 2012 Chapel Hill Consensus Conference definitions for vasculitis*

CHCC 2012 Name	CHCC 2012 Definition
Cryoglobulinemic Vasculitis	Vasculitis with cryoglobulin immune deposits affecting small vessels (predominantly capillaries, venules, or arterioles) and associated with cryoglobulins in serum. Skin and glomeruli are often involved.
IgA Vasculitis (Henoch-Schönlein)	Vasculitis, with IgA1-dominant immune deposits, affecting small vessels (predominantly capillaries, venules, or arterioles). Often involves skin and gut, and frequently causes arthritis. Glomerulonephritis indistinguishable from IgA nephropathy may occur.
Hypocomplementemic Urticarial Vasculitis (Anti-C1q Vasculitis)	Vasculitis accompanied by urticaria and hypocomplementemia affecting small vessels (i.e., capillaries, venules, or arterioles), and associated with anti-C1q antibodies. Glomerulonephritis, arthritis, obstructive pulmonary disease, and ocular inflammation are common.
Variable Vessel Vasculitis	Vasculitis with no predominant type of vessel involved that can affect vessels of any size (small, medium, and large) and type (arteries, veins, and capillaries).
Behçet's Disease	Vasculitis occurring in patients with Behçet's disease that can affect arteries or veins. Behçet's disease is characterized by recurrent oral and/ or genital aphthous ulcers accompanied by cutaneous, ocular, articular, gastrointestinal, and/or central nervous system inflammatory lesions. Small vessel vasculitis, thromboangiitis, thrombosis, arteritis and arterial aneurysms may occur.
Cogan's syndrome	Vasculitis occurring in patients with Cogan's syndrome. Cogan's syndrome is characterized by ocular inflammatory lesions, including interstitial keratitis, uveitis, and episcleritis, and inner ear disease, including sensorineural hearing loss and vestibular dysfunction. Vasculitic manifestations may include arteritis (affecting small, medium or large arteries), aortitis, aortic aneurysms, and aortic and mitral valvulitis.
Single Organ Vasculitis	Vasculitis in arteries or veins of any size in a single organ that has no features that indicate that it is a limited expression of a systemic vasculitis. The involved organ and vessel type should be included in the name (e.g., cutaneous SVV, testicular arteritis, central nervous system vasculitis). Vasculitis distribution may be unifocal or multifocal (diffuse) within an organ. Some patients originally diagnosed with SOV will develop additional disease manifestations that warrant re-defining the case as one of the systemic vasculitides (e.g., cutaneous arteritis later becoming systemic polyarteritis nodosa, etc.).
Vasculitis Associated with Systemic Disease	Vasculitis that is associated with and may be secondary to (caused by) a systemic disease. The name (diagnosis) should have a prefix term specifying the systemic disease (e.g., rheumatoid vasculitis, lupus vasculitis, etc.).
Vasculitis Associated with Probable Aetiology	Vasculitis that is associated with a probable specific aetiology. The name (diagnosis) should have a prefix term specifying the association (e.g., hydralazine-associated microscopic polyangiitis, hepatitis B virus-associated vasculitis, hepatitis C virus-associated cryoglobulinemic vasculitis, etc.).

* ANCA, anti-neutrophil cytoplasmic antibodies; CHCC, Chapel Hill Consensus Conference; MPO, myeloperoxidase; PR3, proteinase 3; SOV, single-organ vasculitis; SVV, small-vessel vasculitis.

Reproduced from Jennette J, Falk R, Bacon P, Basu N, Cid M, Ferrario F, et al. 2012 Revised International Chapel Hill Consensus Conference Nomenclature of Vasculitides. *Arthritis Rheum* 2013;65:1–11. With permission from Wiley.

The hierarchy was expanded to include vasculitis affecting vessels of variable size, single organ vasculitis, and vasculitis associated either with systemic disease or specific aetiologies. A new nomenclature was adopted with a move away from eponyms towards names reflecting pathology or aetiopathogenesis following the introduction of the term GPA for Wegener's granulomatosis [1]. The name eosinophilic granulomatosis with polyangiitis was adopted for Churg–Strauss syndrome and IgA vasculitis for Henoch–Schönlein purpura (IgAV). Definitions were developed for new categories of conditions including single organ vasculitis and vasculitis associated with specific aetiologies, including systemic disease (rheumatoid arthritis, systemic lupus erythematosus) and aetiologies such as infection (cryoglobulinaemia, hepatitis B and C) or drugs (e.g., propylthiouracil).

Critique of the paper

In 1994, consensus was achieved using a modified nominal group process with unanimity by the end of the conference. It is clear from the textural description that consensus was not easy to achieve in some areas, such as the terminology for non-granulomatous vasculitis affecting the upper/lower respiratory tract with or without necrotizing glomerulonephritis, anti-basement membrane antibody, or immune complex deposition. Anti-neutrophil cytoplasmic antibodies was discussed but not included within the definitions, although it was clearly recognized that certain types of vasculitis such as Wegener's granulomatosis and MPA were associated with the presence of anti-neutrophil cytoplasmic antibodies. Vasculitis was classified by vessel size but the definitions of vessel size were not particularly clear nor was it apparent that the group was describing only predominant vessel involvement, not exclusive vessel involvement. The group recognized the importance of histology but did not make it a mandatory feature of the definitions.

The 2012 conference had a broader range of membership and global distribution of members than in 1994, although there was some overlap. The membership of neither conference was totally inclusive and notably did not include ophthalmologists or dermatologists. There are therefore areas which are less well covered and these include a nomenclature system for cutaneous vasculitis and retinal vasculitis.

Significance and importance of the paper

The 1994 conference was the first unified attempt to define the systemic vasculitides and provide a nomenclature system based on a consensus of experts. Until then there had been a plethora of names for many types of vasculitis, leading to confusion. The provision of definitions combined with development of assessment tools made it possible for the field to move forwards and begin to conduct clinical trials using homogenous cohorts of patients. Although not intended to be used as such, the 1994 definitions were used as classification criteria for studies; this was particularly true for MPA, for which there were (and still are) not validated classification criteria. Despite concerns at the time that the definitions would not stand the test of time, by and large they have. Comparison of the definitions between 1994 and 2012 shows relatively little change apart from the addition of statements around the presence or absence of anti-neutrophil cytoplasmic antibodies.

In order to overcome the limitations of misusing definitions as classification criteria, and ACR 1990 vasculitis classification criteria which did not include MPA or anti-neutrophil cytoplasmic antibodies, a classification algorithm was developed by consensus; this has proved successful for use in epidemiology studies in several different populations [2].

Until new validated diagnostic and classification criteria are developed [3], these definitions will continue to be one of the bedrocks on which the whole field of vasculitis is built.

References

1 Falk RJ, Gross WL, Guillevin L, et al. Granulomatosis with polyangiitis (Wegener's): an alternative name for Wegener's granulomatosis. *Ann Rheum Dis* 2011;**70**(4):704.

2 Watts RA, Lane SE, Hanslik T, et al. Development and validation of a consensus methodology for the classification of the ANCA-associated vasculitides and polyarteritis nodosa for epidemiological studies. *Ann Rheum Dis* 2007;**66**(2);222–7.

3 Craven A, Robson J, Ponte C, et al. ACR/EULAR-endorsed study to develop Diagnostic and Classification Criteria for Vasculitis (DCVAS). *Clin Exp Nephrol* 2013;**17**(5):619–21.

Paper 5.7: Development of assessment tools for systemic vasculitis

Reference

Luqmani RA, Bacon PA, Moots RJ, et al. Birmingham Vasculitis Activity Score (BVAS) in systemic necrotizing vasculitis. *QJM* 1994;87(11):671–8.

Purpose

The aim of the study was to develop a clinical scoring tool for the assessment of disease activity in systemic vasculitis and which would accurately reflect the activity of vasculitis in a given patient.

Patients

A total of 213 patients with systemic vasculitis were evaluated: 51 patients with rheumatoid vasculitis, 14 patients with polyarteritis nodosa, 6 patients with MPA, 28 patients with Wegener's granulomatosis, 22 patients with non-renal Wegener's granulomatosis, 11 patients with Takayasu's arteritis, 11 patients with Behçet's disease, 10 patients with giant cell arteritis, and 60 patients with other forms of systemic vasculitis.

Study design

The Birmingham Vasculitis Activity Score (BVAS) is based on clinician assessment of patients and deciding whether clinical features are present and if they are due to active vasculitis. The items to be scored were developed by consensus among a group of physicians (including rheumatologists and nephrologists). The score categorizes abnormalities in nine separate systems: systemic; cutaneous; mucous membranes/eyes; ear, nose, and throat; chest; cardiovascular; abdominal; renal; and neurological. For some systems, additional information is needed, such as a chest radiography, urine analysis, or renal function. Each item was weighted and the degree of weighting was determined by consensus, so myalgia would score 1 but major gastrointestinal bleed due to vasculitis would score 6.

A standard pro forma was developed for recording each item. Points were given for each item, with a maximum number of points per body system and a maximum total score of 63. Items are only recorded if they can be attributable to active vasculitis.

The assessment score was initially assessed for content validity, feasibility, construct validity, reliability, and discriminant validity.

Results

Feasibility

The BVAS was shown to take less than three minutes to compete.

Cross-sectional analysis

Patients judged clinically to be well were shown to have a BVAS = 0, those with active vasculitis prior to treatment had a median score of 7.5, and those with active disease and on treatment had a score of 10. Thirty patients were studied serially and the median BVAS was higher in periods of active disease (BVAS = 15) than in remission (BVAS = 0).

Reliability

Inter-observer variability was determined by two independent observers assessing 14 patients within 20 minutes. The patients were chosen to have a range of disease activity. In 12/14 patients, the two observers agreed closely, with a maximum of two points difference. Construct validity was assessed as follows: 26 consecutive patients were assessed using the BVAS, the vasculitis activity index (VAI), and the Groningen index; the BVAS showed good correlation with the other two scoring systems. However, when the BVAS was compared with the physicians global assessment, no relationship between BVAS and physicians global assessment was found.

Critique of the paper

The methodology used to develop the BVAS was careful and the BVAS was shown to be feasible and reliable. The precise composition of the consensus group used to develop the questionnaire was not stated beyond the inclusion of nephrologists and rheumatologists; thus, it is not clear whether other important and relevant specialists such as ophthalmologists, otorhinolaryngologists, and chest physicians were included. The degree of consensus between members of the group was not reported nor was the precise method of determining the items to be included. The studied patients had a broad range of vasculitic conditions; relatively little data was presented on the performance of the BVAS in each condition, and the number of patients in some subsets was quite small. Over one-quarter of the patients had 'other types' of vasculitis, and a further 25% had rheumatoid vasculitis. The BVAS may perform better in some conditions than others and this was not explored in detail. The process of generating a generic score usable across all types of vasculitis inevitably resulted in the loss of some items which could be important in the assessment of some conditions; for example, there was relatively crude data collection regarding specific pulse loss in large vessel vasculitis.

The BVAS does not address the issue of long-term damage in vasculitis, although the need to develop a score for this was recognized. The BVAS also does not address the issue of patient functional status nor is it designed to be a patient-reported outcome measure.

Significance and importance

This was not the first paper to describe a tool to assess disease activity in systemic vasculitis; previously described tools include the VAI and the Groningen index [1, 2]. The Groningen score was not designed for serial use and is only for use in Wegener's granulomatosis. The VAI has a number of subjective scales. The BVAS therefore had a number of advantages, in particular, feasibility and reliability, which led to its adoption for use in the first wave of European multicentre clinical trials in systemic vasculitis. The development of a reliable method of assessing disease activity in vasculitis directly led to the success of these trials and the establishment of a robust evidence base for the treatment of systemic vasculitis.

The generic nature of BVAS provides overall assessment. It has gone through several amendments but the broad principle remains the same [3]. A disease-specific version for GPA has been developed (BVAS-WG) [4]. The BVAS has been shown to be predictive; a high BVAS at diagnosis predicts poor subsequent outcome in terms of mortality but also predicts responsiveness to therapy [5]. Definitions of remission, relapse, and active disease have been determined in terms of BVAS scores. BVAS also works well in children, and a paediatric-specific score has been developed [6].

References

1 Olsen TL, Whiting-O'Keefe QE, Hellman DB. Validity and precision of a vasculitis activity index (VAI). *Arthritis Rheum* 1992;**35**(9):S164.

2 Kallenberg CGM, Cohen Tervaert JW, Stegeman CA. Criteria for disease activity in Wegener's granulomatosis: a requirement for longitudinal clinical studies. *APMIS* 1990;**19**(Suppl):37–9.

3 Mukhtyar C, Lee R, Brown D, et al. Modification and validation of the Birmingham Vasculitis Activity Score (version 3). *Ann Rheum Dis* 2009;**68**(12):1827–32.

4 Stone JH, Hoffman GS, Merkel PA, et al. A disease-specific index for Wegener's granulomatosis: modification of the Birmingham Vasculitis Activity Score. *Arthritis Rheum* 2001;**44**(4):912–20.

5 Gayraud M, Guillevin L, le Toumelin P, et al. Long-term follow up of polyarteritis nodosa, microscopic polyangiitis, and Churg–Strauss syndrome: analysis of four prospective trials including 278 patients. *Arthritis Rheum* 2001;**44**(3):666–75.

6 Dolezalova P, Price-Kuehne EE, Ozen S, et al. Disease activity assessment in childhood vasculitis: development and preliminary validation of the Paediatric Vasculitis Activity Score (PVAS). *Ann Rheum Dis* 2013;**72**(10):1628–33.

Paper 5.8: Cyclophosphamide as treatment for systemic vasculitis

Reference

Fauci AS, Katz P, Haynes BF, et al. Cyclophosphamide therapy of severe systemic necrotizing vasculitis. *N Engl J Med* 1979;301(5):235–8.

Purpose

To investigate the efficacy of cyclophosphamide therapy in patients with severe vasculitis.

Patients

Patients were diagnosed on clinical grounds. All had active and progressive disease and had received glucocorticoids with significant toxicity.

Study

This was an open-label, unblinded, observational study of 17 patients.

Treatment

Treatment comprised oral cyclophosphamide 2 mg kg^{-1} day^{-1}, combined with oral prednisolone 1 mg kg^{-1} day^{-1}. After induction of remission, cyclophosphamide was continued with alternate-day glucocorticoids. One patient received azathioprine.

Trial end points measured

Trial end points were survival and duration of remission. Remission was defined as disease cessation, which was determined on the basis of no further progression, an improvement in organ function, and a lack of involvement of new organs after the introduction of cytotoxic therapy.

Follow-up

The study included an open-label follow-up. The median follow-up was not stated.

Results

Three patients died during the study. Complete remission occurred in the remaining 14 patients. Glucocorticoids were discontinued in seven patients. The mean duration of remission was 22 months (range, 2–61 months). There were no recurrences during treatment with cyclophosphamide.

Critique of the paper

The paper only includes 17 patients, one of whom was treated with azathioprine. No attempt was made to blind the observers. The paper predates the development of validated scoring systems for vasculitis but despite this demonstrated a significant improvement in survival and remission.

Significance and importance of the paper

This seminal paper by Fauci et al. clearly demonstrated a significant improvement in survival and remission rate compared with that obtained with the existing standard of care using high-dose glucocorticoids. It extended their previous report published in 1973 [1]. The study established the importance of cyclophosphamide in the management of vasculitis and laid the foundation for modern treatment regimens and the European Vasculitis Study Group series of international, multicentre, randomized controls.

Prior to the development of immunosuppressive therapy with glucocorticoids and cyclophosphamide, granulomatosis with polyangiitis (Wegener's; GPA) had a very poor prognosis. The natural history of untreated GPA and MPA is of a rapidly progressive, usually fatal disease; Walton observed a mean survival in patients with GPA of five months, with 82% of patients dying within one year and 89% dying within two years [2]. Oral prednisolone improved the mean survival to 12.5 months [3].

Fauci and colleagues subsequently reported their experience of cyclophosphamide therapy in 85 patients with GPA and followed prospectively over a 21-year period [4]. This study confirmed the efficacy of combination therapy with oral cyclophosphamide and prednisolone. Complete remission was obtained in 79/85 patients, with a mean duration of remission of 48.2 months. Following remission, cyclophosphamide was slowly tapered. Withdrawal of therapy was achieved in 23 patients who were followed for a mean of 35.3 months.

The toxicity of the long-term use of cyclophosphamide, especially the risks of infertility and malignancy, was recognized during the 1980s and 1990s. The Fauci regimen of continuous oral cyclophosphamide as described in these papers led to patients receiving very large cumulative doses. Haemorrhagic cystitis was a particularly frequent complication affecting 34% of patients. Follow-up studies from the National Institutes of Health reported up to a 45-fold increase in the risk of bladder cancer [5].

The recognition of the cumulative toxicity of cyclophosphamide in this cohort of carefully studied patients led to the development of regimens based on the use of lower cumulative doses of cyclophosphamide and on the concept of remission maintenance with immunosuppressive agents other cyclophosphamide. Thus, the way was paved for the European Study Group First wave of clinical trials and, in particular, the CYCAZAREM study. (see paper 5.9 page 181)

References

1 **Fauci AS, Wolff SM.** Wegener's granulomatosis: studies in eighteen patients and a review of the literature. *Medicine* 1973;**52**(6):535–61.

2 **Walton EW.** Giant cell granuloma of the respiratory tract (Wegener's granulomatosis). *BMJ* 1958;**2**(5091):265–70.

3 **Hollander D, Manning RT.** The use of alkylating agents in the treatment of Wegener's granulomatosis. *Ann Intern Med* 1967;**67**(2):393–8.

4 **Fauci A, Haynes BF.** Wegener's granulomatosis: prospective clinical and therapeutic experience with 85 patients for 21 years. *Ann Intern Med* 1983;**98**(1):76–85.

5 **Hoffman G, Kerr G, Leavitt R, et al.** Wegener's granulomatosis: an analysis of 158 patients. *Arch Intern Med* 1992;**116**(6):488–99.

Paper 5.9: Maintenance therapy for systemic vasculitis

Reference

Jayne D, Rasmussen N, Andrassy K, et al. A randomised trial of maintenance therapy for vasculitis associated with antineutrophil cytoplasmic autoantibodies. *N Engl J Med* 2003;349(1):36–44.

Purpose

To evaluate whether exposure to cyclophosphamide could be reduced in patients with generalized AAV by the early substitution of azathioprine at the time of remission.

Patients

The patients examined in this study had been diagnosed with GPA, MPA, or renal-limited vasculitis: renal involvement, other threatened loss of vital organ function, and anti-neutrophil cytoplasmic antibody positivity. Anti-neutrophil cytoplasmic antibody-negative patients were eligible if there was histological confirmation of vasculitis. Patients with serum creatinine >500 μmol/l were excluded. Diagnostic definitions were based on the Chapel Hill Consensus Conference 1994 definitions.

Study

The study comprised a randomized, unblinded trial. Patients were randomized at remission after between three and six months of a cyclophosphamide-based induction regimen. Randomization was to either continuation of cyclophosphamide for 12 months or switch to azathioprine. At 12 months the cyclophosphamide group was switched to the same azathioprine regimen as the azathioprine group had been receiving.

Treatment

Both groups received oral cyclophosphamide (2 mg kg^{-1} day^{-1}) and prednisolone (initially 1 mg kg^{-1} day^{-1}) tapered to 0.25 mg kg^{-1} day^{-1} by 12 weeks. After randomization, patients either received continued cyclophosphamide (1.5 mg kg^{-1} day^{-1}) or azathioprine (2 mg kg^{-1} day^{-1}), with the same dose of prednisolone 10 mg/day. At 12 months both groups received azathioprine 1.5 mg/day and prednisolone 7.5 mg/day.

Trial end points

The primary end point was relapse. Disease activity was assessed using BVAS and the disease extent index. Remission was defined as BVAS indicating no new or worse disease activity, with persistent disease in none or one item. Relapse was defined as recurrence of at least one major item or three minor items in the BVAS. Determinations of remission and relapse were made by the investigator and an independent observer.

Follow-up

Follow-up was performed at 18 months from randomization.

Results

One hundred and fifty-five patients were included in the study; there were no differences between the two groups in demographic, clinical, or laboratory parameters at randomization. Clinical remission was achieved in 144 (93%)—by three months in 119 (77%). These patients were randomized to cyclophosphamide (73) and azathioprine (71). There were seven deaths during the induction phase (two from pneumonia, three from pulmonary vasculitis and infection, and two from cerebrovascular accident).

Eleven patients in the azathioprine group (15.5%) and ten in the cyclophosphamide group (13.7%) relapsed (P = 0.65). Five patients in each group had a major relapse. Relapse was less common in among patients with MPA (4/52; 8%) than among those with GPA (17/92; 18%); no other variable affected relapse rate.

Adverse events were common in both groups, with neutropaenia occurring in 55% of patients. There was no difference in adverse event rate between the groups.

Critique of the paper

This was a well-conducted clinical trial. The patients included were representative of the most common presentations of AAV. Patients with severe disease were excluded but were eligible for another trial (MEPEX) investigating the role of plasma exchange in patients with severe life-threatening disease [1]. There may also have been under-recruitment of patients with minimal renal disease, as these patients were eligible for the NORAM trial, in which induction therapy with methotrexate was compared with cyclophosphamide [2]. This trial used oral cyclophosphamide rather than an intravenous-pulse cyclophosphamide regimen because, at the time the trial was designed, this was the most widely used induction regimen in Europe, although by the time of publication reports had emerged suggesting that the intravenous regimen was safer but associated with a higher relapse rate. The follow-up period was 18 months, for only 6 months of which were all the patients taking azathioprine.

Significance and importance of the paper

This study was part of the first wave of European studies, which included MEPEX and NORAM, which have laid the foundation for the evidence-based treatment of AAV. This paper showed that it was possible to reduce the duration of cyclophosphamide treatment without loss of short-term disease control. The toxicity of cyclophosphamide is determined primarily by the cumulative dose of cyclophosphamide and therefore regimens using lower cumulative doses should be safer. This study also confirmed the effectiveness of an induction regimen based on oral cyclophosphamide therapy, with remission being achieved by 93% of patients. It also showed that, in the short term, azathioprine was an effective remission maintenance agent. These three findings rapidly formed the basis of the standard of care for patients presenting generalized AAV and were incorporated into national and international guidance [3–5]. Recently, data on the long-term follow-up of these patients have been reported; with a median follow-up of 8.5 years, there was a non-significant increased relapse rate in the azathioprine group compared with the cyclophosphamide group [6].

The effectiveness of cyclophosphamide was also confirmed in a trial of oral versus pulse cyclophosphamide; the trial showed that pulse IV cyclophosphamide was as effective as oral cyclophosphamide at remission induction but used a lower total cyclophosphamide dose. However, there was a slightly increased risk of minor relapses with the cyclophosphamide regimen, again probably associated with the lower cumulative dose of cyclophosphamide used in the pulse IV regimen [7].

The cyclophosphamide regimens based on these studies have been used as the standard against which new therapies such as rituximab have been compared (see Paper 5.10) and used on an empirical basis in other types of vasculitis such as rheumatoid vasculitis [8].

References

1 **Jayne DR, Gaskin G, Rasmussen N, et al**. Randomized trial of plasma exchange and high dosage methylprednisolone as adjunctive therapy for severe renal vasculitis. *J Am Soc Nephrol* 2007;**18**(7):2180–8.

2 **de Groot K, Rasmussen N, Bacon P, et al**. Randomized trial of cyclophosphamide versus methotrexate for induction of remission in early systemic antineutrophil cytoplasmic antibody associated vasculitis. *Arthritis Rheum* 2005;**52**(8):2461–8.

3 **Lapraik CJ, Watts RA, Scott DG, et al**. BSR/BHPR guidelines for the management of adults with ANCA-associated vasculitis. *Rheumatology* 2007;**46**(10):1615–16.

4 **Mukhtyar C, Guillevin L, Cid M, et al**. EULAR recommendations for the management of primary small and medium vasculitis. *Ann Rheum Dis* 2009;**68**(3):310–17.

5 **Ntatsaki E, Carruthers D, Chakravarty K, et al**. BSR and BHPR guidelines for the management of adults with ANCA associated vasculitis. *Rheumatology* 2014;**53**(12):2306–9.

6 **Walsh M, Faurschou M, Berden A, et al**. Long-term follow-up of cyclophosphamide compared with azathioprine for initial maintenance therapy in ANCA-associated vasculitis. *Clin J Am Soc Nephrol* 2014;**9**(9):1571–6.

7 **de Groot K, Harper L, Jayne DR, et al**. Pulse versus oral cyclophosphamide for induction of remission in anti neutrophil cytoplasmic antibody associated vasculitis: a randomized trial. *Ann Intern Med* 2009;**150**(10):670–80.

8 **Ntatsaki E, Mooney J, Scott DGI, et al**. Systemic rheumatoid vasculitis in the era of modern immunosuppressive therapy. *Rheumatology* 2014;**53**(1):145–52.

Paper 5.10: Biologic therapy for systemic vasculitis

Reference

Two papers on the use of rituximab in AAV were published in simultaneously in 2010.

The RITUXVAS trial

Jones RB, Cohen Tervaert JW, Hauser T, et al. Rituximab versus cyclophosphamide in ANCA-associated renal vasculitis. *N Engl J Med* 2010;363(3):211–20.

The RAVE trial

Stone JH, Merkel PA, Spiera R, et al. Rituximab versus cyclophosphamide for ANCA-associated vasculitis. *N Engl J Med* 2010;363(3):221–32.

Purpose

The purpose of both the RAVE and RITUXVAS trials was to investigate the efficacy of rituximab in the management of AAV.

Patients

RITUXVAS

This trial examined 44 patients with newly diagnosed AAV and renal involvement and who were from eight centres. There were 22 GPA, 16 MPA, and 6 renal-limited vasculitis patients in the study. Renal involvement was defined as necrotizing glomerulonephritis on renal biopsy, red blood cell casts, or haematuria (>30 red blood cells/high-powered field).

RAVE

Nine centres enrolled 197 anti-neutrophil cytoplasmic antibody-positive patients with either GPA or MPA. Patients were eligible if they were positive for anti-neutrophil cytoplasmic antibodies by ELISA for PR3 or MPO and had a BVAS-WG score of 3 or more. Patients with newly diagnosed and relapsing disease were eligible.

Study design

RITUXVAS

This was an open-label, two-group, parallel-design, randomized trial. Patients were allocated in a 3:1 ratio.

RAVE

This was a multicentre, randomized, double-blind, double-dummy, non-inferiority trial. Patients were randomized 1:1, stratified by clinical type and anti-neutrophil cytoplasmic antibody type.

Disease activity was assessed by BVAS-WG and the physician's global assessment.

Treatment

RITUXVAS

In this trial, treatment comprised rituximab 375 mg/m^2 weekly for four weeks, with IV cyclophosphamide pulses at the first and third rituximab infusions, or IV cyclophosphamide for 3–6 months, followed by azathioprine. Patients in the rituximab group did not receive azathioprine as maintenance therapy. All patients received intravenous methylprednisolone (1 g) followed by the same oral glucocorticoid regimen; 1 mg/kg per day initially, with a reduction to 5 mg/day at the end of six months.

RAVE

In this trial, treatment comprised rituximab 375 mg/m^2 weekly for four weeks compared with oral cyclophosphamide 2 mg kg^{-1} day^{-1}. The rituximab group received daily placebo cyclophosphamide. Treatment lasted six months. Both treatment groups received the same glucocorticoid regimen: one to three pulses of methylprednisolone (1 g) followed by oral prednisolone 1 mg kg^{-1} day^{-1}, tapered so that all patients who had achieved remission were withdrawn from prednisolone. Patients in the cyclophosphamide group who achieved remission were changed to oral azathioprine (2 mg kg^{-1} day^{-1}), and those in the rituximab group from placebo cyclophosphamide to placebo azathioprine.

Trial end points measured

RITUXVAS

The primary outcomes were remission and severe adverse events at 12 months (Figure 5.5). Remission was defined as an absence of clinical disease activity, as indicated by a BVAS score of 0 maintained for two months. Sustained remission was defined as a BVAS of 0 for at least six months. Relapse was defined as the recurrence or new appearance of any disease activity attributable to active vasculitis. Deaths and malignancies occurring after 12 months were also recorded.

RAVE

The primary end point was disease remission defined as BVAS-WG = 0, without prednisolone usage at six months. Relapse was defined as an increase in BVAS-WG of 1 point or more.

Follow-up

RITUXVAS

Patients were followed for 12 months.

RAVE

Patients were followed for six months.

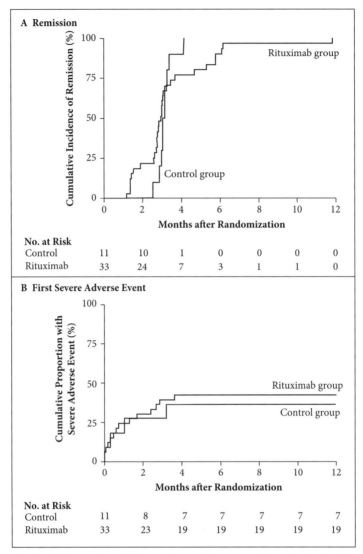

Fig. 5.5 Cumulative incidence of remission and cumulative proportion of patients with a severe adverse event. Panel A shows the time to remission. Remission time was the time at which a Birmingham Vasculitis Activity Score of 0 was first recorded. Data for patients who died were censored at the time of death. Panel B shows the time to the first severe adverse event.

From New England Journal of Medicine, Rachel B. Jones et al, Rituximab versus Cyclophosphamide in ANCA-Associated Renal Vasculitis, 363, Copyright © 2010 Massachusetts Medical Society. Reprinted with permission from Massachusetts Medical Society.

Results

RITUXVAS

Sustained remission occurred in 25/33 patients in the rituximab group (76%) and in 9/11 in the control group (82%). The absolute difference in sustained remission was −6 percentage points (95% CI, −33 to 21; P = 0.68). Six patients in the rituximab group and one in the control group died. Among the survivors, there was no difference in the t = rates of sustained remission (93% vs 90%, respectively). The median time to remission was 90 days in the RTX group and 94 days in the control group.

There was no difference in the rates of adverse events between the two groups. Rates of infection were similar in the RTX group and the control group (36% vs 27%, respectively).

RAVE

Baseline disease activity, organ involvement, and proportion of patients with relapsing disease were similar in the two groups. Sixty-three patients in the rituximab group (64%) and 52 (53%) in the control group achieved the primary end point. This met the predetermined criteria for non-inferiority (P < 0.001). For relapsing patients in the rituximab group, 34/51 patients (67%) achieved remission, as compared with 21/50 (42%) in the control group (P = 0.01). There were no significant differences between the treatment groups in adverse events.

Critique of the papers

Both papers reported that rituximab was effective in achieving remission but not superior to a conventional cyclophosphamide-based regimen. The follow-up in both papers was short (6 months in the RAVE trial, and 12 months in the RITUXVAS trial) and therefore no data was presented about either long-term adverse effects (such as infection or hypogammaglobulinaemia) or relapse rates. The rituximab-treated patients in the RITUX-VAS study did not receive any maintenance therapy.

Both studies used a rituximab regimen of 375 mg/m^2 weekly for four weeks, based on the regimen used to treat lymphoma patients, rather than the alternative of 1 g repeated once after two weeks, which is used to treat rheumatoid arthritis. The latter may be more convenient for patients and less costly. No data on cost effectiveness was presented.

The studies did not address maintenance with rituximab. There are several possible approaches such as retreat on clinical relapse, retreat on elevation of anti-neutrophil cytoplasmic antibody titre, or a programme of infusions, for example, every six months for two years; these approaches are being explored in several ongoing trials.

Significance and importance of the papers

These two papers reported the first randomized trials to show that B-cell depletion using rituximab was an effective treatment for AAV. Until then there had been a number of individual cases and case series suggesting efficacy. Cyclophosphamide is associated with significant long-term toxicity, much of which is cumulative and dose dependent; therefore, there is an urgent need to develop regimens which are as effective but less toxic. The observations reported in these studies provide a means by which cumulative cyclophosphamide doses may be further reduced. The observation in RAVE that rituximab was more effective than use of further cyclophosphamide in relapsing patients is particularly important as this is a group of patients at high risk of receiving high cumulative doses of cyclophosphamide. The use of rituximab in AAV has been incorporated into national guidelines [1].

There remain, however, a number of questions, in particular, regarding dosing; in a retrospective review of 65 patients, the two regimens for rituximab in AAV were compared and found to be of equal efficacy [2]. There was no difference in the duration of B-cell depletion or the therapeutic effect, despite the fact that the mean serum concentration after using the 'lymphoma regimen' is higher than that achieved with the 'RA regimen'. The latter results in a lower total dose of rituximab over a shorter period of time but is more convenient for patients and cheaper.

The RA regimen has advantages in term of cost and patient convenience and is quite widely used. Further, the optimum strategy to prevent relapses has not been defined. Data from an observational study suggested that a two-year, fixed-interval rituximab retreatment regimen was associated with a reduction in relapse rates during the retreatment period and a more prolonged period of remission during subsequent follow-up than a strategy based on retreatment at relapse [3]. In the absence of biomarkers that accurately predict relapse, routine rituximab retreatment may be an effective strategy for remission maintenance [3]. Recent data from the French MAINRITSAN trial indicate that repeat dosing at fixed intervals is associated with a lower relapse rate than conventional azathioprine therapy after 39 months of follow-up [4].

These two studies were influential in the introduction of rituximab into the routine treatment of AAV and have been adopted into national guidelines in several countries including the United Kingdom [1].

References

1 **Ntatsaki E, Carruthers D, Chakravarty K, et al**. BSR and BHPR guidelines for the management of adults with ANCA associated vasculitis. *Rheumatology* 2014;**53**(12):2306–9.

2 **Jones RB, Ferraro A, Chaudry A, et al**. A multicenter survey of rituximab therapy for refractory antineutrophil cytoplasmic antibody-associated vasculitis. *Arthritis Rheum* 2009;**60**(7):2156–68.

3 **Smith RB, Jones R, Guerry M, et al**. Rituximab for remission maintenance in relapsing ANCA-associated vasculitis. *Arthritis Rheum* 2012;**64**(11):3760–9.

4 **Terrier B, Pagnoux C, Karras A, et al**. Rituximab versus azathioprine for maintenance in antineutrophil cytoplasmic antibodies associated vasculitis: follow-up at 39 months. *Arthritis Rheum* 2013;**65**(Suppl 10):2783.

Chapter 6

Osteoarthritis

Iain Goff and Fraser Birrell

Introduction

The challenge in selecting ten landmark papers in osteoarthritis is as great for selecting the papers to leave out as for choosing those to include. We consulted widely, speaking with members of the British Society for Rheumatology Osteoarthritis Special Interest Group, which includes clinicians, allied health professionals, and biomechanicists, as well as with pure scientists. However, ultimately, the selection is our own and, in the finest tradition, we should like credit for papers that inspire the reader to share them with other, and accept personal responsibility for any striking omissions.

In particular, we would like to highlight that no genetic studies have been included. It may well turn out that certain studies like arcOGEN turn out to be landmarks [1]. However, at the time of writing, the loci identified have not yet led to practical biomarkers or the development of novel treatments. It is on a similar basis that seminal work on the identification of metalloproteinases by Tim Cawston and others has not been included, although if the editors had included a chapter on mechanistic understanding of all types of arthritis, this strand would have been hard to leave out.

There are other highly influential epidemiology studies, including very early comparisons between symptoms and structural changes, such as, for example the study by Lawrence et al. [2]. Careful reading of this study reveals an early appreciation that pain and structural changes are more strongly associated in OA than in RA, almost 50 years before this view became widely accepted.

Nick Bellamy should certainly be recognized for a highly systematic development and validation of a disease specific health status tool in WOMAC (e.g. [3]). But he and Michel Lesquesne have not made our top ten, as their work represents vital underpinning rather than discovery.

There was much enthusiasm for the inclusion of an injection study. However, we are aware that intra-articular injection of corticosteroid remains an underused option in clinical practice. Given our increasing understanding of the limited efficacy and toxicity of other treatment options, notably paracetamol, which is increasingly being correctly classified as a weak non-steroidal anti-inflammatory drug, injection may become a more core therapy in the future, in which case one or more of the injection studies may be seen as landmarks, especially if high-resolution musculoskeletal ultrasound is used to predict response to therapy in this context.

There are two other particular studies, which again with time might become landmarks, if they lead to licensed disease modifying therapy for OA. First is the SEKOIA trial [4], which provided the first widely accepted proof of concept for OA disease modification. Unfortunately, with respect to the development of strontium ranelate as a licensed therapy for OA, at the time of writing, a query has been raised about the cardiovascular risk of this agent. This concern is based on an excess of non-fatal MIs in an aggregate analysis of the Phase 3 trials for osteoporosis and has not been demonstrated in either SEKOIA or in postmarketing surveillance (in contrast to definite signals for the over-the-counter labelled agents paracetamol and diclofenac). Therefore, it is highly doubtful whether the manufacturer will seek an OA license. The other bone agent showing promise in knee OA is zoledronate. In a small 12-month study, there was an inconsistent improvement in both pain and bone marrow lesions at 6 months but not 12 months [5].. This suggests refinement of patient selection and/or treatment dose or frequency may lead to a therapy helping both symptoms and structural progression.

We are aware that there is a preponderance of papers in our selection pertaining to osteoarthritis of the knee. Rather than highlighting our biases, this is a genuine reflection of the body of evidence in osteoarthritis research. The knee has been the focus of so much research in part due to the prevalence of knee OA as a clinical problem but also because of the accessibility of this joint to performing clinical and radiographic assessment. A major assumption made in trying to generalize the results of these studies is therefore that OA of the knee is a suitable model for OA at other body sites; time will tell whether this assumption is reasonable.

References

1 **arcOGEN Consortium; arcOGEN Collaborators**. Identification of new susceptibility loci for osteoarthritis (arcOGEN): a genome-wide association study. *Lancet* 2012;**380**(9844):815–23.

2 **Lawrence JS, Bremner JM, Bier F**. Osteo-arthrosis: Prevalence in the population and relationship between symptoms and X-ray changes. *Ann Rheum Dis* 1966;**25**(1):1–24.

3 **Bellamy N, Buchanan WW, Goldsmith CH, et al**. Validation study of WOMAC: a health status instrument for measuring clinically important patient relevant outcomes to antirheumatic drug therapy in patients with osteoarthritis of the hip or knee. *J Rheumatol* 1988;**15**(12):1833–40.

4 **Reginster JY, Badurski J, Bellamy N, et al**. Efficacy and safety of strontium ranelate in the treatment of knee osteoarthritis: results of a double-blind, randomised placebo-controlled trial. *Ann Rheum Dis* 2013;**72**(2):179–86.

5 **Laslett LL, Doré DA, Quinn SJ, et al**. Zoledronic acid reduces knee pain and bone marrow lesions over 1 year: a randomised controlled trial. *Ann Rheum Dis* 2012;**71**(8):1322–8.

Paper 6.1: The first description of nodal osteoarthritis

Reference

Heberden, W. Commentaries on the history and cure of diseases. London: T. Payne; 1802.

Background

William Heberden the Elder was born in 1710 in Southwick, London, undergoing early schooling at St Saviour's Grammar School. His academic promise was spotted early and, when he was aged only 14, he was sent to study at St John's College, Cambridge. He was first awarded his MA before becoming a fellow of St John's College in 1731 and obtaining his MD in 1739. He worked as a physician in Cambridge for 10 years before going on to establish a large and fashionable practice in London, where he remained for the remainder of his career.

Heberden became one of the pre-eminent physicians of his era, renowned for his thorough clinical approach, but was also famously described by George Crabbe as 'tender, ardent and kind'. By the time of his death in 1801, he had lived through one of the most vibrant centuries of medical history. The eighteenth century saw the widespread adoption of the scientific method into medical practice, the invention of the stethoscope, the advent of vaccination, and the development of pathology, epidemiology, and public health as specialties.

Methods

Throughout his career, Heberden took meticulous notes and reflections on the clinical cases he encountered, recording them at the patients' bedsides in Latin in a pocketbook. Many of his observations were discussed at his annual series of public lectures on *materia medica* and which contained the enduring theme that the physician should always be guided by his own detailed observation of the patient. He continued this advice when helping to establish the Medical Transactions of the Royal College, a forum where physicians could share their observations of patients. After his death in 1801, Heberden's surviving son William Heberden Jr, also a successful physician, collected his father's reflections, translated them into English, and published them in two volumes (English and Latin) in 1802. At 483 pages long, the 'Commentaries' covers a wide range of topics but is particularly noted for the original description of angina pectoris and the differentiation of chickenpox as a separate disease from smallpox.

Results

At only 78 words long, *Digitorum nodi* (Chapter 28) is one of the shorter chapters in the book:

> What are those little hard knobs, about the size of a small pea, which are frequently seen upon the fingers, particularly a little below the top, near the joint? They have no connexion with the gout, being found in persons who never had it: they continue for life; and being hardly ever attended with pain, or disposed to become psoriasis, are rather unsightly and inconvenient, though they must be some little hindrance to the free use of fingers.

Critique of the paper

While descriptive and based on observation during his practice rather than on any formal trial design, this original question is important in its differentiation of osteoarthritis of the hand from the commonly encountered gout and the lack of association with psoriasis. The text describes the clinical features of osteophytes around the distal interphalangeal joints, as well as recognizing that established nodal hand OA is often associated with minimal pain.

Significance and importance of the paper

While OA is ubiquitous in animals with synovial joints and is identifiable in fossilized and mummified remains, it was not differentiated from other causes of musculoskeletal aches and pains by ancient or medieval medical practitioners. The significance of William Heberden's observation was the recognition of different disease processes affecting the joints and which behave differently and have other disease associations (e.g. the lack of psoriasis in nodal hand OA). Key to his work was the close clinical observation and meticulous attention to detail when recording his findings, and this is a message that clinical teachers continue to impart to this day. Though clinical observation was not a new concept, Heberden elevated it to the level of craft, which gained him international renown, and honorary membership of the Paris Royal Society of Medicine.

The impact of Heberden's description of the hands in OA is still evident in the ongoing use of the eponymous term 'Heberden's nodes', coined shortly after the publication of his 'Commentaries' and learned by clinicians worldwide. Along with his descriptions of other illnesses that most probably represent rheumatoid arthritis and complex regional pain syndrome, his detailed observations led to him being adopted as the patron of the Heberden Society, now the British Society for Rheumatology.

It could be argued that eponymous names are a sentimental sign of respect for a dead colleague; however, William Heberden was an ardent educator throughout his career in medicine, and a medical leader lauded by his peers. Although the papers he published while alive did not have the same enduring impact as his posthumous 'Commentaries on the history and cure of diseases', his example of detailed clinical examination and note keeping, combined with his compassionate treatment of patients, make him thoroughly deserving of historical acclaim.

Paper 6.2: Arthroplasty of the hip

Reference

Charnley J. Arthroplasty of the hip. A new operation. *Lancet* 1961;277(7187):1129–32.

Purpose

To describe short-term results from a novel hip replacement procedure.

Patients

The study examines three groups of patients with 'gross disablement': those with rheumatoid arthritis, patients over 65 with severe OA, and middle-aged patients with severe bilateral OA.

Study design

The report describes an unblinded, uncontrolled observational study of a new surgical procedure.

Treatment

Charnley describes the three key features of his hip arthroplasty operation that set it apart from the others of its day: thus use of a small-headed metallic femoral prosthesis, the technique of cementing the prosthesis into the femoral canal, and the technique of articulating the prosthesis with a thick, polytetrafluoroethylene acetabular cup.

Trial end points measured

The trial end points included reduction in pain, range of movement, and mortality/morbidity. Charnley also remarks on the mechanical durability of the prostheses as indicated by radiographs.

Follow-up

Open-label follow-up for up to one year was described.

Results

Immediate post-operative results were positive, with patients reporting early pain relief. They spent three weeks in a splint and were allowed to fully weight bear at five weeks; the average hospital stay was eight weeks.

There was one death in the follow-up group at one year, due to a coronary event six weeks post-surgery. The only other serious side effect reported was DVT, although Charnley did not report how often this occurred. There were instances of post-operative infection, although again the number was not made clear. All but one of these were in what he described as 'difficult salvage cases', where previous attempts at arthroplasty procedures had taken place.

In terms of pain relief and function, the results of this unblinded and uncontrolled study appear impressive. At three weeks post-operation, upon removal of their splints, most patients were able to execute a straight leg raise and had no pain or muscular spasm on passive hip movement. While those with the most restriction in range of movement pre-operatively remained restricted (up to 30 degrees), these movements were pain-free.

With regard to the durability of the prostheses, radiographs at one year post-surgery showed negligible, if any, wear, despite patients having been fully weight bearing for ten months at this point. There were no reports of loosening of the femoral prosthesis.

Critique of the paper

This is not the type of robust clinical trial that would be required for publication in *The Lancet* today. The details of the outcomes of the surgical procedure are not consistent, although it is not dissimilar to other papers of the era. When looking back, it seems a shame that a comparative trial of different procedures/prostheses (or even sham surgery) was not considered, especially in light of the results from later, well-controlled trials of surgery, such as that conducted in 2002 by Moseley et al. (see Paper 6.8) [1]. However, we must judge Charnley by the standards of the day: he must be recognized for his innovation and commitment to publish and share surgical outcome data—a tradition now continued by the National Joint Registry.

Significance and importance of the paper

The earliest attempts at curing OA of the hip surgically simply involved excision of part or all of the joint material and were developed based on the practice already in use of joint excision as an alternative to amputation of a limb. Henry Park and Percival Pott, working at the Royal Infirmary in Liverpool, had described the 'cure by means of Callus', in which damaged joints were excised and the subsequent ankylosis led to an inflexible but stable and functional limb.

Anthony White (1782–1849) of the Westminster Hospital in London is credited with the first excision arthroplasty of the hip in 1821, although he did not publish the results of his procedure. Like the previously described joint excisions, this procedure relieved pain and facilitated mobility, although in the early stages this was at the expense of stability, which only came much later when a fibro-cartilaginous union developed and, in some cases, complete ankylosis.

The subsequent evolution of hip arthroplasty involved the interposition between the femoral head and the acetabulum of various materials, including fascia lata, pig's bladder, and gold foil, all of which had variable success. It was not until 1891 that the true birth of arthroplasty occurred, with Professor Themistocles Gluck replacing the femoral head of a patient with one crafted from ivory. Though this did not turn out to be the right material to choose, the race was on in earnest to refine the procedure.

By the time John Charnley was practising, there were two hip replacement procedures which had become established, although both had well-known flaws. The Smith–Peterson method involved placing a loose-fitting metal cup over the femoral head, which had been reduced in size and where the acetabulum had been enlarged by removal of the eburnated lining. The loose-fitting nature of the prosthesis meant that the hip was not as stable as a native joint, although over time the gaps did fill with fibrous material. While this improved stability, it tended to lead to a significant degree of stiffness and loss of function.

The Judet joint on the other hand used a hemispherical femoral prosthesis that was secured in place by driving the attached spike down the stump of the femoral neck. The acetabulum was widened to be just large enough to accept the prosthesis but there was no other alteration made. This led to a joint that was stable very early post-surgery but at the

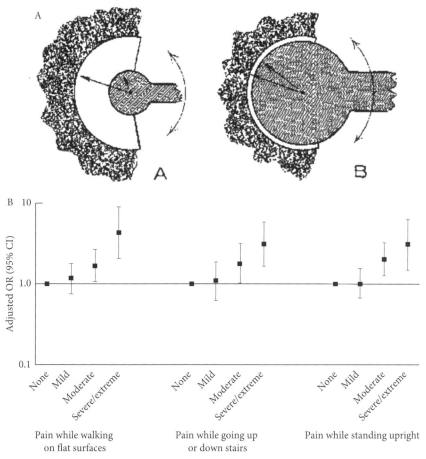

Fig. 6.1 A. Illustrating how rotation of the socket against the bone is less likely with a small head and thick socket than with a large head and thin socket as a result of differences in the moment of the frictional force as a result of differences in radii of the parts. B. Odd of radiographic knee osteoarthritis for individual pain items on the Western Ontario and McMaster Universities score.

expense of increased frictional forces within the joint. Judet joints were notorious for their squeaking noises, a sign of high friction between the femoral prosthesis and the acetabulum, although the squeak was not present when normal articular cartilage remained (e.g. in procedures performed for sub-capital femoral neck fractures). This increased friction led to accelerated wear of the joint and was also known to cause the bond between the femoral spike and the surrounding bone to break, allowing the prosthesis to rotate. These problems acted as a catalyst for an ongoing search for lower-friction materials that could be used instead.

It should be noted that Charnley had to do early revision procedures on the first 200 or so patients who had his prosthesis, as the medium-term data did show high wear and failure rates within two to three years, and a harder polyethylene had to be used.

The use of a metallic femoral prosthesis articulating with a high-density plastic acetabular implant remains the standard today. The practice of cementing the femoral prosthesis into the shaft of the femur to allow earlier mobilization, reduce infection rates, and prevent loosening in the long term continues today. Finally, the use of a small-headed femoral prosthesis, the mechanics of which Charnley eloquently explained in this paper, is still the most common design for prosthetic femoral implants (Figure 6.1). He even took pains to explain why large-headed femoral implants would be likely to lead to increased wear rates, a lesson so dramatically illustrated in recent controversy over large-head, metal-on-metal hip replacements, which have been associated with an increased appearance of ectopic bone and higher failure rates.

The technique of hip replacement surgery developed and refined by Charnley remains essentially unchanged to this day, making this one of the landmarks in the management of osteoarthritis, one which has stood the test of time.

Reference

1 Moseley JB, O'Malley K, Petersen NJ, et al. A controlled trial of arthroscopic surgery for osteoarthritis of the knee. *N Engl J Med* 2002;**347**(2):81–8.

Paper 6.3: Prevalence of symptoms and structural changes of osteoarthritis in the population

Reference

Kellgren JH, Lawrence JS. Osteoarthrosis and disc degeneration in an urban population. *Ann Rheum Dis* 1958;17(4):388–97.

Purpose

To describe the prevalence of symptoms and signs of osteoarthritis and correlate clinical osteoarthritis with radiographic and serologic markers.

Patients

Patients were diagnosed on clinical grounds. All had active and progressive disease and had received glucocorticoids with significant toxicity.

Study design

This is a cross-sectional epidemiological study with a random selection of the population in the Lancashire town of Leigh, where Kellgren and Lawrence had previously conducted an epidemiologic study of rheumatic complaints in the adult population in 1949–1950. One in ten of the population aged 55–64 years was approached to take part in the study and had been identified from those who had been in the 50–59-year age group in the previous study five years earlier.

Methods

Participants were subjected to a thorough clinical examination, radiographs of their hands, feet, knees, pelvis, cervical spine, and lumbar spine were taken, and blood was drawn for the sheep cell agglutination test.

Preliminary approaches were taken by conducting house-to-house visits, where an explanation of the study took place and an initial examination of the hands was performed, along with questioning about past and present rheumatic complaints and any disability. Participants were then invited to attend a special examination centre, where a much more detailed questionnaire was completed, and a thorough physical examination, radiographs, and blood tests were performed. For each physical sign (e.g. tendon nodules, Heberden's nodes, etc.) the examiner would comment on it either being absent or present in doubtful, slight, or severe degree. A similar approach was taken to the overall clinical grading of OA at each joint, and examiners were also asked to comment on the personality type of each individual (normal, neurotic, or psychotic).

Follow-up

There was no follow-up as part of this study.

Results

Two hundred and four men and 277 women were approached to take part in the study; of these, 173 men and 207 women attended the clinical assessment centre and had radiographs taken. The prevalence of radiographic osteoarthritis (Kellgren–Lawrence grade 2 or above) at any site X-rayed was 83% in men and 88% in women. Assuming no OA in the group who declined X-rays, the prevalence in the whole population sampled was 70% for men and 66% for women; the true value was likely to have been somewhere between these figures (70%–83% men, 66%–88% women). While any site OA was similar between males and females, disc degeneration was more common in men (69%–83%) than in women (53%–73%).

The observations previously made of associations between OA and previous joint injury, occupation, and obesity were all found to be statistically significant. There was a previously unseen observation of an association between obesity and OA of the DIP joints of the fingers (Figure 6.2), suggesting a metabolic component to this particular pattern of arthritis.

Critique of the paper

The use of radiographs in a true population cohort is the key defining feature of this study. This approach allowed the investigators to confirm several assertions, which were previously only tentative. These include the observation that when it is present, OA tends to affect multiple joints; the association of OA with injury, occupation, and obesity; and the distinctive pattern of OA joint involvement, particularly in women.

In confirming assertions made in previous research, this study does raise questions that have gone on to further our understanding of OA at a molecular level. For example, the increased incidence of DIP involvement in obesity, together with the female pattern of joint distribution in obese men, suggests a metabolic and hormonal influence on the phenotype of OA in individuals. While the results of this study in an industrial Lancashire town cannot necessarily be extrapolated to all regions, it is important for its systematic approach to the epidemiological study of OA in the population.

Significance and importance of the paper

At the time this paper was published, a significant number of observations had already been made describing the nature and range of presentations of OA. [1–3] The radiographic and pathologic features of osteophytosis, cartilage loss, subchondral sclerosis, and cyst formation had been described by various authors, and the first atlas of the radiographic features of OA had been published [4]. It had been observed that primary generalized OA was a distinct clinical entity, with an association with the female sex, and a posited genetic contribution. It was also known that obesity played a role in the development of OA, and that previous joint injury was a predisposing factor.

This study was significant for being random-population based rather than limited to patients presenting with musculoskeletal symptomatology. Prior epidemiological studies

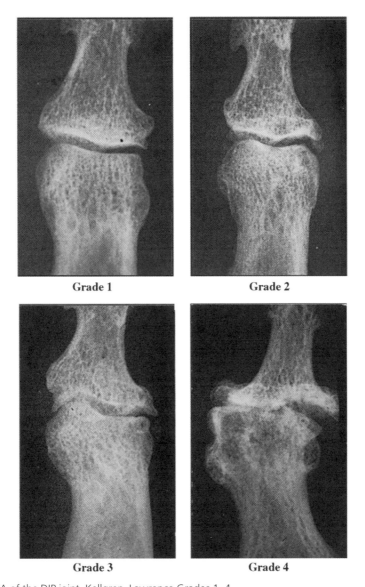

Grade 1   Grade 2

Grade 3   Grade 4

Fig. 6.2 OA of the DIP joint, Kellgren–Lawrence Grades 1–4.
Reprinted from The Lancet, Vol. 277, John Charnley, ARTHROPLASTY OF THE HIP A New Operation, 1129–1132, Copyright (1961), with permission from Elsevier.

of OA relied on self-reported symptoms, and clinical examination. This was the first population study to correlate self-reported symptoms with both clinical examination and imaging, allowing both confirmation of the presence of radiographic disease and grading of severity. Additionally, the authors set out to understand the pathophysiology of OA by correlating its presence with a range of possible influences such as weight, occupation, and previous joint injury.

References

1 Hanlon CR, Estes WL Jr. Osteo-arthritis aggravated by trauma. *Am J Surg* 1949;**78**(5):556–69.

2 Kellgren JH, Moore R. Generalized osteoarthritis and Heberden's nodes. *Br Med J* 1952;**1**(4751):181–7.

3 Kellgren JH, Lawrence JS. Radiological assessment of osteo-arthrosis. *Ann Rheum Dis* 1957;**16**(4):494–502.

4 Kellgren JH, Lawrence JS. The epidemiology of chronic rheumatism. Atlas of standard radiographs of arthritis. Oxford: Blackwell Scientific Publications; 1963.

Paper 6.4: Effect of age on the prevalence of osteoarthritis

Reference

Felson DT, Naimark A, Anderson J, et al. The prevalence of knee osteoarthritis in the elderly. The Framingham Osteoarthritis Study. *Arthritis Rheum* 1987;30(8):914–18.

Purpose

To investigate whether the prevalence and severity of OA continued to increase in the elderly, or if once present it remained stable.

Patients

The sampling frame was the Framingham study: a large, prospective, longitudinal cohort study that was designed to identify the factors associated with the presence and development of arteriosclerotic and hypertensive disease. The plan was to recruit 6,000 participants aged 30–59, following them up every two years for a period of 20 years to gather a range of data associated with cardiovascular disease. In 1948, with the backing of the United States Public Health Service, data collection began in the town of Framingham, Massachusetts, USA. While recruitment targets were short of their original aspirations, the cohort did prove to be stable enough to allow researchers to begin studying other diseases within the group. In 1983–1985, the eighteenth biennial follow-up period, Felson et al. used the study cohort to investigate the prevalence of osteoarthritis of the knee in the elderly population.

Study design

This paper describes an observational cohort study in a defined population sample unselected for the presence of knee pain or radiographic change.

Methods

A medical history, clinical examination of the knees, and radiographs of both knees were obtained. The medical history included questions about whether subjects had ever had pain in or around the knee on most days over a one-month period, while the physical examination was conducted by the Framingham study physicians.

Antero-posterior standing radiographs of both knees were obtained and were read by an experienced musculoskeletal radiologist who was blinded to the participants' ages and assigned a Kellgren–Lawrence grade (0–4), which was based on the presence and size of osteophytes, joint space narrowing, subchondral sclerosis, and subchondral cysts, to each knee (Figure 6.3). A grade of ≥2 was used as the definition of prevalent OA. To minimize any drift in scoring of the films, they were scored by the same reader on two occasions, one month apart. A second researcher also scored the entire dataset, to ensure that the results were robust; both inter- and intra-rater reliability were excellent (Figure 6.4).

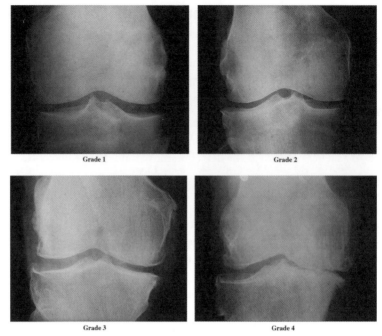

Fig. 6.3 OA of the knee, Grades 1–4.

Reproduced from Felson DT, Naimark A, Anderson J, Kazis L, Castelli W, Meenan RF, The prevalence of knee osteoarthritis in the elderly. The Framingham Osteoarthritis Study. Arthritis and Rheumatism. 1987;30(8):914–8 with permission from Wiley.

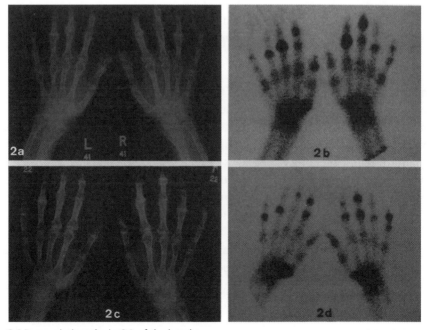

Fig. 6.4 Bone scintigraphy in OA of the hand.

Follow-up

This study did not include follow-up as it examined outcomes at a single time point.

Results

A total of 1,805 subjects were recruited to participate, of which 1,424 (78.9%) attended for radiographs to be taken (59% female and 41% male). The majority of those not attending were unable to because of mobility problems, although comparison of the groups showed similar percentages complaining of knee pain. The non-radiograph group were older and more likely to be female, reflecting the demographic of those in care homes.

In the study population as a whole, there was a highly statistically significant ($P < 0.001$), age-associated, increase in the prevalence of OA, and this increase remained when the cut-off grade for radiographic OA was increased to Grade 3 and above, and when analysed in 5-year age groupings. Twenty-seven per cent of those aged 65–69 had radiographic OA versus 51% in those over 85 years. Analysis according to gender showed that in women there was an age-associated increase in the prevalence of OA, though this trend was non-significant in men.

There was no significant difference between men and women in the prevalence of OA, although women were more likely to have symptomatic OA (11.4% vs 6.8%, $P = 0.003$). Symptoms were found in both groups to be more prevalent with the increasing grade of OA, although on the dichotomous measure that they used only 40% of those with Grade 3–4 radiographic changes and who had had knee pain on most days of the preceding month.

Critique of the paper

This is a robust epidemiological study on a true population sample, providing novel data, but no epidemiological study is perfect. While the authors comment on the fact that even in participants with higher grades of OA the majority denied frequent pain, the use of a single question with a dichotomous answer is unlikely to capture the true symptom burden of those with OA. Subsequent studies have looked at the subject of symptoms and severity of OA in much greater detail. The study was also limited, as a large group of potential participants were excluded because of their poor mobility. While it is argued that this group could have either more or less OA, the fact that they are significantly older suggests that they are likely to have more pathologic change than the group who attended for radiographs. It is likely, therefore, that Felson's observed rates of OA are actually an underestimate of the true prevalence.

Significance and importance of the paper

This study demonstrated that not only does the prevalence of osteoarthritis increase with age but the severity of osteoarthritis increases through the age bands as well. The finding suggests that cartilage degradation and bony change are ongoing processes, which are associated with the ageing process. At the time, this was a major advance in the understanding of OA, showing that, rather than being a dichotomous disease which is either present or absent, it is a continuous process of cartilage degradation and subchondral bone adaptation.

A second significant finding of this study was the link between increasing presence of symptoms and increasing radiographic severity of OA. Although a single yes–no question was used about the presence of pain on most days in the preceding month, there was a clear stepwise increase in those answering 'yes' with each radiographic increment. As one would expect, recent reports of associations between cardiovascular outcomes, knee osteoarthritis, and hip osteoarthritis have also been shown for the hand in the Framingham cohort (Haugen et al, 2103), which has been so pivotal in our understanding of both cardiovascular risk factors and osteoarthritis prevalence [1, 2].

References

1 Nüesch E, Dieppe P, Reichenbach S, et al. All cause and disease specific mortality in patients with knee or hip osteoarthritis: population based cohort study. *BMJ* 2011;**342**:d1165.
2 Haugen IK, Ramachandran VS, Misra D, et al. Hand osteoarthritis in relation to mortality and incidence of cardiovascular disease: data from the Framingham Heart Study. *Ann Rheum Dis* 2013;**74**(1):74–81.

Paper 6.5: Predicting progression of osteoarthritis using imaging

Reference

Dieppe P, Cushnaghan J, Young P, et al. Prediction of the progression of joint space narrowing in OA of the knee by bone scintigraphy. *Ann Rheum Dis* 1993;52(8):557–63.

Purpose

To determine if subchondral bone activity as determined by scintigraphy could be used to predict disease progression in osteoarthritis of the knee.

Patients

One hundred patients with knee pain and radiographically proven osteoarthritis affecting at least one knee were involved in this study.

Study design

This is an observational cohort study of patients with knee pain and proven osteoarthritis. Radiographs and bone scintigraphy at baseline and follow-up were scored by blinded observers to determine the severity of radiographic change, and the presence and pattern of scintigraphic activity.

Methods

Participants had PA and lateral radiographs of the knees, scored for individual radiographic features of osteoarthritis. Gamma camera images at 3–5 minutes and 3–4 hours post injection of technetium-99m were recorded and scored for both the presence of bone uptake and, if present, the pattern of uptake.

Clinical data such as the duration and severity of symptoms, clinical features of crepitus, bony swelling, soft tissue swelling, and disability were estimated based upon walking distance and the need for walking aids.

Progression of osteoarthritis was defined as either the need for joint replacement surgery, or a tibio-femoral joint space loss of greater than 2 mm.

Follow-up

Participants were followed for five years.

Results

Ninety-four patients were recruited to the study; of these, 66% had medial compartment osteoarthritis, 41% had lateral compartment osteoarthritis, and 71% had patella–femoral osteoarthritis. The 65 women and 29 men had a mean (SD) age of 64.2 (11.6) years at study entry in 1986, and a mean BMI of 26.2 (5.1), with 27% classed as obese (BMI >30). Tri-compartmental radiographic change was present in 44 (23%) of knees, while the remainder had one (26 (14%)) or two compartments (44 (23%)) affected.

Seventy-five patients completed follow-up; of these, 15 progressed in the five-year study duration to the point of needing total knee replacement. Of the remainder, the symptoms were evenly spread between being worse (34 knees), the same (42 knees), or better than before (41 knees).

Positive bone scintigraphy at baseline was found to be predictive of knees that subsequently progressed to either joint replacement or radiographic joint space narrowing. Some form of radiographic deterioration was seen in 60% of those with positive scintigraphy at baseline, and all those who met the study criteria for progression had positive scintigraphs. While the positive predictive value of scintigraphy was relatively low at 39%, it had a negative predictive value of 100%, with no patients having negative scintigraphy progressing to radiographic progression.

Critique of the paper

A key criticism of this paper is the use of total knee replacement as an outcome measure. The justification for joint replacement surgery is principally for pain relief, which is a very subjective measure. While patients with worse joint damage are more likely to have pain, this study is not large enough to ensure differences in pain tolerance and perception did not skew the data. Equally subjective is the potential variation in the interpretation of bone scintigraph images, which can be influenced by minor alterations in positioning of joints. Despite these criticisms, every effort was taken to blind assessors to the symptoms and clinical features of each patient and also to the order in which radiographs were taken.

Significance and importance of the paper

This is the first paper to demonstrate that increases in the metabolic activity of subchondral bone are predictive of progression of osteoarthritis. Importantly, it also shows that the absence of subchondral bone activity indicates a low (zero) probability of progression in this cohort. While previous research had shown that scintigraphy could predict disease progression in nodal osteoarthritis of the hand [1, 2], it did not discriminate between activity in subchondral bone and synovium. By looking at the pattern of technetium-99m uptake in the knees of these participants, this study sheds light on the pathogenesis of osteoarthritis by demonstrating metabolic activity of the bone as being integral to disease progression, an insight that has now been elucidated considerably by MRI studies of bone marrow lesions.

While bone scintigraphy will never be the investigation of choice for population prediction of OA progression due to its variable reliability and high radiation dose, the study established the principle that progression in OA can be predicted. This is valuable information for future research into both pathogenesis and treatments.

References

1 Hutton CW, Higgs ER, Jacobson PC, et al. 99mTc HMDP bone scanning in generalised arthritis. II. The four hour bone scan image predicts radiographic change. *Ann Rheum Dis* 1986;**45**(8): 622–6.

2 Macfarlane DG, Buckland Wright JC, Emery P, et al. Comparison of clinical, radionuclide, and radiographic features of osteoarthritis of the hands. *Ann Rheum Dis* 1991;**50**(9):623–6.

Paper 6.6: Aerobic exercise and resistance exercise versus an education programme in knee osteoarthritis

Reference

Ettinger WH, Burns R, Messier SP, et al. A randomized trial comparing aerobic exercise and resistance exercise with a health education program in older adults with knee osteoarthritis: the Fitness Arthritis and Seniors Trial (FAST). *JAMA* 1997;277(1):25–31.

Purpose

To compare the effects of two types of exercise (aerobic and resistance) with a control group, over an 18-month period, in a group of over-60s with knee OA.

Patients

Advertisement of the study took place via the local media, local physicians, community mailings, and telephone calls. Those responding to the initial advert were questioned via telephone about their knee pain and were invited to have knee radiographs taken. Participants were aged over 60 years, had knee pain on most days, had radiographic evidence of OA, and had some form of functional limitation. Recruitment took place over a 15-month period from May 1992.

Study design

The report described a two-centre, three-arm, single-blind, randomized controlled study of two exercise interventions versus a health education programme.

Treatment

Subjects were randomized to one of three study arms: an aerobic exercise programme, a resistance exercise programme, or a health education programme (control group). Each intervention arm received an exercise plan which required aerobic or resistance training to take place three times per week. Following a three-week supervised induction and a three-month initial training period, participants were discharged to complete the remainder of the study as a home-based exercise programme. The control group received three 90-minute education sessions consisting of video material regarding osteoarthritis and exercise, a question and answer session about the topic, and printed material to take home. Telephone follow-up took place once every three weeks, and the total number of contacts with the study team was the same in both the intervention and control groups.

Trial end points measured

A range of baseline data was collected from all study groups, including a disability questionnaire, a graded treadmill test, strength testing, timed functional measures, and a pain questionnaire. These measures were repeated at 3, 6, and 18 months from commencement of the study, by assessors who were blinded to the participants' study arm.

Follow-up

Participants were followed for 18 months.

Results

Of 4,575 potential participants screened, 1,164 were found to have knee OA, and 439 met criteria for inclusion and were randomized to one of the three study arms. There were no significant differences between the groups for baseline data or study completion rates.

Compliance rates with exercise were found to be the same in both intervention groups, with an overall compliance of 68% in the aerobic group and 70% in the resistance group. There was a decline in compliance over time in both intervention groups: 85% at 3 months, 70% at 9 months, and 50% at 18 months.

Both intervention groups saw statistically significant improvements in the primary study outcome measure of disability (10% for aerobic and 8% for resistance exercise), although the aerobic exercise group showed improvements in more of the disability sub-scores. The exercise groups also showed improvements in a range of other parameters: the aerobic group showed improvements in pain, all performance measures, VO_2 max, and knee flexion strength, whereas the resistance group showed improvements in pain, in all performance measures except stair climb, and in knee flexion strength. There was no difference in X-ray progression between any of the intervention and control arms.

Subgroup analysis showed that the beneficial effects of exercise were seen in both sexes, in different racial groups, and in high-risk groups such as the elderly (over 70 years) and obese participants. Analysis of the participants' exercise diaries showed that there was a clear dose-response effect, with increasing amounts of exercise being associated with greater improvements in pain scores, disability, and six-minute walk distance.

Critique of the paper

This was the first robust study to confirm the beneficial effects of exercise on patients suffering pain due to OA of the knee. While the benefits were modest, it must be taken into account that the exercise regimens were themselves very gentle, with the emphasis being on consistent participation rather than vigorous exertion. Despite this, there was a clear improvement with increased exercise exposure, and the true potential for exercise to improve symptoms was not discovered by this study. At some point the benefits of increasing exercise levels may be outweighed by increased injury rates and reduced compliance; however, the principle of exercise helping with OA was confirmed in this paper.

While this study would appear to be particularly prone to selection bias, with more motivated participants entering the study, subgroup analysis seemed to show that all subgroups were able to benefit from the interventions. In fact it could be argued that the control group were not truly representative of the normal population, as they too received education on the health benefits of exercise and were given regular telephone support. As a consequence, this study may actually underestimate the effects of exercise on symptoms and disability in OA; however, this problem is inherent in pragmatic studies like this, which cannot be blinded or have a true placebo arm.

Significance and importance of the paper

It is now generally accepted that moderate cardiovascular exercise on a regular basis is beneficial to long-term health through multifactorial mechanisms. At the time this paper was published, the American College of Rheumatology had published guidelines advocating exercise as one of the mainstays of management of OA of the knee; however, this recommendation was based upon studies which were both small and short term. There was no robust evidence to support this recommendation, and questions remained over the potential for exercise to cause additional deterioration in joints which were already damaged.

This study set out to address questions concerning the safety and acceptability of exercise as a treatment for osteoarthritis of the knee, along with answering the fundamental question of its efficacy for improving pain and disability in patients with knee OA. What types of exercise are most beneficial—aerobic or resistance? Will older people comply with a prescribed exercise programme? Are there benefits other than those physically measured—is there psychosocial improvement? Is long-term exercise harmful to people with OA of the knee? The principal aim of this study was to compare the effects of two types of exercise (aerobic and resistance) with a control group, over an 18-month period, in a group of over-60s with knee OA.

In showing longer term efficacy of exercise, without any detrimental effect on progression, this was one of the more influential studies in determining that exercise should be a core component of managing the symptoms of osteoarthritis.

Paper 6.7: Glucosamine sulphate for symptoms and progression of knee osteoarthritis

Reference

Reginster JY, Deroisy R, Rovati, et al. Long-term effects of glucosamine sulphate on osteoarthritis progression: a randomised, placebo-controlled clinical trial. *Lancet* 2001; 357(9252):251–6.

Purpose

To investigate the efficacy of glucosamine sulphate in symptoms and radiographic progression in knee osteoarthritis.

Patients

Patients over 50 years of age with primary knee OA (Kellgren–Lawrence grade ≥2) were recruited via the outpatient clinic of the University Hospital Centre, Liege, Belgium.

Study design

A double-blind, randomized, placebo-controlled trial of glucosamine sulphate for the treatment of OA of the knee was used.

Treatment

Treatment comprised administration of a glucosamine sulphate oral powder (Rottapharm) or a placebo, at a dose of 1,500 mg daily.

Trial end points measured

Primary outcome measures included structural (median and minimal joint space widths in the medial compartment) and symptomatic (WOMAC score) components, with secondary outcome measures including withdrawal from the study, the use of rescue medication, adverse drug reactions, and abnormalities of blood parameters, including blood glucose. These were recorded at baseline and yearly for three years, with intention-to-treat analysis used in order to minimize the impact of patients who withdrew from the study.

Follow-up

The study included a three-year blinded follow-up. An unblinded extension analysis looking at rates of knee arthroplasty in the original treatment groups was been published separately [1].

Results

Based upon a power calculation requiring 60 patients per group (80% power, 5% significance; estimated 40% dropout), a total of 212 patients were randomized.

The demographics between the recruited groups was similar (age, sex, and BMI), with both having mild-to-moderate radiographic OA and with no significant differences in symptoms or medication intake. A total of 139 patients completed the study (71 placebo and 68 glucosamine), with both groups reporting a similar intake of study drug (>70% intake in 81% vs 91%; non-significant).

Median joint space width (JSW) of the medial compartment of the knee was measured by digital analysis of radiographs and showed significant differences between the study groups. Intention-to-treat analysis demonstrated a change in median JSW of −0.31 mm in the placebo group and −0.06 mm in the active drug group (P = 0.043; difference = 0.24 mm). Minimum JSW showed similar differences, with changes of −0.4 mm in the placebo group versus −0.07 mm in the glucosamine group (P = 0.003). The reductions in both median JSW and minimal JSW from baseline were statistically significant in the placebo group but not in the active drug group.

Analysis of the WOMAC scores demonstrated a deterioration of 9.8% in the symptoms of those participants taking placebo but an improvement of 11.7% in the symptom score in the glucosamine group (P = 0.02). These changes applied to both the pain and function aspects of the WOMAC score, although there were non-significant differences in the stiffness subscale (Figure 6.5).

From a safety point of view, there was little difference between the study groups. Most participants took a rescue medication during the study, on average once every six days.

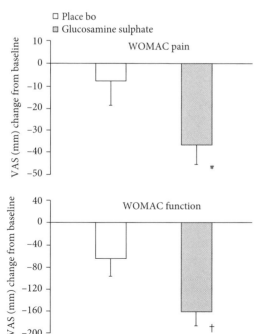

Fig. 6.5 Intention-to-treat mean (SE) sum of VAS change subscales after 3 years. Upper: WOMAC pain Lower: WOMAC physical function. *p=0.047; †p=0.020. VAS=visual analogue scale. Reprinted from The Lancet, Vol. 357, Jean Yves Reginster et al, Long-term effects of glucosamine sulphate on osteoarthritis progression: a randomised, placebo-controlled clinical trial, 251–256, Copyright (2001), with permission from Elsevier.

Similarly, most reported at least one adverse drug side effect (93% in placebo group; 94% in glucosamine group), the majority of which were transient, and mild to moderate in severity. Markers of metabolic activity, including plasma glucose concentration, showed no significant difference between study groups.

Critique of the paper

This was the first study to show evidence of OA being a disease that is modifiable by the use of oral medication. The authors used a range of validated measures, including digital JSW measurement, minimal JSW, and WOMAC, to characterize the changes between placebo and treatment groups, and found glucosamine sulphate to be superior in all primary outcome measures. While this study only looked at the knee joint and thus cannot be extrapolated to all joints, the results hold potential promise for similar improvements in other weight-bearing joints.

However, there have been major criticisms made of this study. These include the agent not having a plausible mechanism of action or achieving sufficient concentrations in vivo; the primary analysis being based on mean JSW; possible confounding by analgesia of radiographic outcomes (as a standard frame was not used to achieve a reproducible knee position); lack of correlation between changes in structure and changes in function in those receiving active treatment; the data being too homogenous to have occurred in a genuine study; lack of independent replication—the only replication study being funded by the same company [2], whereas non-industry funded studies have been negative for symptoms and structure outcomes [3].

Significance and importance of the paper

While this paper is one of the most controversial ever published, it is fair that it be regarded as a landmark. Despite OA being the commonest form of arthritis in the population, the management of it has revolved around symptom control with medications along with surgery when required. While research into the inflammatory arthritides has led to the development of small molecule, and subsequently biologic, DMARDs capable of inducing disease remission, there has been no such breakthrough in OA. This paper was the first study published in a high impact, peer-reviewed journal to show evidence that OA is a modifiable disease in which both symptoms and progression can be improved by patients taking an oral preparation. It has certainly stimulated great interest, and debate and refutation of hypotheses and studies is a fundamental part of the scientific process.

References

1 **Bruyere O, Pavelka K, Rovati LC, et al**. Total joint replacement after glucosamine sulphate treatment in knee osteoarthritis: results of a mean 8-year observation of patients from two previous 3-year, randomised, placebo-controlled trials. *Osteoarthritis Cartilage* 2008;**16**(2):254–60.

2 **Pavelká K, Gatterová J, Olejarová M, et al**. Glucosamine sulfate use and delay of progression of knee osteoarthritis: a 3-year, randomized, placebo-controlled, double-blind study. *Arch Intern Med* 2002;**162**(18):2113–23.

3 **McAlindon TE, Bannuru RR, Sullivan MC, et al**. OARSI guidelines for the non-surgical management of knee osteoarthritis. *Osteoarthritis Cartilage* 2014;**22**(3):363–88.

Paper 6.8: Arthroscopy versus sham arthroscopy in knee osteoarthritis

Reference

Moseley JB, O'Malley K, Petersen NJ, et al. A controlled trial of arthroscopic surgery for osteoarthritis of the knee. *N Engl J Med* 2002;347(2):81–8.

Purpose

To investigate the efficacy in knee osteoarthritis of arthroscopic lavage, and arthroscopic lavage plus debridement.

Patients

One hundred and eighty secondary-care patients were referred to the Department of Orthopaedics at the Veterans Affairs Medical Center in Houston. Subjects were eligible if they had knee OA according to American College of Rheumatology criteria and had moderate pain (>4/10). One hundred and sixty-five patients completed the trial.

Study design

The study comprised a three-arm, sham-controlled, randomized, double-blind trial of surgical intervention for knee osteoarthritis.

Treatment

Treatment comprised arthroscopic lavage, arthroscopic lavage plus debridement, or a 'placebo procedure' (sham arthroscopy).

Trial end points measured

Outcomes included the pain and function scales from AIMS-2 and from the SF-36. The authors developed their own 12-item self-reported 'Knee- Specific Pain Scale' and 'Physical Functioning Scale'; the latter included the time (in seconds) that a patient required to walk 30 m/100 ft and to climb up and down a flight of stairs as quickly as possible.

Follow-up

At all review time points up to two years, data were collected by personnel unaware of the intervention assigned, and subjects were asked which treatment they thought they had received.

Results

The authors report 'at no point did either of the intervention groups report less pain or better function than the placebo group' and

the 95 percent confidence intervals for the differences between the placebo group and the intervention groups exclude any clinically meaningful difference. ... For example, mean (±SD) scores on the Knee-Specific Pain Scale (range, 0 to 100, with higher scores indicating more severe pain) were similar in the placebo, lavage, and débridement groups: 48.9 ± 21.9, 54.8 ± 19.8, and 51.7 ± 22.4.

Critique of the paper

This is a beautiful study, as robust as one can hope for given the challenges of conducting research in osteoarthritis and especially for a surgical intervention. Consent included agreeing that 'On entering this study, I realize that I may receive only placebo surgery. I further realize that this means that I will not have surgery on my knee joint. This placebo surgery will not benefit my knee arthritis.' Randomization was stratified based on severity, in blocks of six, into the three groups. Every consideration was given to the possibility of unblinding: subjects undergoing the sham procedure were still put to sleep with intravenous tranquillizer, they had three 1 cm skin incisions consistent with arthroscopy, and the surgeon not only asked for instruments and manipulated the knee but even splashed saline to simulate the sound of lavage; in addition, subjects that had undergone the sham procedure were given post-op care that was identical to that given to subjects that had undergone the actual procedure. Unblinding was also assessed at every time point: the sham group were no more likely than the two active arms to identify they were in the sham group (e.g. 13.8% vs 13.2% at week 2).

Significance and importance of the paper

The earlier discussion of the Charnley paper on hip arthroplasty (see Paper 6.2) highlighted the weaknesses of uncontrolled interventional studies; nevertheless, it is still common for healthcare professionals to say that it is 'unethical' to do a randomized controlled trial of surgical interventions. In fact, this remarkable study from the Veterans Affairs Medical Center in Houston demonstrates that it is not only possible to conduct robustly blinded studies in this setting but that it is unethical not to. The authors highlight that, at the time of the study, 650,000 knee lavage or debridement procedures per year were being performed in the USA, at a cost of $3.25 billion. They state that the physiological basis for the relief of pain was unclear and that there had been a lack of controlled studies prior to this one.

This study is definitely a landmark. By showing that it is both possible and necessary to perform well-controlled, long-term follow-up studies in surgery, it has changed the landscape of surgical research forever. Given the 1.6% incidence of complications after knee arthroscopy and the rate of 650,000 procedures per annum prior to this study [1], it is likely that this study has prevented 10,400 complications per annum and over 50 deaths per annum in the USA alone.

Reference

1 **Martin CT, Pugely AJ, Gao Y, et al**. Risk factors for thirty-day morbidity and mortality following knee arthroscopy: a review of 12,271 patients from the national surgical quality improvement program database. *J Bone Joint Surg Am* 2013;**95**(14):e98.

Paper 6.9: Association of pain and radiographic change

Reference

Duncan R, Peat G, Thomas E, et al. Symptoms and radiographic osteoarthritis: not as discordant as they are made out to be? *Ann Rheum Dis* 2007;66(1):86–91.

Purpose

To answer the question 'does radiographic osteoarthritis occur more frequently in those with severe or persistent pain compared with those with mild or intermittent pain?' In doing so, the hope was to demonstrate a link between severity of pain and degree of disability with radiographic changes of OA.

Patients

Three general practices in North Staffordshire, UK, were approached, and all patients over the age of 50 years were sent a short survey asking whether they had experienced knee pain in the preceding 12 months. If knee pain was reported, patients were invited to a research clinic, at which a range of investigations were performed.

Study design

The report describes a prospective observational cross-sectional study of patients with knee pain and who were from the general population.

Methods

Patients were interviewed about their pain, examined, had digital photographs and radiographs taken, had anthropometry conducted, and were given a self-completion questionnaire. This paper is part of a larger study and only reports on some of these measures.

The specific radiographic views collected in this study were postero-anterior standing semi-flexed, lateral supine semi-flexed, and skyline. Radiographic OA was deemed to be present if the Kellgren–Lawrence grade was ≥2 on any of the views taken. While lateral knee views were not included in the original KL grading scale, the presence of posterior osteophytes was scored in the same manner as on PA views.

The severity of knee pain, stiffness, and disability was measured using the 24-item Western Ontario and McMaster Universities (WOMAC) Osteoarthritis Index; each item had five response options (none, mild, moderate, severe, and extreme). The total subscale scores for pain (5 items, total score 0–20), stiffness (2 items, total score 0–8), and disability (17 items, total score 0–68) could be totalled or analysed separately. The team also conducted interviews to assess not only the severity of pain experienced but also the frequency and persistence.

Results

Between August 2002 and September 2003, 819 people attended the clinical assessment centre; of these, 745 were eligible to be included in the study (407 women, 338 men; mean age 65.2 (SD 8.6) years; mean BMI 29.6 (SD 5.2)). A total of 509 (68.3%) participants had radiographic evidence of OA: combined tibio-femoral and patello-femoral OA, 40.4%; isolated patello-femoral OA, 23.9%; and isolated tibio-femoral OA, 4.0%.

Radiographic OA was most common in those with a long history of knee pain, or a high level of pain and disability, with an odds ratio of 2.8 (CI 1.4–5.6) between those in the reference group and those with persistent, high-intensity pain. There was a statistically significant association between increasing severity of symptoms and higher radiographic grades of OA, and this association remained upon adjusting for age and sex. There were significant associations between all of the WOMAC pain items and the higher radiographic grades and, although stiffness and function did not meet statistical significance, the trend was towards an association.

Critique of the paper

This paper tackled the long-held myth in osteoarthritis that there is no association between the presence of pain and the presence of radiographic change. The authors did this by carefully analysing the methodological deficiencies of previous studies and designing a study to eliminate the flaws. Without needing for complex statistical or epidemiological techniques, they elegantly demonstrated that there is a strong association between pain and structural change in a true cross-sectional population study. While the results they presented for knee pain cannot be assumed to be representative of OA at all body sites, their approach to investigating the presence of radiographic disease sets an example to future researchers in the field.

Significance and importance of the paper

For many years, there was a documented discordance between the presence of radiographic osteoarthritis in a joint and patient's reports of pain (e.g. [1–3]). The reasons for this discrepancy were hotly debated but the assertion was particularly based upon the presence of knee pain in those with no radiographic evidence of OA. Research into this issue looked at factors such as depression and poor quadriceps strength as possible confounders and overlooked the fact that there are non-OA causes of knee pain.

Duncan et al. reviewed the literature, with a particular focus on the methodology of the previous studies, and found three factors which may have skewed the results towards there being no association between pain and radiographic change. First, previous studies had a tendency to dichotomize pain as being present or absent rather than grading it according to severity. Second, the radiographic analysis of the knee joint had been incomplete, omitting views of the patello-femoral joint and not looking at lateral views of the tibio-femoral joint. Finally, the studies had not been adjusted for biopsychosocial factors, on the false assumption that these had no relation to the disease progression.

Although there have been other papers since to address this issue, and careful re-examination of the data presented in original population studies (e.g. [4]) confirms there is a stronger association between pain and structural change in osteoarthritis than in rheumatoid arthritis, this paper was pivotal in changing the prevailing paradigm.

References

1 **Cobb S, Merchant WR, Rubin T**. The relation of symptoms to osteoarthritis. *J Chronic Dis* 1957;**5**(2):197–204.

2 **Cicuttini FM, Baker J, Hart DJ, et al**. Association of pain with radiological changes in different compartments and views of the knee joint. *Osteoarthritis Cartilage* 1996;**4**(2):143–7.

3 **Hannan MT, Felson DT, Pincus T**. Analysis of discordance between radiographic change and knee pain in osteoarthritis of the knee. *J Rheumatol* 2000;**27**(6):1513–7.

4 **Lawrence JS, Bremner JM, Bier F**. Osteo-arthrosis. Prevalence in the population and relationship between symptoms and x-ray changes. *Ann Rheum Dis* 1966 **25**(1):1–24.

Paper 6.10: Efficacy and toxicity of paracetamol

Reference

Doherty M, Hawkey C, Goulder M, et al. A randomised controlled trial of ibuprofen, paracetamol or a combination tablet of ibuprofen/paracetamol in community-derived people with knee pain. *Ann Rheum Dis* 2011;70(9):1534–41.

Purpose

To investigate the efficacy and safety of paracetamol and ibuprofen, alone and in combination, in knee osteoarthritis.

Patients

The study involved participants aged >40 years with knee pain 30–80 mm on 100 mm VAS and who were recruited via several routes, including by postal questionnaire, by local advertisements, and by general practitioners.

Study design

This report describes a randomized, double-blind, four-arm, active controlled study which lasted for a duration of three months.

Treatment

Treatment comprised the administration three times per day of two blinded capsules which delivered doses of ibuprofen 400 mg tds, paracetamol 1 g tds, ibuprofen 200 mg + paracetamol 500 mg tds, or ibuprofen 400 mg/paracetamol 1 g tds.

Trial end points measured

The primary outcome measures for this study were short-term change in the pain subscale of WOMAC at day 10, and longer-term change in symptom control, measured on a five-point ordinal scale at 13 weeks. The primary safety end point was the incidence of moderate and severe adverse events reported during the study period.

Follow-up

The study included a three-month follow-up.

Results

For this study, 892 participants were recruited from eight recruiting centres and randomly assigned to one of the four treatment arms. Groups were well balanced, with a mean age of 60.6 years, and were 51% male. After formal grading, radiographic osteoarthritis (Kellgren–Lawrence grade ≥2) was identified in 559 (63%) of participants, and 758 (85%) participants fulfilled the ACR criteria for clinical diagnosis of knee osteoarthritis.

Six hundred and fifteen participants completed the 13-week study, with a similar number of withdrawals across three of the groups but a higher number in the paracetamol arm. At day 10, there were significantly more responders taking two combination tablets versus paracetamol (P = 0.0063). At the study end point, the percentage of responders was 55.5% for two combination tablets, 57.7% for one combination tablet, 52.8% for ibuprofen, and 49.1% for paracetamol.

In terms of primary outcome measures, the higher-dose combination medication was superior to paracetamol for pain, stiffness, and function at day 10 and week 13, and superior to paracetamol, ibuprofen, and low-dose combination for functional scores at week 13. The low-dose combination medication was superior to paracetamol for pain at week 13.

In terms of safety, there were 18 serious adverse events through the study, 3 of which were felt to be treatment related. As a combined group, moderate and serious adverse events were relatively common, occurring at a rate of 1.1 per patient day. The most frequently encountered of these were gastrointestinal disturbances, including diarrhoea, dyspepsia, nausea, and abnormalities of liver function. When comparing groups, the high-dose combination medication had significantly more side effects than ibuprofen (51% vs 42% of patients) but other group comparisons were non-significant.

Haemoglobin concentrations showed reductions in all groups at day 10, which became more prevalent through the study to week 13. A reduction of 1 g/dl was observed in the paracetamol group of 7.3% at day 10, and 23% at week 13; 11.3% and 19.6%, respectively, in the ibuprofen group; 10.8% and 24.1%, respectively in the low-dose combination group; and 17.5% and 38.4%, respectively, in the high-dose combination group. Larger haemoglobin reductions were significantly more likely in the combination-tablet groups, with 2 g/dl reductions of 1.8% seen in the low-dose combination group, and 6.9% seen in the high-dose combination group (vs 0.9% for both paracetamol and ibuprofen monotherapy). Rises in platelet count and reduced MCV levels were felt to indicate GI blood loss as the cause of the haemoglobin reduction.

Critique of the paper

This study enrolled people in the community with knee pain rather than selecting for patients who presented with OA knee; nonetheless, 85% of the patients met the criteria for a clinical diagnosis of knee osteoarthritis, so the results are generalizable to both those with knee pain taking over-the-counter medication and those with diagnosed OA. The landmark findings of this study concern the effects of combining non-prescription doses of over-the-counter medicines. The investigators showed that a combination of paracetamol and ibuprofen in a dose of 1 g paracetamol:400 mg ibuprofen three times daily gave some of the best outcomes in terms of pain and function (although not better than ibuprofen 400 mg tds alone) but that this came at a cost.

The gastrointestinal toxicity of NSAIDs has been known for a long time and a range of therapeutic options, including the use of COX-2 inhibitors, addition of a PPI, and switching to paracetamol as an alternative, have been tried to negate this toxicity. This study demonstrates that the risk of haemoglobin reduction with paracetamol monotherapy was similar to that with ibuprofen 400 mg tds but that paracetamol was not as effective as an analgesic as ibuprofen.

It also shows, worryingly, that the use of combinations of ibuprofen and paracetamol increased haemoglobin reduction synergistically, despite not delivering a significant improvement in analgesia when compared to ibuprofen alone.

Significance and importance of the paper

The spectrum of rheumatic disease seen and managed in secondary care in the UK is influenced by the excellent primary care services available in the NHS and which work as gatekeepers to specialist services. Patients requiring specialist treatment for OA tend to have more severe pain, increased functional impairment, and more advanced radiographic changes than the background population. Patients in secondary care have formed the basis for much of the OA research performed in the past but they do not necessarily represent the general population. The vast majority of patients with joint pains (with or without proven OA), are managed in primary care and a significant proportion (28%–33%) self-manage using a range of strategies, including non-prescription medications [1–3].

The recommendation from NICE for paracetamol as the first-line oral analgesic for osteoarthritis was based on the modest efficacy data but perceived safety of this agent [4]. This study has robustly demonstrated equivalent toxicity of paracetamol as monotherapy compared to low-dose ibuprofen, lower efficacy than low-dose ibuprofen and synergistic toxicity in combination without increased analgesic effect. Given these and our increased understanding that paracetamol should be correctly classified as a non-steroidal anti-inflammatory with all of the other toxicities in observational studies one would expect, including cardiovascular events, hypertension and renal impairment, it is increasingly clear that paracetamol no longer has a key role in the management of osteoarthritis and should be avoided completely in combination with other NSAIDs. The key question for the MHRA must be whether diclofenac, which was made available over the counter in 2009 when its cardiovascular risk profile was already being recognized, and paracetamol should continue to be available without prescription.

References

1 **Dieppe P, Basler HD, Chard J, et al**. Knee replacement surgery for osteoarthritis: effectiveness, practice variations, indications and possible determinants of utilization. *Rheumatology* 1999;**38**(1):73–83.

2 **Peat G, McCarney R, Croft P**. Knee pain and osteoarthritis in older adults: a review of community burden and current use of primary health care. *Ann Rheum Dis* 2001;**60**(2):91–7.

3 **Jinks C, Jordan K, Ong BN, et al**. A brief screening tool for knee pain in primary care (KNEST). 2. Results from a survey in the general population aged 50 and over. *Rheumatology* 2004;**43**(1):55–61.

4 **National Institute for Health and Care Excellence**. Osteoarthritis: the care and management of osteoarthritis in adults. <http://www.nice.org.uk/guidance/CG59>, accessed 26 January 2015.

Chapter 7

Gout and crystal arthropathies

Lorna Clarson and Edward Roddy

Introduction

Gouty arthritis was first described by Hippocrates in the fifth century BC as the 'arthritis of the rich', although archaeologists identified deposits of uric acid in the joints of mummified Egyptians dating back approximately 4,000 years. The term gout, from the Latin 'gutta' (meaning drop) originated from the belief that health and disease arose from the balance between the four bodily humours (black bile, yellow bile, blood, and phlegm), gout being caused by humours falling to the affected body part causing inflammation and swelling [1]. The Greek word *podagra* or 'foot-grabber' refers to the predilection of gout for the foot and dates back to the second century AD [2].

It was not until the 1800s that Sir Alfred Garrod differentiated gouty arthritis using the presence of serum hyperuricaemia and later suggested that hyperuricaemia could be controlled by limiting dietary intake of purines [3, 4].

Treatment for acute gout with colchicine, extracted from autumn crocus, was thought to have been in use from the sixth century AD; however, prophylactic treatments for gout were much later in their evolution. Salicylates were used as uricosurics in the 1800s; however, the high doses required to induce this effect rendered their use impractical and they were replaced by other uricosuric drugs such as probenecid, sulfinpyrazone, and benzbromarone [5]. These were superseded by allopurinol, the first xanthine oxidase inhibitor, in the 1960s, with the only widely available alternative to allopurinol, febuxostat, not introduced until 2005. Work continues with interleukin receptor antagonists, and uricase treatments, but these are not yet in common usage [6, 7].

Deposition of calcium pyrophosphate (CPP) crystals (CPPD) is a common age-related phenomenon. CPP crystals were first identified in synovial fluid aspirated from the acutely inflamed knees of patients with radiographic chondrocalcinosis (CC), leading to the use of the term 'pseudogout' because of its clinical similarity to acute gout [8]. A number of clinical syndromes associated with CPPD such as 'pseudo-rheumatoid arthritis', 'pseudo-osteoarthritis' (with or without inflammation), and 'pseudo-neuropathic' arthritis were then described, in addition to 'lanthanic' (asymptomatic) radiographic CC [9]. Pyrophosphate arthropathy referred to the coexistence of CPPD with structural osteoarthritis. It is not known whether these syndromes are truly clinically distinct subsets and, as a result, the European League Against Rheumatism proposed a new terminology in 2011 [10]. In this simplified nomenclature, CPPD is used as an umbrella term for all instances of CPP crystals, CC refers to cartilage calcification of any cause, acute CPP crystal arthritis replaces acute pseuodogout, and osteoarthritis with CPPD refers to concurrence of CPPD in a joint with structural changes of osteoarthritis (previously 'pyrophosphate arthropathy'), whether symptomatic or asymptomatic.

These papers were selected because they report findings which made a substantial contribution to either our understanding or management of crystal arthropathies.

The first three papers focus on novel discoveries in the pathogenesis of crystal arthropathies. These include the first description of negatively birefringent monosodium urate (MSU) crystals in both the synovial fluid and tophi of patients with gout [11], and the techniques which subsequently allowed the same authors to identify CPP crystals [8]. This discovery, using polarized light microscopy, established gout as a crystal-induced arthritis and provided a reliable technique for diagnosis of the condition. Following this is the first description of the mechanism underlying the renal urate transporter (URAT1), a urate–anion exchanger regulating blood urate levels, and the site of action of uricosuric drugs, providing important insights into urate homeostasis and a target for the potential development of new drugs against hyperuricaemia [12]. The final paper focusing on pathogenesis, describes the NALP3 inflammasome, an intracellular receptor through which crystals stimulate the activation of interleukin-1β and thus trigger inflammation and joint synovitis in gout and CPPD [13]. Increased understanding of the mechanism underlying crystal-induced inflammation via the inflammasome has led to interest in treating crystal-induced inflammation with IL-1 antagonists.

The next papers report two of the most important epidemiological studies investigating associations with gout. The first reports findings from the Health Professionals Follow-up Study, a large longitudinal study which prospectively followed male health professionals in the US and investigated the association between dietary intake and incident gout. Although suspicion of dietary influences on risk of gout can be traced back as far as Hippocrates, there was little epidemiological evidence underpinning these associations, and this and subsequent papers from this study have provided important insights into the aetiology of gout [14]. The second paper reports results from a large prospective cohort, nested within the Framingham study. It was the first paper to identify increased incidence of cardiovascular disease in patients with gout, reawakening clinical and academic interest in long-term adverse health outcomes associated with gout [15].

The next three papers describe important findings in the treatment of gout. The discovery of the xanthine oxidase inhibitor allopurinol, amongst other drugs, was rewarded with a Nobel prize for two of the authors, Elion and Hitching. The paper chosen is the first to describe the clinical results of long-term allopurinol therapy in the treatment of gout [16]. The discovery of this drug revolutionized the experience of patients with gout by providing what has become the most commonly prescribed urate-lowering medication to this day [17]. The next paper reports a trial comparing the efficacy of allopurinol with a new xanthine oxidase inhibitor, febuxostat, offering evidence to inform choice of therapy in patients with gout [18]. The third paper demonstrated that gout could be considered a 'curable' condition, since patients' burden of both urate crystals and frequency of flares of acute gout could be reduced by maintaining serum urate (SUA) levels below 6 mg/dl (360 μmol/l) [19], a target adopted into national and international guidance on the management of gout [20, 21].

The final two papers focus on important research specific to CPPD. The first explored both the pathogenesis and heritability of CPPD, identifying the ankylosis human multipass transmembrane protein (ANKH) gene, which encodes a membrane inorganic pyrophosphate transport channel, and demonstrated that an *ANKH* mutation increases extracellular inorganic pyrophosphate and predisposes to the formation of CPP crystals [22]. The final paper provides the first detailed examination of the clinical and radiological features of CPPD, along with predisposing factors and associations [23].

In our opinion, all of these papers have irrevocably changed the way that we understand and manage crystal-related arthropathies, and their findings are still applied in practice, either directly or indirectly today.

References

1 **Copeman WSC**. A short history of the gout and the rheumatic diseases. Los Angeles: University of California Press; 1964.

2 **Porter R, Rousseau GS**. *Gout: the patrician malady*. New Haven and London: Yale University Press; 1998.

3 **Garrod AB**. Observations on certain pathological conditions of the blood and urine, in gout, rheumatism, and Bright's disease. *Med Chir Trans* 1848;**31**:83.

4 **Garrod AB**. A treatise on gout and rheumatic gout (rheumatoid arthritis), 3rd edn. London: Longman Green; 1876.

5 **Yu TF, Gutman AB**. Study of the paradoxical effect of salicylate in low, intermediate and high dosage on the renal mechanisms of excretion of urate in man. *J Clin Invest* 1959;**38**(8):1298–315.

6 **So A, De Smedt T, Revaz S, et al**. A pilot study of IL-1 inhibition by anakinra in acute gout. *Arthritis Res Ther* 2007;**9**(2):R28.

7 **Pui CH**. Rasburicase: a potent uricolytic agent. *Expert Opin Pharmacother* 2002;**3**(4):433–42.

8 **Hollander JL, Jessar RA, McCarty DJ**. Synovianalysis: an aid in arthritis diagnosis. *Bull Rheum Dis* 1961;**12**:263–4.

9 **McCarty DJ**. Calcium pyrophosphate dihydrate crystal deposition disease—1975. *Arthritis Rheum* 1976;**19**(Suppl 3):275–85.

10 **Zhang W, Doherty M, Bardin T, et al**. European League Against Rheumatism recommendations for calcium pyrophosphate deposition. Part I: terminology and diagnosis. *Ann Rheum Dis* 2011;**70**(4):563–70.

11 **McCarty DJ, Hollander JL**. Identification of urate crystals in gouty synovial fluid. *Ann Intern Med* 1961;**54**(3):452–60.

12 **Enomoto A, Kimura H, Chairoungdua A, et al**. Molecular identification of a renal urate anion exchanger that regulates blood urate levels. *Nature* 2002; **417**(6887):447–52.

13 **Martinon F, Petrilli V, Mayor A, et al**. Gout-associated uric acid crystals activate the NALP3 inflammasome. *Nature* 2006;**440**(7081):237–41.

14 **Choi HK, Atkinson K, Karlson EW, et al**. Purine-rich foods, dairy and protein intake, and the risk of gout in men. *N Engl J Med* 2004;**350**(11):1093–103.

15 **Abbott RD, Brand FN, Kannel WB, et al.** Gout and coronary heart disease: the Framingham Study. *J Clin Epidemiol* 1988;**41**(3):237–42.

16 **Rundles RW, Metz EN, Silberman HR.** Allopurinol in the treatment of gout. *Ann Intern Med* 1966;**64**(2):229–57.

17 **Annemans L, Spaepen E, Gaskin M, et al.** Gout in the UK and Germany: prevalence, comorbidities and management in general practice 2000–5. *Ann Rheum Dis* 2008;**67**(7):960–6.

18 **Becker MA, Schumacher HR Jr, Wortmann RL, et al.** Febuxostat compared with allopurinol in patients with hyperuricemia and gout. *N Eng J Med* 2005;**353**(23):2450–61.

19 **Li-Yu J, Clayburne G, Sieck M, et al.** Treatment of chronic gout. Can we determine when urate stores are depleted enough to prevent attacks of gout? *J Rheumatol* 2001;**28**(3):577–80.

20 **Zhang W, Doherty M, Pascual E, et al.** EULAR Standing Committee for International Clinical Studies Including Therapeutics. EULAR evidence based recommendations for gout. Part II: Management. Report of a task force of the Standing Committee for International Clinical Studies Including Therapeutics (ESCISIT). *Ann Rheum Dis* 2006;**65**(10):1312–24.

21 **Khanna D, Fitzgerald JD, Khanna PP, et al.** 2012 American College of Rheumatology guidelines for management of gout. Part 1: systematic non-pharmacologic and pharmacologic therapeutic approaches to hyperuricemia. *Arthritis Care Res* 2012;**64**(10):1431–46.

22 **Pendleton A, Johnson MD, Hughes A, et al.** Mutations in *ANKH* cause chondrocalcinosis. *Am J Hum Genetics* 2002;**71**(4):933–40.

23 **Dieppe PA, Alexander GJM, Jones HE, et al.** Pyrophosphate arthropathy: a clinical and radiological study of 105 cases. *Ann Rheum Dis* 1982;**41**(4):371–6.

Paper 7.1: Identification of urate crystals in gouty synovial fluid

Reference

McCarty DJ, Hollander JL. Identification of urate crystals in gouty synovial fluid. *Ann Intern Med* 1961;54(3):452–60.

Purpose

Crystals had been noted in the synovial fluid of patients with gout in earlier reports; however, these findings were believed to be infrequent and of little diagnostic importance to the clinician. The aim of this investigation was to determine the frequency of occurrence of crystals in the synovial fluid of patients with gout and to demonstrate that these crystals were composed of urate.

Patients

Eighteen patients presenting to a rheumatology clinic with clinically diagnosed or suspected gout underwent arthrocentesis.

Study design

This was an open observational study.

Methods

Synovial fluid was examined using both ordinary light microscopy (OLM) and polarized light microscopy (PLM) at magnifications of 100×, 250×, and 500× for the presence of crystals. For both OLM and PLM, a drop of fluid was placed directly on to a glass slide from the aspirating syringe without a coverslip. PLM uses a polarizing light filter to squeeze light into a single plain before passing it through the synovial fluid. The light is then examined through a second filter. Light slows as it passes through crystals, is split into different planes (birefringent—two planes) by the atoms within their structures, and refracts with an angle proportional to its change in velocity. On leaving the crystal, the light accelerates back to the same speed but the waves are unsynchronized since they have travelled at different speeds through the crystal. Thus, when they pass through the second polarizing filter and are combined back into one plane, they produce new wavelengths and associated colours which are individual to particular crystals.

The composition of the crystals was investigated using a uricase digestion test, as follows: up to 0.5 ml of synovial fluid was combined with uricase diluted 1:10 in saline, using a ratio of one part uricase to five parts joint fluid, and then incubated in a waterbath at 45°C for four hours. A random drop of this solution was then examined under PLM for the presence of crystals.

Results

The knee was the most frequently aspirated joint (n = 10), followed by the first metatarsophalangeal joint (n = 6), and the elbow and pre-patellar bursa in the two remaining patients.

Aspiration was undertaken during an acute attack of gout in nine patients, after an acute attack had settled but while joint effusion persisted in six, and from chronic tophaceous joints in three.

Crystals were identified in the synovial fluid of 13 patients by OLM (all 4 patients with chronic tophaceous gout and 9 of the 14 non-tophaceous patients) and 15 patients by PLM (all 4 with tophaceous gout, and 11 with non-tophaceous gout). Eight of the nine patients experiencing an acute attack had crystals in their synovial fluid identified by PLM.

PLM demonstrated that the crystals found in both synovial fluid and tophi, although morphologically different, were both negatively birefringent. Negatively birefringent crystals were not seen in synovial fluid aspirated from the joints of patients with rheumatoid, osteoarthritis, traumatic arthritis, or asymptomatic hyperuricaemia. The addition of PLM increased accurate detection of crystals from 61% using OLM alone, with both false positives and false negatives, to 83%.

The uricase digestion test was applied to all 15 samples which contained crystals identified by PLM. Crystals were destroyed in all 15 of these samples after exposure to the uricase, confirming them to be composed of MSU. However, crystals were also destroyed in two control samples diluted with saline and heated to 45°C in the waterbath but not exposed to uricase.

Critique of the paper

This was a small but well-designed study, and although synovial fluid for only 18 patients with suspected gout was analysed, this analysis was exhaustive, not only identifying the presence of crystals in the synovial fluid of patients with gout but their absence in patients with non-crystal-related arthritis and asymptomatic hyperuricaemia, and their composition of MSU. These findings and the comparison of both ordinary and polarizing light microscopy in order to improve reliable identification of MSU crystals made a convincing case for the diagnostic significance of MSU crystals in synovial fluid, one which remains unrefuted.

Significance and importance of the paper

This paper demonstrated that negatively birefringent MSU crystals are frequently present in synovial fluid aspirated from the joints of patients with gout. Such crystals were not present in synovial fluid from patients with rheumatoid arthritis, osteoarthritis, traumatic arthritis, or asymptomatic hyperuricaemia. The authors suggested that identification of negatively birefringent crystals in synovial fluid has the same diagnostic significance as finding a tophus and proposed that aspiration of gouty joints with microscopic examination of synovial fluid for crystals, by PLM if possible, should become a standard diagnostic procedure. Identification of crystals in synovial fluid by PLM went on to become, and still remains, the gold standard diagnostic test for gout [1].

Interestingly, crystals were seen by OLM in fluid obtained from two patients who had been thought to have otherwise typical acute gouty arthritis; these crystals were not birefringent on PLM and not digested by uricase. The authors presciently suggested that these individuals might have a hitherto unrecognized metabolic abnormality mimicking acute gout and subsequently identified CPP crystals in synovial fluid obtained from acutely inflamed knees of patients with radiographic CC [2].

This is the first report confirming that negatively birefringent MSU crystals are present in both the synovial fluid and tophi of patients with gout and that they should be considered important in the diagnosis and pathogenesis of the disease. Furthermore, similar techniques were used to allow Hollander and McCarty to first describe CPP crystals in the literature. This paper provided insight into the pathogenesis of both gout and CPPD.

References

1 **Hollander JL, Jessar RA, McCarty DJ**. Synovianalysis: an aid in arthritis diagnosis. *Bull Rheum Dis* 1961;**12**:263–4.

2 **Zhang W, Doherty M, Pascual E, et al**. EULAR Standing Committee for International Clinical Studies Including Therapeutics. EULAR evidence based recommendations for gout. Part I: Diagnosis. Report of a task force of the Standing Committee for International Clinical Studies Including Therapeutics (ESCISIT). *Ann Rheum Dis* 2006;**65**(10):1301–11.

Paper 7.2: Molecular identification of a renal urate anion exchanger that regulates blood urate levels

Reference

Enomoto A, Kimura H, Chairoungdua A, et al. Molecular identification of a renal urate anion exchanger that regulates blood urate levels. *Nature* 2002;417(6887):447–52.

Purpose

To investigate the molecular basis of human renal handling of urate.

Methods

Since urate exists primarily as a weak acid within the body, it was thought likely that the structure of any urate transporter would be similar to that of other organic anion transporters (OATs). The OAT system of the proximal tubules of the human kidney is known to play an important role in the elimination of an assortment of potential toxins and are thought to be the final part of an active transport system whereby a Na^+ gradient drives the uptake of α-ketoglutarate (an intermediary in the Krebs cycle, and a nitrogen transporter), which is exchanged for various organic anions specific to individual OATs [1]. For this reason, DNA sequences similar to those of the genes for known human OATs were identified from the human genome database, and a sequence similar to that for the OAT4 transporter (an apical anion/dicarboxylate exchanger found in renal proximal tubules) was found. The structure of this gene (*SLC22A12*) was predicted, and the complementary DNA (named *URAT1* and composed of 2,642 base pairs) was isolated from human kidney RNA using rapid amplification techniques.

Immunohistochemical analysis and high-magnification microscopy was used to investigate the precise site of the URAT1 protein in the human kidney. Western blot analysis (using protein-specific antibodies to detect the presence of particular membrane proteins) was also used to test affinity for an anti-URAT1 antibody in the human kidney.

URAT1 complementary RNA was then injected into Xenopus oocytes, and time-dependent transport of ^{14}C-labelled urate, along with the transport of typical substrates of known anion and cation transporters across this new transporter, was measured. The mode of transport of urate across the newly identified URAT1 transporter was investigated by a series of substitution experiments measuring urate transport via URAT1 in the presence or absence of extracellular sodium, potassium, and chloride ions and in differing pH environments. Potential inhibitors of URAT1-mediated urate uptake, such as the organic anions lactate, nicotinate, and succinate, and drugs such as uricosurics, and diuretics, were also investigated using similar techniques.

The final investigation reported in this paper attempted to link URAT1 with urate transport in humans with idiopathic renal hypouricaemia, a rare disorder linked to a defect in the renal tubular transport of uric acid resulting in increased excretion of uric acid, by injecting a portion of mutated cRNA into oocytes and measuring urate transport activity.

Results

The predicted amino acid sequence of URAT1 shared 42% similarity with that of OAT4 (an apical anion/dicarboxylate exchanger found in renal proximal tubules). The hydropathy plot identified 12 membrane-spanning clusters of hydrophobic amino acids consistent with transmembrane proteins, similar to other OATs.

Immunohistochemical analysis showed URAT1 to be present in epithelial cells of the proximal tubules in the renal cortex but high-magnification microscopy revealed that URAT1 was only present in the luminal membrane of the epithelium of the proximal tubules and not found in the distal tubules. Western blot analysis revealed affinity for an anti-URAT1 antibody in the human kidney.

When *URAT1*-complementary RNA was injected into Xenopus oocytes, although time-dependent transport of ^{14}C-labelled urate across this transporter could be demonstrated, transport of various other substrates typical of other organic anion or cation transporters could not. This, in combination with the location of URAT1 in the proximal epithelial cells of the human kidney, suggested that URAT1 is the mechanism by which extracellular urate is reabsorbed from the tubular lumen to the intracellular cytosol and occurs at the level of the proximal tubule.

URAT1-specific transport of urate was measured in the presence or absence of extracellular sodium, potassium, and chloride ions. Although efflux of inorganic halide ions was stimulated by extracellular urate, demonstrating an exchange mechanism for urate, this was not thought to be the mode of urate transport across URAT1 as in other OATs. Similarly, intracellular and extracellular pH did not influence urate transport across URAT1, in contrast to urate transporters identified from other animals.

URAT1-mediated transport of urate was selectively inhibited by the presence of organic anions such as lactate, nicotinate, and succinate. Aromatic monocarboxylates (e.g. nicotinate) were more effective in the inhibition of URAT1-mediated urate uptake than aliphatic monocarboxylates (e.g. lactate) but, unlike other OATs, URAT1 was not inhibited by para-aminohippurate, demonstrating no role for this particular compound in urate homeostasis. URAT1-mediated urate uptake was also inhibited by diuretics and known uricosuric drugs, including probenecid, benzbromarone, sulfinpyrazone, phenylbutazone, indomethacin, and losartan, with benzbromarone the most potent inhibitor.

Intracellularly loaded anions such as lactate and nicotinate strongly stimulated urate uptake, with the most powerful being pyrazinecarboxylic acid (PZA), an active metabolite of the anti-tuberculosis drug pyrazinamide, already known to alter renal urate clearance. The effect of intracellularly loaded NaCl and KCl was statistically significant but much less than that of PZA, suggesting that organic anions were the major counteranion in the URAT1-mediated exchange of urate rather than inorganic anions such as chloride. A stimulatory effect of anions relevant to the human renal proximal tubule, particularly intracellularly preloaded sodium nicotinate, on URAT1-mediated urate uptake, was shown, as was efflux of nicotinate via URAT1 stimulated by extracellular urate. Thus, for the first time, a mechanism by which urate is exchanged for anions at the proximal tubule via URAT1 was proposed: intracellular accumulation of those anions (from the glomerular filtrate, peritubular capillaries, and cell metabolism) favours the uphill reabsorption of urate in exchange for these anions, which move down an electrochemical gradient into the tubular lumen (Figure 7.1).

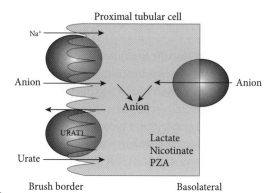

Fig. 7.1 Proposed model of indirect coupling of sodium and urate transport via URAT1.

Similarly, drugs or compounds with an affinity for URAT1 will be uricosuric when acting from the lumen, and anti-uricosuric (driving urate influx) when acting from the intracellular space. Further investigations showed that a patient with a known selective defect in renal urate resorption resulting in idiopathic renal hypouricaemia was shown to have mutations in the portion of DNA which coded for URAT1 and that injecting a portion of mutated cRNA into oocytes halted urate transport activity.

Critique of the paper

This detailed and well-designed investigation identified URAT1 as the transporter responsible for tubular reabsorption of urate and demonstrated a mutation in *URAT1* in a patient with idiopathic renal hypouricaemia. Although in this study the function of URAT1 and the genetic variant encoded were identified and examined in a Japanese population alone, subsequent studies have confirmed these findings in other populations.

Significance and importance of the paper

It was already known that urate is present at higher levels in human blood than in other mammals as a result of the evolutionary loss of hepatic urate oxidase, which functions to degrade uric acid produced by the catabolism of purines. It was also thought that the kidney played an important role in urate homeostasis and that reduction in the efficiency of this mechanism contributed to the development of hyperuricaemia and gout. However, the molecular basis for human renal handling of urate remained unclear.

By demonstrating that the presence of URAT1 can halt urate transport and result in the accumulation of urate in humans, the authors identified a key difference between urate homeostasis in humans, where fractional excretion is typically less than 10%, and other mammals, where the urate excretion rate exceeds the rate at which it is being filtered.

Prior to this discovery, other transporters in cells of various tissues, such as galectin 9, had been suggested to function as a urate transporter; however, they lacked the typical architecture of a transporter, and transmembrane transport could not be demonstrated. URAT1 not only demonstrates architecture that would be expected of a transmembrane transporter but also selective substrate specificity not seen in other multispecific organic anion and cation transporters.

This is the first identification of the renal urate transporter (URAT1), a urate–anion exchanger regulating blood urate levels and the site of action of uricosuric drugs, providing not only much-needed insight into the mechanism of human urate homeostasis but also a target for the potential development of new drugs against hyperuricaemia.

Reference

1 **Sekine T, Miyazaki H, Endou H**. Molecular physiology of renal organic anion transporters. *Am J Physiol Renal Physiol* 2006;**290**(2):F251–61.

Paper 7.3: Gout-associated uric acid crystals activate the NALP3 inflammasome

Reference

Martinon F, Petrilli V, Mayor A, et al. Gout-associated uric acid crystals activate the NALP3 inflammasome. *Nature* 2006;440(7081):237–41.

Hypothesis

While it was known that deposition of MSU and CPP crystals in joints and soft tissues were responsible for gout and acute CPP crystal arthritis respectively, little was understood of the mechanism underlying crystal-induced inflammation. Inflammation in other auto-inflammatory conditions was known to be caused by increased production of the inflammatory cytokine interleukin-1β (IL-1β) in three steps: (1) production of a pro-IL-1β protein, (2) cleavage of pro-IL-1β to produce active IL-1β, and (3) release of active IL-1β into the extracellular environment. Processing of pro-IL-1β in Step 2 involves activation of the 'inflammasome', a multiprotein complex linking the identification of intracellular danger signals by nucleotide-binding oligomerization domain (NOD)-like receptors to the activation of pro-inflammatory cytokines. Once activated, the inflammasome is formed by a member of the NALP protein family (NALP 1, 2, or 3) and the adaptor protein ASC that connects NALPs with caspase-1, allowing cleavage of the pro-IL-1β into active IL-1β. However, prior to the work of the authors, signals and mechanisms leading to inflammasome activation were poorly understood, although constituents of the inflammasome considered specific to the intracellular threat, and thus also to the pathogenesis of particular diseases, had been detected. The NALP3 inflammasome had also been shown to activate in response to cellular stress, danger signalling, and degradation products of bacterial cell walls. Since MSU crystals are released from dying cells, the authors investigated whether it is the NALP3 inflammasome which is activated by MSU crystals.

Methods

Monocytes from the THP1 cell line were incubated with MSU crystals and observed for maturation of IL-1β. A caspase-1 inhibitor was then added to test the proposed caspase-1 dependency of the pro-IL-1β cleavage. These experiments were repeated using CPP crystals, non-pathogenic crystals, including allopurinol crystals and diamond crystals, and particulate elements such as aluminium powder to attempt to test the specificity of this crystal-induced inflammatory pathway. Peritoneal macrophages from mice deficient in various key proteins of the inflammasome complex, or other pro-inflammatory pathways were then analysed after stimulation with MSU and CPP crystals.

Results

Maturation and secretion of IL-1β was seen after stimulation of monocytes by only 10 μg/ml of MSU or CPP crystals but not by non-pathogenic crystals or the particulate elements tested, demonstrating the specificity of this pathway. Furthermore, presence of a caspase-1 inhibitor completely blocked MSU-induced IL-1β maturation, confirming the role of caspase-1 in cleavage of the pro-IL-1β. MSU and CPP were shown to be more potent activators of the inflammasome than those already known, such as adenosine triphosphate (ATP) and crude lipopolysaccharide.

Peritoneal macrophages derived from caspase-1-deficient mice did not produce mature IL-1β, nor did those derived from mice deficient in the adaptor protein ASC, demonstrating that ASC was the particular adaptor protein involved in recruiting caspase-1. IL-1β release was also impaired in NALP3-deficient mice. Furthermore, IL-1β induction by ATP was also shown to be dependent on NALP3, demonstrating that NALP3 is the particular NALP protein involved in this mechanism. Blocking receptor P2X7 (an ATP-specific cation channel) inhibited inflammasome activation driven by ATP but did not affect MSU-induced activation, demonstrating that the two pathways are independent.

Tumour necrosis factor (TNF) secretion was also induced by exposure to MSU and CPP crystals. Release of TNF is known to be independent of caspase-1, suggesting that crystals also induce inflammation by mechanisms other than the inflammasome. Production of TNF was found to be slow and preceded by the release of IL-1β, suggesting that TNF secretion may be initiated by mature IL-1β. Blocking maturation of IL-1β reduced production of TNF induced by MSU and CPP. This suggested processing of IL-1β is a proximal event in the inflammatory cascade triggered by crystal deposition.

Pretreatment of THP1 monocyte cells with colchicine, a common treatment for acute crystal-induced arthritis, prior to exposure to MSU or CPP crystals blocked the processing of IL-1β. However, colchicine did not inhibit activation of IL-1β by extracellular ATP, suggesting that colchicine acts upstream of inflammasome activation.

Recruitment of peritoneal neutrophils in mice following injection of MSU or CPP crystals consistent with that seen in acute crystal arthritis was also observed. However, recruitment of neutrophils was significantly reduced when MSU or CPP crystals were injected in mice deficient in either caspase-1 or the adaptor protein ASC, demonstrating the role of the inflammasome in crystal-induced inflammation *in vivo*.

Critique of the paper

This is a methodologically sound and detailed paper reporting a thorough investigation of the components, triggers and actions of the NALP3 inflammasome *in vivo* using an animal model, and presenting new targets for the development of novel therapies for gout.

Significance and importance of the paper

The finding that maturation of IL-1β induced by MSU and CPP crystals requires the presence of the components of the inflammasome, that is, NALP3, ASC, and caspase-1, revealed the NALP3 inflammasome as the mechanism underlying crystal-induced inflammation in both acute gout and acute CPP crystal arthritis (Figure 7.2). This is further supported by the observation that colchicine blocks IL-1β maturation induced by MSU and

CPP crystals, since colchicine is known to reduce inflammation in both acute gout and acute CPP crystal arthritis. The authors hypothesize that since colchicine inhibits microtubule assembly, it acts at the level of neutrophilic crystal endocytosis or presentation to the inflammasome. However, the mechanism by which endocytosed crystals are detected by the inflammasome remains unclear. This mechanism must be sensitive to subtle differences in the structure of crystals since MSU crystals are extremely similar in structure to allopurinol crystals which do not activate the inflammasome.

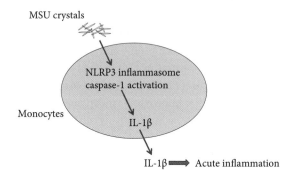

Fig. 7.2 Proposed mechanism of activation of the NALP3 inflammasome by MSU crystals.

This paper was the first to elucidate the mechanism by which inflammation is induced by MSU and CPP crystals. The discovery that crystal-mediated IL-1β maturation requires the presence of the components of the NALP3 inflammasome, that is, NALP3, ASC, and caspase-1, not only allowed clearer understanding of the cellular triggers for acute inflammation in gout and acute CPP crystal arthritis but also identified new targets for the development of novel therapies for acute crystal synovitis, such as antagonists of IL-1. Subsequently, randomized controlled trials have reported the effectiveness of rilonacept and canakinumab for the treatment of acute gout and case reports describe successful treatment of acute CPP crystal arthritis with anakinra [1–4].

References

1 Schlesinger N, Alten RE, Bardin T, et al. Canakinumab for acute gouty arthritis in patients with limited treatment options: results from two randomised, multicentre, active-controlled, double-blind trials and their initial extensions. *Ann Rheum Dis* 2012;**71**(11):1839–48.

2 Terkeltaub RA, Schumacher HR, Carter JD, et al. Rilonacept in the treatment of acute gouty arthritis: a randomized, controlled clinical trial using indomethacin as the active comparator. *Arthritis Res Ther* 2013;**15**(1):R25.

3 McGonagle D, Tan AL, Madden J, et al. Successful treatment of resistant pseudogout with anakinra. *Arthritis Rheum* 2008;**58**(2):631–3.

4 Announ N, Palmer G, Guerne PA, Gabay C. Anakinra is a possible alternative in the treatment and prevention of acute attacks of pseudogout in end-stage renal failure. *Joint Bone Spine* 2009;**76**(4):424–6.

Paper 7.4: Dietary risk factors for gout

Reference

Choi HK, Atkinson K, et al. Purine-rich foods, dairy and protein intake, and the risk of gout in men. *N Engl J Med* 2004;350(11):1093–103.

Purpose

The historical view of gout as the 'disease of Kings' and its association with an intemperate lifestyle led to the commonly held assumption that excessive consumption of dietary purines and alcohol were widely to blame [1]. Urate is the end product of purine metabolism in humans; thus, patients with gout have traditionally been advised to avoid habitual intake of purine-rich foods such as meats, seafood, purine-rich vegetables, and animal protein. However, there had been little research investigating either the role of dietary factors in the pathogenesis of hyperuricaemia and gout or the effectiveness of dietary modification in the treatment of gout.

Population studied

The authors prospectively evaluated the relationship between reported intake of purine-rich food, dairy, and protein, and the incidence of gout in a cohort of 47,150 male health professionals with no prior history of gout.

The analysis was undertaken in the Health Professionals Follow-Up Study (HPFS), an ongoing longitudinal study in the United States of over 50,000 male dentists, optometrists, vets, and other health-care professionals, all of whom were aged between 40 and 75 years of age in 1986.

Methods

Eligible participants were sent a questionnaire about diet, past medical history, and medication. Responders without a history of gout at baseline were sent a semi-quantitative food-frequency questionnaire (previously validated against two 1-week diet records in this cohort) asking about consumption of over 130 different food and drink items during the last year. A further questionnaire was sent again in 1990 and 1994 to update records. Responses were used to calculate nutritional intake by multiplying the frequency of consumption of specified units of each of the foods or drinks by the recorded nutrient content of a specified portion of that particular dietary item. Information about weight, regular use of medications, and medical conditions was collected at baseline and every two years thereafter. Loss to follow-up was low, at <10%.

Participants were also asked, on every biennial questionnaire, specifically about diagnosis of gout given by a physician. In 2001, participants who reported incident gout between baseline and 1998 (n = 1,332) were sent a supplementary questionnaire to ascertain whether they met the American College of Rheumatology (ACR) preliminary survey criteria for the acute arthritis of primary gout (Table 7.1) [2].

Table 7.1 American College of Rheumatology preliminary survey criteria for the acute arthritis of primary gout; 6 of 11 needed to fulfil criteria*

6 of 11 clinical criteria:	
1	More than one attack of acute arthritis
2	Maximum inflammation developed within 1 day
3	Oligoarthritis attack
4	Redness observed over joints
5	First MTP joint painful or swollen
6	Unilateral first MTP joint attack
7	Unilateral tarsal joint attack
8	Tophus (suspected or proven)
9	Hyperuricaemia
10	Asymmetric swelling within a joint
11	Complete termination of an attack

MTP, metatarsophalangeal.

Reproduced from Wallace SL, Robinson H, Masi AT, Decker JL, McCarty DJ, Yu TF. Preliminary criteria for the classification of the acute arthritis of primary gout. *Arthritis Rheum* 1977;20:895–900. With permission from Wiley.

Cox proportional hazards regression was used to estimate multivariate risk of developing incident gout according to various cumulative average dietary intakes, from the return of the baseline questionnaire in 1986 to the first of diagnosis of gout, death, or the end of the study. Those who did not return the supplementary gout questionnaire had their follow-up censored at the date of diagnosis of gout.

Average daily servings of each individual food item were calculated, the average daily intake of similar items was combined into four food groups (total meat, seafood, purine-rich vegetables, and dairy), and total daily intake for each group was recorded. Average intake of foods was categorized into quintiles, and the model was adjusted for age (continuous), alcohol consumption (in seven categories), body mass index (BMI) (in six categories), use of diuretics (yes/no), hypertension (yes/no), chronic renal failure (yes/no), and fluid intake (in quintiles).

Results

In this study, 47,150 male health professionals with no prior history of gout were followed for 12 years. During follow-up, there were 730 incident cases of gout confirmed by the ACR criteria. Incidence of gout increased with age in participants in this study, with an incidence of between 1 case per 1,000 person-years in the under-45 age group to 1.8 cases per 1,000 person-years of follow-up between the ages of 55 and 64.

The baseline characteristics of the participants in each group were similar in mean age, and BMI. Average daily intake of alcohol tended to decrease with increasing intake of protein or dairy products. A history of hypertension was slightly more common in those in the highest quintile of protein intake than in the others.

The multivariate relative risk (RR) of incident gout was 1.41 in those in the highest quintile of meat consumption compared to the lowest quintile (95% confidence interval (CI), 1.07–1.86). The increase in multivariate RR conferred by each additional daily portion was 1.21 (95% CI, 1.04–1.41). Individually, only intake of beef, pork, or lamb as the main meal was shown to increase risk of incident gout.

Increased intake of seafood also increased risk of incident gout. The RR was 1.51 in the highest quintile of seafood consumption compared to the lowest quintile (95% CI 1.17–1.95). The RR conferred by each additional weekly serving of seafood was 1.07 (95% CI, 1.01–1.12). Increased intake of all individual seafood items was associated with an increased risk of gout.

Total level of consumption of purine-rich vegetables was not associated with increased risk of gout nor were any of the individual purine-rich vegetable items.

A strong inverse relationship between the consumption of dairy products, especially low-fat dairy, and incident of gout was demonstrated, with the risk of gout in those in the highest quintile of total dairy consumption approximately half that of those in the lowest quintile (multivariate RR 0.56, 95% CI, 0.42–0.74). The RR of incident gout was 0.82 (95% CI, 0.75–0.90) for each additional daily portion consumed. When examined individually, this inverse relationship was confined to low-fat dairy products (highest vs lowest quintile multivariate RR 0.58, 95% CI, 0.45–0.76), with an additional 21% reduction in risk for each additional daily serving (multivariate RR 0.79 95% CI, 0.71–0.87), although not for high-fat dairy products (multivariate RR 1.00, 95% CI, 0.77–1.29). Individually, two or more 240 ml glasses of skimmed milk per day almost halved the risk of incident gout (multivariate RR 0.54, 95% CI 0.40–0.73) as compared to those who consumed less than one glass per month.

Total protein intake (as a percentage of all energy intake) and animal protein intake were not associated with an increased risk of gout, whereas those in the highest quintiles of both vegetable protein intake and dairy protein intake had a reduced risk of incident gout, compared with those in the lowest quintile (vegetable protein intake multivariate RR 0.73, 95% CI, 0.56–0.96; dairy protein intake 0.52, 95% CI, 0.40–0.68).

Most associations remained unaltered by the influence of BMI and alcohol consumption, with the exception of seafood intake. The risk associated with seafood consumption was significantly stronger in those with a BMI of less than 25 than in those with a BMI of 25 or greater.

Repeating the analysis using dietary intake at baseline and dietary intake as updated every four years, the results were unaltered. Similarly as the analysis was repeated using progressively more strict definitions of gout, from self-reported diagnosis of gout (n = 1,332) to gout defined by the ACR criteria (n = 730) to those with tophaceous or crystal proven gout (n = 118), the magnitude of all of the associations strengthened as the case definition became more specific, while those that had not been found to be statistically significant in the original analysis remained so.

Critique of the paper

This was a well-designed prospective study, conducted in a large cohort of patients. However, it should be noted that the study population was composed of male health professionals who may not be representative of the wider population of gout patients and may not accurately reflect the associations of dietary components in the incidence of gout in women.

Significance and importance of the paper

Although the link between purine-rich diets and hyperuricaemia, rather than gouty arthritis, in both animals and humans had been established in metabolic experiments, little was known about the precise nature of the purine content of foods and how the differing bioavailability of various purines affects their contribution to the risk of hyperuricaemia and gout. Furthermore, the majority of patients who develop hyperuricaemia do not go on to develop clinical gout; so, simply proving the contribution of particular foods to hyperuricaemia does not necessarily elucidate whether that particular food increases the risk of clinical gout. This large, prospective study examined each of the purported 'high-risk' food groups individually, adjusting for a wide range of likely confounders and only using incident cases of gout as the outcome of interest, allowing determination of the increased risk of gout conferred by each additional unit of the food consumed.

The results reported raise many more interesting questions which require further investigation. For example, men who were not overweight were at increased risk of gout related to seafood intake, whereas those who were overweight were not. It is unclear whether this relates to differences in metabolism, differences in excretion of purines between these groups, or a combination of these two factors. Similarly, no association between purine-rich vegetable intake and the risk of gout was found, which may suggest that the bioavailability for purine to uric acid metabolism differs between purine sources and that this influences the contribution made by dietary constituents to the risk of developing gout.

This study also identified potentially protective foods, including dairy products, particularly low-fat dairy products and vegetable proteins. It is not fully understood why dairy products should protect against incident gout. Milk proteins such as casein and lactalbumin are known to have a uricosuric effect, reducing uric acid levels in healthy subjects [3]. The authors postulated that, since dairy products are low in purine content, this urate-lowering effect is not cancelled out by a high concomitant purine load.

A higher total intake of animal or vegetable protein was not associated with increased risk of gout, with vegetable sources of protein appearing protective, although not to the same extent as dairy products. This supports previous reports that high protein diets are associated with increased urinary excretion of uric acid and may reduce SUA levels and that a proportional increase in protein intake can lead to a reduction in the rate of recurrent attacks of gout [4, 5]. It is likely that protein content is not a good proxy for purine content.

The obvious implication of this paper for clinical practice is that it provides evidence to support dietary modification in the treatment of gout. However, it should be remembered that the study tells us about the risk of gout incidence associated with excessive consumption of dietary purines and its findings should only be extrapolated to the treatment of clinically evident gout with caution. Further research into the effectiveness of dietary modification as a treatment strategy is needed.

This was the first prospective study to examine the relationship between dietary constituents and risk of incident gout and provide preliminary epidemiological evidence on which to base clinical advice and patient education about lifestyle modification. The authors went on to use data from the HPFS to examine other risk factors for gout, such as alcohol and fructose intake [6, 7], obesity [8], hypertension [8], and diuretic use [8], all of which appear to predispose to incident gout [8], and consumption of vitamin C and coffee, which appear to be protective [9, 10].

References

1 **Adams F (trans)**. The genuine works of Hippocrates, vols I and II. New York: Wood; 1886.

2 **Wallace SL, Robinson H, Masi AT, et al**. Preliminary criteria for the classification of the acute arthritis of primary gout. *Arthritis Rheum* 1977;**20**(3):895–900.

3 **Ghadirian P, Shatenstein B, Verdy M, et al**. The influence of dairy products on plasma uric acid in women. *Eur J Epidemiol* 1995;**11**(3):275–81.

4 **Gibson T, Rodgers AV, Simmonds HA, et al**. A controlled study of diet in patients with gout. *Ann Rheum Dis* 1983;**42**(2):123–7.

5 **Matzkies F, Berg G, Madl H**. The uricosuric action of protein in man. *Adv Exp Med Biol* 1980;**122**A:227–31.

6 **Choi HK, Atkinson K, Karlson EW, et al**. Alcohol intake and risk of incident gout in men: a prospective study. *Lancet* 2004;**363**(9417):1277–81.

7 **Choi HK, Curhan G**. Soft drinks, fructose consumption, and the risk of gout in men: prospective cohort study. *BMJ* 2008;**336**(7639):309–12.

8 **Choi HK, Atkinson K, Karlson EW, Curhan G**. Obesity, weight change, hypertension, diuretic use, and risk of gout in men: the health professionals follow-up study. *Arch Intern Med* 2005;**165**(7):742–8.

9 **Choi HK, Gao X, Curhan G**. Vitamin C intake and the risk of gout in men: a prospective study. *Arch Intern Med* 2009;**169**(5):502–7

10 **Choi HK, Willett W, Curhan G**. Coffee consumption and risk of incident gout in men: a prospective study. *Arthritis Rheum* 2007;**56**(6):2049–55.

Paper 7.5: Gout and coronary heart disease: the Framingham Study

Reference

Abbott RD, Brand FN, Kannel WB, et al. Gout and coronary heart disease: the Framingham Study. *J Clin Epidemiol* 1988;41(3):237–42.

Background

Gout had been linked to increased risk of atherosclerosis in prior studies, although conflicting findings were reported. Effect of SUA levels on coronary heart disease, including some cases of clinical gout, had also been investigated; however, this relationship was potentially confounded by the use of diuretics. For this reason, the authors sought to examine the relationship between gout and incident coronary heart disease, in patients with no history of diuretic use or cardiovascular disease.

Purpose

To investigate the relationship between gout and incident coronary heart disease, in patients with no history of diuretic use or cardiovascular disease.

Population studied

Patients enrolled in the Framingham Study, a prospective longitudinal study investigating risk factors for coronary heart disease, began to collect data in 1948, with 5,209 participants aged 30 to 62 years of age followed biennially for the development of coronary heart disease, for up to 32 years.

Study design

This was a longitudinal observational study using the Framingham Study population.

Methods

At each biennial follow-up, subjects were asked specifically about the incidence of gout during the previous two years. Gout was defined as any episode of acute joint paint accompanied by swelling and heat, lasting from a few days to two weeks, followed by complete remission of symptoms, or exhibiting prompt response to colchicine or any drug taken hourly and producing nausea, vomiting, or diarrhoea, if the drug could not be named. Only cases where the participant had not been exposed to diuretics were considered in the further analysis.

All participants were examined for risk factors associated with both gout and coronary heart disease, including systolic blood pressure, total cholesterol, smoking history, BMI, and diabetes. For patients with gout, these risk factors were measured at the biennial examination where incidence of gout was first recorded and, for those patients, this was considered their baseline measurement.

For comparison, a group of those within the study of a similar age who did not go on to develop gout were also examined for the same risk factors; however, their measurements were taken at the seventh biennial examination, and this was considered their baseline measurement.

Both the participants with gout and those without were free of coronary heart disease at the time of their baseline measurement and it was from this point that incidence of coronary heart disease was measured at each subsequent biennial examination. Coronary heart disease was considered to be (1) a diagnosis of myocardial infarction or angina pectoris, or (2) clinical evidence of any of these at the cardiovascular assessment performed at each biennial follow-up. Only participants free of coronary heart disease at each biennial examination continued to be observed for a new event during the remaining follow-up time and so participants were essentially censored at incidence of coronary heart disease, whether they had developed gout or not.

Logistic regression and analysis of covariance were used to compare the risk factors measured, adjusted for age. Risk of incident coronary heart disease in those who had gout compared with those who did not was calculated using Cox proportional hazards regression. Time to diagnosis of coronary heart disease was calculated from incidence of gout in those who developed gout or from the seventh biennial examination in those who did not, until first incidence of coronary heart disease, death, or loss to follow-up, whichever occurred first.

Results

The authors report that 5,186 of the 5,209 participants in the Framingham Study were free of gout at baseline. Twenty men and 3 women reported a history of gout not associated with diuretics at baseline, and a further 74 of 2,316 men and 16 of 2,870 women went on to develop gout during follow-up. Incidence of gout was six times greater in men than women (total 2-year incidence rate per 1,000 subjects for men was 3.2 and for women was 0.5), with no clear relationship with age demonstrated in either gender.

Average age of those with gout was 53.3 years for men, and 58.7 years for women, and for those without gout was 54.6 years for men, and 55.3 years for women. For men, risk factors differed significantly between those with gout and those without. Systolic blood pressure, alcohol intake, and BMI were higher in those with gout than those without (P < 0.01), whereas total cholesterol was lower in men with gout (P < 0.05). There was no relationship between gout and cigarette use or diabetes in men. In women, there were no significant differences between those with and without gout in risk factors, although the authors acknowledge this may be a consequence of the small number of female subjects.

Incident coronary heart disease was reported in 37/94 men and 3/19 women with gout, and 509/1,764 men and 428/2,424 women without gout. Average age at experiencing a coronary event in patients with gout was 62.1 years in men and 69.0 years in women, and in patients without gout was 66.7 years for men and 69.0 years for women. Two-year age-adjusted incidence rate of coronary heart disease per 1,000 subjects in men with gout was

5.8, compared to 3.8 in men without gout, which corresponded to an adjusted hazard ratio of 1.6 (95% CI, 1.1–2.5). Two-year age-adjusted incidence rate per 1,000 subjects of angina pectoris in men with gout was 3.1 compared to 1.7 in men without gout, corresponding to an adjusted excess risk of 1.8 (95% CI, 1.1–3.2). No statistically significant increased risk of myocardial infarction was found in men and there was no increased risk of any of the adverse coronary outcomes associated with gout in women.

Critique of the paper

This prospective cohort study used a population free of vascular disease at inception to investigate the true incidence of vascular disease in patients with gout, although as an epidemiological study causation could not be inferred. Adjustment was made for the majority of important confounders, and although presence of co-morbidities, risk factors, and outcomes was reliably ascertained using biennial cardiovascular assessment, it is possible that this may have introduced an element of surveillance bias affecting the estimate of risk associated with gout itself.

Significance of the paper

An earlier report based on the Framingham Study had stated that hyperuricaemia was not a significant predictor of coronary heart disease, once other cardiovascular risk factors were accounted for, in contrast to this paper, which reports that an increased risk of coronary heart disease in men is associated with gout, even after adjustment for other cardiovascular risk factors. A significant body of evidence has subsequently confirmed that both hyperuricaemia and gout are in fact important risk factors for cardiovascular disease [1–5].

Other epidemiological studies had reported that patients with gout were at increased risk of cardiovascular disease [6]. However, this risk was thought to be largely attributable to the higher prevalence of other vascular risk factors such as hypertension and obesity in patients with gout, as compared to controls, rather than being considered intrinsic to gout itself. The Framingham Study was the first to demonstrate that the increased risk of coronary heart disease persisted even after adjustment for these potential confounders.

Although causation cannot be inferred from a study of this design, the authors suggested that gout should act as a marker of susceptibility to coronary heart disease and went on to suggest thorough cardiovascular assessment of all patients with gout. This suggestion has since been incorporated into national and international guidelines on the management of gout [7–9]. However, the authors were unable to assess the effect of treatment of gout on cardiovascular risk in this cohort and, to date, this question remains unanswered. Subsequent studies have demonstrated an association between gout and cardiovascular mortality [1]. Several mechanisms for this association have been suggested, including immobility related to joint pain and additional cardiovascular risk conferred by medications such as non-steroidal anti-inflammatory drugs, which are commonly used to manage acute attacks of gout [10]. However, it has more recently been suggested that this risk is likely to result from a combination of the effect of hyperuricaemia, an acknowledged cardiovascular risk factor in its own right, and persistent systemic inflammation present in patients with clinical gout, which together cause atherogenesis via a mechanism of endothelial dysfunction and impaired blood flow, thus leading to a pro-atherogenic state [11].

This is the first paper to estimate excess risk of coronary heart disease in patients with gout compared to those without, attempting to remove the element of confounding introduced by treatment with diuretics and other cardiovascular risk factors. This paper also provides evidence on the comparative prevalence of cardiovascular risk factors in patients with and without gout, supporting links with long-term adverse outcomes and prompting increased attention to the condition from both the medical and academic community.

References

1 **Clarson L, Chandratre P, Hider S, et al**. Increased cardiovascular mortality associated with_gout: a systematic review and meta-analysis. *Eur J Prev Cardiol* 2013;2047487313514895.

2 **Gelber AC, Klag MJ, Mead LA, et al**. Gout and risk for subsequent coronary heart disease: the Meharry-Hopkins study. *Arch Intern Med* 1997;**157**(13):1436–40.

3 **Krishnan E, Baker JF, Furst DE, et al**. Gout and the risk of acute myocardial infarction. *Arthritis Rheum* 2006;**54**(8):2688–96.

4 **Kuo CF, Yu KH, See LC, et al**. Risk of myocardial infarction among patients with_gout: a nationwide population-based study. *Rheumatology* 2013;**52**:111–7.

5 **Seminog OO, Goldacre MJ**. Gout as a risk factor for myocardial infarction and stroke in England: evidence from record linkage studies. *Rheumatology (Oxford)* 2013;**52**(1):2251–9.

6 **Klein R, Klein BE, Cornoni JC, et al**. Serum uric acid. Its relationship to coronary heart disease risk factors and cardiovascular disease, Evans County, Georgia. *Arch Intern Med* 1973;**132**(3): 401–10.

7 **Zhang W, Doherty M, Pascual E, et al**. EULAR evidence based recommendations for gout. Part II: Management. Report of a task force of the Standing Committee for International Clinical Studies Including Therapeutics (ESCISIT). *Ann Rheum Dis* 2006;**65**(10):1312–24.

8 **Khanna D, Fitzgerald JD, Khanna PP, et al**. 2012 American College of Rheumatology guidelines for management of gout. Part 1: systematic non-pharmacologic and pharmacologic therapeutic approaches to hyperuricemia. *Arthritis Care Res* 2012;**64**(10):1431–46.

9 **Jordan KM, Cameron JS, Snaith M, et al**. British Society for Rheumatology and British Health Professionals in Rheumatology guideline for the management of gout. *Rheumatology* 2007;**46**(8):1372–4.

10 **McGettigan P, Henry D**. Cardiovascular risk with non-steroidal anti-inflammatory drugs: systematic review of population-based controlled observational studies. *PLoS Med* 2011;**8**:e1001098.

11 **Brook RD, Yalavarthi S, Myles JD, et al**. Determinants of vascular function in patients with chronic gout. *J Clin Hypertens* 2011;**13**(3):178–88.

Paper 7.6: Allopurinol therapy for gout

Reference

Rundles RW, Metz EN, Silberman HR. Allopurinol in the treatment of gout. *Ann Intern Med* 1966;64(2):229–57.

Purpose

Although the pathogenesis of gout was becoming clearer, preventative treatment for gout remained confined to the use of uricosurics such as probenecid which were not always effective or well tolerated. In a previous paper in 1963, Elion et al. had described both the structure of allopurinol (4-hydroxypyrazolo(3,4-d)pyrimidine) and its function as an inhibitor of the enzyme xanthine oxidase, known to be the catalyst for the oxidation of hypoxanthine and xanthine, products of purine catabolism, to uric acid [1]. Previous papers also reported its effects on dose, tolerance, hyperuricaemia, and gout; however, the work by Rundles et al. was the first paper to report clinical findings on safety and efficacy from long-term human exposure to allopurinol.

Patients

The study described 46 patients with previously documented acute gout, chronic gout, or both. Eight patients who had infrequent attacks of acute gout or mild chronic joint symptoms were classified as having 'mild' disease. A further eight were classified as having 'moderate' disease, which was defined as frequent attacks of gout or renal stones. The remaining 30 patients were classified as having 'severe' disease, characterized by young age at onset, poor control with standard agents, and the presence of complications such as large tophi, joint destruction, and nephropathy.

Study design

This was an open-label observational study.

Treatment

The dose of allopurinol was adjusted to achieve normalization of serum uric acid.

Study end points measured

Clinical data were collected on joint destruction, the frequency and severity of flares, the presence and size of tophi, and nephropathy. Response to allopurinol was graded into 'excellent', 'good', and 'fair'. An 'excellent' response was recorded where a patient achieved a complete cessation of symptoms and signs of gout, and a 'good' response when a substantial reduction in the frequency and severity of attacks of acute gout and in the burden of chronic symptoms was achieved. 'Fair' was recorded if any improvement in the clinical manifestations of gout was seen.

Baseline blood and urine tests were carried out prior to commencing allopurinol therapy and then regularly thereafter to monitor blood cell counts and renal and hepatic function, as well as serum and urinary uric acid levels and urinary levels of oxypurines (xanthine and hypoxanthine).

All participants taking allopurinol 'long term' were examined regularly (every one to three months) for cumulative and chronic drug toxicity, by means of blood counts and film examination, blood urea nitrogen, serum glucose, serum lactate, liver function tests, serum protein electrophoresis, and urinalysis.

The absorption, excretion, and metabolism of allopurinol was studied by oral administration of radiolabelled allopurinol, in conjunction with Gertrude Elion, who first investigated the use of allopurinol and whom was later awarded the Nobel Prize for Medicine. These findings were reported in detail elsewhere but the preliminary findings were reported in this paper [2].

Follow-up

Patients were followed up for a mean of just over 12 months (range, 2–30 months).

Results

Patients were aged between 18 and 73 years (average age, 50 years), with 40 male participants and 6 female participants. Duration of gout ranged from 18 months to 29 years (average, 11.5 years).

The average SUA level prior to the initiation of allopurinol was 9.3 mg/100 ml and typically began to fall within two days of commencing allopurinol therapy. Maximum urate suppression for a particular dose of allopurinol was reached between seven and ten days. Allopurinol treatment was continued for up to 30 months in some individuals, with an average duration of therapy of just over 12 months for the whole group. Urate was suppressed to within normal range in all patients and could be maintained at set levels by adjustment of the dose of allopurinol. Reduction in SUA was accompanied by a fall in urinary uric acid, and both increased concurrently on cessation of allopurinol therapy.

The dose of allopurinol required to achieve normouricaemia in participants ranged from 200–1,000 mg/day, with an average of 500 mg/day, usually given in two or three divided doses. In patients with mild gout, 200–300 mg/day of allopurinol was sufficient to achieve normouricaemia, with doses of 400–600 mg/day required in those with moderate to severe gout. Doses in excess of 600 mg/day were rarely necessary and, after a period of allopurinol therapy, the dose required to maintain normouricaemia tended to decrease.

The degree of clinical improvement also varied according to severity of disease, since 15 of the 16 patients with mild or moderate gout experienced good or excellent results. Optimal control was maintained in 12 patients by the continuation of allopurinol therapy, and 2 patients with excellent control after several months on allopurinol remained well controlled for up to 24 months after stopping allopurinol. Those with severe gout took longer to respond to allopurinol. Twenty of these 30 patients achieved 'good' responses, and 7 of the remaining patients who achieved only 'fair' results had only had a short trial of therapy or had another complicating condition. Six patients could not complete the study follow-up, three patients had a drug reaction early in the course of treatment, and three patients with severe gout died during the study.

In those with severe gout, acute attacks of gout persisted even after attainment of normouricaemia if colchicine, probenecid, or anti-inflammatory medications were abruptly discontinued after the initiation of allopurinol. Less acute attacks were precipitated if allopurinol was first used as an adjunct to previous therapy rather than as a substitute. However, after persistence of weeks or months, the frequency and severity of acute attacks began to reduce and an improved response to colchicine and anti-inflammatory drugs was seen. In most participants, the dose of colchicine or anti-inflammatories was then successfully reduced or stopped altogether. In 8 of the 30 patients with severe gout, normouricaemia and clinical remission from symptoms was maintained using allopurinol alone. Improvements in general well-being were also reported following initiation of allopurinol, and patients with hand and wrist involvement began to report reduction in pain, stiffness, and limitation in mobility.

Reduction in size of tophi was also shown, with complete disappearance of small tophi on ears, hands, and feet reported after three to six months. None of the participants developed new tophi during treatment. One participant was also found to have evidence of healing of areas of bony destruction on X-ray after treatment with allopurinol.

Combination therapy with allopurinol and uricosurics was also examined and it was determined that, while the average SUA level reduced significantly following initiation of allopurinol, urinary uric acid clearance remained similar. The concurrent use of probenecid, even in the presence of normouricaemia, increased the average urinary uric acid clearance rate.

Overall, allopurinol was well tolerated by participants in the study, and even those taking daily doses of 1 g or more for prolonged periods did not report gastrointestinal side effects and experienced no effect on peripheral or central nervous system function, or renal or hepatic impairment. Electroencephalograms were undertaken where uric acid was suppressed below 3 mg/100 ml and no abnormalities were detected.

Five patients, all of whom had severe gout and renal impairment, developed a drug reaction to allopurinol, three within a month of initiation and two between 6 and 22 months. Three patients had a milder rash with scaling and itching, whereas two experienced a more severe skin eruption associated with fever, malaise, and aching. Symptoms began to regress within two to three days of discontinuing the drug and rapidly recurred when reinstated in three of these patients.

After an average follow-up of just over 12 months (range, 2–30 months) on allopurinol, no evidence of cumulative or chronic drug toxicity was found, even in participants known to have pre-existing bone marrow or renal impairment. No evidence of iron deficiency was found in any of the participants in this study, despite previous suggestions that xanthine oxidase had a role in absorption of iron from the gut and reducing ferric iron in ferritin during its mobilization from the liver.

Critique of the paper

This investigation was undertaken using a small number of patients and with a relatively short follow-up period, although it should be noted that this paper reports only the preliminary findings of the study. Despite this, the robust study methodology and detailed data collection, alongside subsequent longer-term reports, resulted in the justifiable widespread use of allopurinol as the most common form of urate-lowering therapy in gout, and it remains so to date.

Significance of the paper

This paper reports reduction in SUA, acute attacks of gout, and tophus size in 46 patients with gout treated with allopurinol.

While contemporaneous literature suggested that acute attacks of gout are precipitated by the initiation of allopurinol therapy, the authors contended that this is not directly attributable to the allopurinol, particularly if colchicine and uricosurics already prescribed are continued, despite at least two participants experiencing acute attacks shortly after allopurinol was initiated. Acute attacks of gout following initiation of allopurinol and also once normouricaemia was achieved were suggested to result from the persistence of urate deposits, with attacks decreasing in severity and frequency as crystal burden is reduced. Allopurinol-induced acute attacks are now thought to arise as a result of urate-lowering bringing about partial dissolution of MSU crystals, which are then more easily shed from articular cartilage into the joint space, where they provoke an intense acute inflammatory response [3]. Other clinical observations from this study have also been borne out by subsequent research and recommendations. First, the study found that allopurinol should be continued for life in patients with gout, since relapse frequently occurs following cessation of allopurinol therapy. Furthermore, the study found that several months of treatment with allopurinol may be required before improvements are seen. These findings underpin guidance on management of recurrent gout with urate-lowering therapy [4–6].

The side effects of allopurinol remain the subject of discussion today, with severe but not life-threatening reactions reported in two patients in this study, and milder skin reactions in three others. While Klinenberg et al. reported a severe reaction in one patient who developed fever, pruritus, and leucopenia following initiation of allopurinol [7], and Hande et al. later described the rare but potentially life-threatening allopurinol hypersensitivity syndrome (AHS) [8], no evidence of adverse haematopoietic effects was found in this study. All five patients who developed toxic reactions had impaired renal function, which has subsequently been confirmed in controlled studies as an important risk factor for AHS [8].

The authors conclude that, in patients with occasional acute gout, symptomatic and prophylactic use of colchicine or uricosurics are probably sufficient but that for patients with severe and poorly controlled gout, impaired renal function or nephropathy, allopurinol should be considered the drug of choice and initiated in conjunction with colchicine in many cases. This is the foundation of current recommendations on initiation of allopurinol [4–6].

This report demonstrates a new prophylactic therapy for patients with hyperuricaemia and gout, targeting a novel mechanism. Hitchings and Elion were awarded the Nobel Prize for Medicine in 1988 for the discovery of this and six other drugs, and allopurinol remains to this day the most widely used treatment in the prophylaxis of gout [9].

References

1 **Elion GB, Callahan S, Nathan H, et al**. Potentiation by inhibition of drug degradation: 6-substituted purines and xanthine oxidase. *Biochem Pharmacol* 1963;**12**(1):85–93.

2 **Elion GB, Kovensky A, Hitchings GH**. Metabolic studies of allopurinol, an inhibitor of xanthine oxidase. *Biochem Pharmacol* 1966;**15**(7):863–80.

3 **Roddy E, Mallen CD, Doherty M**. Gout. *BMJ* 2013;**347**:f5648.

4 **Zhang W, Doherty M, Pascual E, et al**. EULAR evidence based recommendations for gout. Part II: Management. Report of a task force of the Standing Committee for International Clinical Studies Including Therapeutics (ESCISIT). *Ann Rheum Dis* 2006;**65**(10):1312–24.

5 **Khanna D, Fitzgerald JD, Khanna PP, et al**. 2012 American College of Rheumatology guidelines for management of gout. Part 1: systematic non-pharmacologic and pharmacologic therapeutic approaches to hyperuricemia. *Arthritis Care Res* 2012;**64**(10):1431–46.

6 **Jordan KM, Cameron JS, Snaith M, et al**. British Society for Rheumatology and British Health Professionals in Rheumatology guideline for the management of gout. *Rheumatology* 2007;**46**(8):1372–4.

7 **Klinenberg JR, Goldfinger SE, Seegmiller JE**. The effectiveness of the xanthine oxidase inhibitor allopurinol in the treatment of gout. *Ann Intern Med* 1965;**62**(4):639–47.

8 **Hande KR, Noone RM, Stone WJ**. Severe allopurinol toxicity. Description and guidelines for prevention in patients with renal insufficiency. *Am J Med* 1984;**76**(1):47–56.

9 **Annemans L, Spaepen E, Gaskin M, et al**. Gout in the UK and Germany: prevalence, comorbidities and management in general practice 2000–5. *Ann Rheum Dis* 2008;**67**(7):960–6.

Paper 7.7: Febuxostat compared with allopurinol in patients with hyperuricemia and gout

Reference

Becker MA, Schumacher HR Jr, Wortmann RL, et al. Febuxostat compared with allopurinol in patients with hyperuricemia and gout. *N Eng J Med* 2005;353(23):2450–61.

Purpose

Febuxostat was the first novel drug for the prophylaxis of gout since the description of allopurinol in 1966, and prior to its release patients either unresponsive to or unable to tolerate allopurinol were left with the limited options offered by uricosuric agents. Febuxostat, also a xanthine oxidase inhibitor, offered a potential alternative to allopurinol. The purpose of this study was to compare the safety and efficacy of febuxostat with that of allopurinol in patients with gout and hyperuricaemia.

Patients

Patients with an SUA ≥8.0 mg/dl (480 μmol/l) and who satisfied the ACR preliminary criteria for the acute arthritis of primary gout were included [1]. Exclusion criteria included serum creatinine >1.5 mg/dl (133 μmol/l); estimated creatinine clearance <50 ml/1.73 m^2 body surface area; pregnancy/lactation; use of urate-lowering treatment, azathioprine, 6-mercaptopurine, thiazides, aspirin, or prednisolone >10 mg daily; BMI >50 kg/m^2; xanthinuria, active liver disease, or hepatic dysfunction; change in hormone replacement therapy or oral contraceptive therapy within the last three months; or a history of alcohol abuse or alcohol intake of more than 14 drinks per week.

Study design

The Febuxostat versus Allopurinol Controlled Trial was a Phase 3, randomized, double-blind, multicentre trial.

Treatment

Subjects were randomized to one of three groups: febuxostat 80 mg per day, febuxostat 120 mg per day, or allopurinol 300 mg per day. Those already taking urate-lowering therapy underwent a two-week washout period prior to randomization. All patients were given prophylaxis against acute attacks during this washout period and for the first eight weeks of the double-blind treatment, comprising either 250 mg naproxen twice per day or 0.6 mg colchicine once per day. Treatment of subsequent flares was at the investigators' discretion.

Study end points measured

Patients were examined at two and four weeks, and monthly thereafter with vital signs, SUA, and renal function measured, compliance with study drugs assessed, and concomitant medication use, gouty flares, and adverse events recorded. The primary efficacy end point was an SUA level of <6.0 mg/dl at each of the last three monthly measurements. Those who left the study prior to three clinic visits were considered not to have reached this end point. Secondary efficacy end points included the proportion of participants with an SUA level <6.0 mg/dl at each clinic visit, and the percentage reduction in SUA measurement at each visit when compared with each participants baseline measurement. Clinical end points included proportion of subjects requiring treatment for acute flares of gout between weeks 9 and 52, as well as change in number and size of tophi at each visit.

Efficacy was analysed by sequential comparison: each febuxostat group was compared to the allopurinol group for non-inferiority; then, each febuxostat group shown to be non-inferior to the allopurinol group was tested for superiority to the allopurinol group.

Follow-up

The trial lasted 52 weeks.

Results

Of 1,283 patients screened for eligibility, 762 were randomized to one of the three groups: febuxostat 80 mg per day (n = 256), febuxostat 120 mg per day (n = 251), or allopurinol 300 mg per day (n = 253), with 760 receiving at least one dose of the study drug.

There were no significant differences among the three treatment groups at baseline.

The primary end point (SUA level <6.0 mg/dl at the last three measurements) was reached by 53% taking febuxostat 80 mg per day, 62% taking 120 mg febuxostat per day, but only 21% of those taking allopurinol (P < 0.001 for each febuxostat group compared to the allopurinol group). This finding remained when the proportions achieving the primary end point were stratified by baseline SUA level. The proportion of participants with SUA level <6.0 mg/dl was significantly higher in both of the groups receiving febuxostat compared with those receiving allopurinol by the first visit after randomization at week 2 of the study (febuxostat 80 mg, 80%; febuxostat 120 mg, 88%; allopurinol, 42%). This difference remained at all visits up to and including those in week 52 (febuxostat 80 mg, 81%; febuxostat 120 mg, 82%; allopurinol, 39%). Mean percentage reduction in SUA from baseline was also higher in both of the febuxostat groups than in the allopurinol group. In post hoc analyses, the proportions of subjects with final SUA levels <5.0 or <4.0 mg/dl were significantly greater in both of the febuxostat groups compared to the allopurinol groups (P < 0.001).

During weeks 0–8, when prophylaxis against acute gouty flare was given, a significantly greater proportion of those receiving febuxostat 120 mg experienced a flare (36%), compared with those receiving febuxostat 80 mg (22%) or allopurinol (21%; P < 0.001 for both comparisons). Between weeks 9 and 52, there was an increased incidence of gout flare in all groups, with similar proportions of participants in each group requiring treatment for flares of gout (febuxostat 80 mg, 64%; febuxostat 120 mg, 70%; allopurinol, 64%). Incidence of flare decreased with time, and between weeks 49 and 52 occurred in 8% of those receiving febuxostat 80 mg, 6% of those receiving febuxostat 120 mg, and 11% of those receiving allopurinol.

There were no statistically significant differences among the groups in terms of the reduction in the number of tophi or the percentage reduction in tophus area.

The incidence of all adverse events was similar in all three treatment groups. The most frequent treatment-related adverse events were liver-function abnormalities (febuxostat 80 mg, 4%; febuxostat 120 mg, 5%; allopurinol, 4%) and diarrhoea (3% in all groups). Most adverse events were considered to be of mild-to-moderate severity. Serious adverse events occurred in 51 participants, distributed evenly across groups, 34 of whom were able to continue in the study while the event resolved, and experienced no recurrence. Four patients died: two who had received febuxostat 80 mg (one from congestive heart failure and one from respiratory failure) and two who had received febuxostat 120 mg (one from metastatic colon cancer and one from cardiac arrest). All four deaths were judged to be unrelated to the study drugs.

The tolerability of the drugs appeared similar, with discontinuation in 34% (n = 88) of those receiving febuxostat 80 mg, 39% (n = 98) of those receiving febuxostat 120 mg, and 26% (n = 66) of those receiving allopurinol.

Critique of the paper

This study used randomization to assign patients to each treatment group, and all three groups were of reasonable and similar size and composition. Although the methods used to compare outcomes, safety, and tolerability of febuxostat with allopurinol were generally sound, it should be considered when interpreting these results that both febuxostat groups were compared with a fixed dose of 300 mg of allopurinol rather than a dose that had been individually titrated to adequately achieve target urate suppression, as is considered best practice.

Significance of the paper

Administration of both allopurinol and febuxostat resulted in rapid (within two weeks) and sustained reduction of SUA levels. Although significantly more of the patients taking febuxostat (at either dose) than those taking allopurinol achieved SUA <6.0 mg/dl, clinical outcomes (reduction in number of flares and tophus area) were similar in all groups.

Only 21% of the allopurinol group achieved three successive urate measurements of 6.0 mg/dl or less but this is likely to reflect the study protocol to administer a fixed dose of 300 mg per day rather than an upward titration of dose according to repeated urate measurement as is recommended by best practice [2–4].

Studies had already shown that maintenance of SUA levels below 6.0 mg/dl reduces the number of gout flares experienced, and the size and number of tophi [5–7]. Similar improvements in these clinical outcome measures were seen in all three groups in this trial but a statistically significant difference between those with a mean post-baseline SUA of less than 6.0 mg/dl and more than 6.0 mg/dl was only seen in the last 4 weeks, suggesting that this relatively short trial of 52 weeks follow-up was of insufficient length to assess differences in clinical outcomes.

This paper presents evidence that febuxostat is an efficacious and safe alternative to allopurinol for urate-lowering therapy. Febuxostat (at a dose of either 80 mg or 120 mg daily) produces a greater reduction in SUA than allopurinol at a fixed dose of 300 mg daily. However, it should be noted that best-practice titration of allopurinol beyond doses of 300 mg daily was not permitted during this trial and, to date, febuxostat has not been compared to such dose-titration regimes.

References

1 **Wallace SL, Robinson H, Masi AT, et al**. Preliminary criteria for the classification of the acute arthritis of primary gout. *Arthritis Rheum* 1977;**20**(3):895–900.

2 **Zhang W, Doherty M, Pascual E, et al**. EULAR evidence based recommendations for gout. Part II: Management. Report of a task force of the Standing Committee for International Clinical Studies Including Therapeutics (ESCISIT). *Ann Rheum Dis* 2006;**65**(10):1312–24.

3 **Khanna D, Fitzgerald JD, Khanna PP, et al**. 2012 American College of Rheumatology guidelines for management of gout. Part 1: systematic non-pharmacologic and pharmacologic therapeutic approaches to hyperuricemia. *Arthritis Care Res* 2012;**64**(10):1431–46.

4 **Jordan KM, Cameron JS, Snaith M, et al**. British Society for Rheumatology and British Health Professionals in Rheumatology guideline for the management of gout. *Rheumatology* 2007;**46**(8):1372–4.

5 **Li-Yu J, Clayburne G, Sieck M, et al**. Treatment of chronic gout. Can we determine when urate stores are depleted enough to prevent attacks of gout? *J Rheumatol* 2001;**28**(3):577–80.

6 **Shoji A, Yamanaka H, Kamatani N**. A retrospective study of the relationship between serum urate level and recurrent attacks of gouty arthritis: evidence for reduction of recurrent gouty arthritis with antihyperuricemic therapy. *Arthritis Rheum* 2004;**51**(3):321–5.

7 **Perez-Ruiz F, Calabozo M, Pijoan JI, et al**. Effect of urate-lowering therapy on the velocity of size reduction of tophi in chronic gout. *Arthritis Rheum* 2002;**47**(4):356–60.

Paper 7.8: Can acute attacks of gout be prevented by optimum suppression of urate?

Reference

Li-Yu J, Clayburne G, Sieck M, et al. Treatment of chronic gout. Can we determine when urate stores are depleted enough to prevent attacks of gout? *J Rheumatol* 2001;28(3):577–580.

Hypothesis

Although urate-lowering therapy for gout was widely available, knowledge of the optimum level of SUA for control of the condition was limited. It had been hypothesized by others that reduction in SUA to below 6 mg/dl or 360 µmol/l (considered to be below the saturation point of blood with urate) was sufficient to deplete crystal stores and prevent flares; however, this hypothesis had not been tested.

Patients

Participants (all male) had hyperuricaemia at baseline, were treated with allopurinol, and had gout confirmed by identification of MSU crystals in a sample of synovial fluid aspirated from the knee.

Study design

This was a prospective observational study. Patients were recalled in 1999 (ten years after the study was initiated), and all recorded measurements of SUA were reviewed. All of those who had attained an SUA measurement of ≤6.0 mg/dl and maintained this level for at least 12 months were asked to undergo a further aspiration of synovial fluid from the knee, and a smaller percentage of those with an SUA of >6.0 mg/dl also had a repeat aspiration of the knee joint.

SUA and creatinine were also measured on the day of arthrocentesis. Duration of gout, frequency and sites of prior attacks, dosage and duration of drug therapies, and joints in which MSU crystals had previously been identified were ascertained by participant interview and review of medical records.

Treatment

Participants and their physicians were advised that dosage of allopurinol should be titrated until SUA was suppressed and maintained below 6 mg/dl.

Follow-up

Patients were followed prospectively at intervals for two to ten years.

Results

The 57 men were divided into two groups based upon the SUA level at follow-up in 1999: Group A (n = 38), in whom SUA remained >6 mg/dl, and Group B (n = 19), in whom SUA was maintained at ≤6 mg/dl for at least 12 months.

The groups were similar in age and gout duration. Over the follow-up period, Group A was prescribed lower doses of allopurinol (100–300 mg daily) than Group B (300–600 mg) was and the duration of allopurinol therapy was shorter in Group A (2 months–13 years vs 5–20 years). Gout flare frequency in the most recent year was higher in Group A (mean, 6; range, 4–12) than in Group B (mean, 1; range, 0–3). Forty-two per cent of those in Group B had not had an acute gout flare for at least two years. Tophi were more prevalent at follow-up in Group A (37%) than in Group B (16%), although the prevalence of tophi at baseline was not reported.

Sixteen participants (42%) in Group A consented to a repeat arthrocentesis of their knee. Fourteen (88%) were found to have MSU crystals in the synovial fluid. Of the 16 Group B participants who underwent repeat arthrocentesis, MSU crystals were found in synovial fluid in 7 (44%).

Critique of the paper

This was a small study, using a solely male population; however, despite this, loss to follow-up was minimal, the methodology was sound, and follow-up was sufficiently long and detailed to support the validity of the authors' conclusions.

Significance of the paper

This prospective observational study demonstrated that better control of gout can be achieved when SUA levels are maintained below 6 mg/dl. Flare frequency and tophus were seen less commonly at follow-up in those maintaining SUA levels below target. Importantly, whereas all participants had MSU crystals seen in synovial fluid aspirated from the knee at baseline, those who maintained SUA below 6 mg/dl were half as likely to have MSU crystals on repeat knee arthrocentesis at follow-up as those in whom SUA remained above this level, demonstrating that maintenance of SUA levels below 6 mg/dl frequently leads to depletion of MSU crystal stores. However, the observation that, of those who achieved a target SUA level, 44% still had evident MSU crystals in aspirated knees, with 42% having had no attacks for at least two years, suggests that MSU crystal depletion may take longer than previously thought. The authors acknowledge that they were unable to assess the effect of urate-lowering on crystal deposition in joints and soft tissues, as X-rays of symptomatic joints were not taken as part of the study follow-up, although more sophisticated assessment is now possible through modern imaging techniques such as ultrasound, and dual-energy computed tomography (DECT) [1, 2].

A further important observation concerns suboptimal management of patients with gout, even within the confines of a study protocol. Several studies have subsequently replicated this finding [3–5]. The majority of patients did not maintain an SUA level of <6 mg/dl as requested by the study investigators. This is likely to have resulted from both infrequent measurement of SUA levels and inadequate titration of medication by the responsible clinicians but possibly also poor adherence of the patients to urate-lowering medications, although data on compliance with allopurinol are not presented.

This paper demonstrates that MSU crystal stores were depleted in the majority of patients in whom SUA levels were supressed to ≤6 mg/dl for several years. This was the first time a target level for SUA had been set and additionally demonstrated a reduction in both crystal burden and number of flares experienced in the majority of patients. International management guidelines have subsequently adopted the cut-off of 6 mg/dl (360 μmol/l) as the minimum target for urate-lowering therapy [6, 7].

References

1 **Chowalloor PV, Keen HI**. A systematic review of ultrasonography in gout and asymptomatic hyperuricaemia. *Ann Rheum Dis* 2013;**72**(5):638–45.

2 **Dalbeth N, Choi HK**. Dual-energy computed tomography for gout diagnosis and management. *Curr Rheumatol Rep* 2013;**15**(1):301

3 **Pal B, Foxall M, Dysart T, et al**. How is gout managed in primary care? A review of current practice and proposed guidelines. *Clin Rheumatol* 2000;**19**(1):21–5.

4 **Roddy E, Zhang W, Doherty M**. Concordance of the management of chronic gout in a UK primary-care population with the EULAR gout recommendations. *Ann Rheum Dis* 2007;**66**(10):1311–5.

5 **Singh JA, Hodges JS, Toscano JP, et al**. Quality of care for gout in the US needs improvement. *Arthritis Rheum* 2007;**57**(5):822–9.

6 **Zhang W, Doherty M, Pascual E, et al**. EULAR evidence based recommendations for gout. Part II: Management. Report of a task force of the Standing Committee for International Clinical Studies Including Therapeutics (ESCISIT). *Ann Rheum Dis* 2006;**65**(10):1312–24.

7 **Khanna D, Fitzgerald JD, Khanna PP, et al**. 2012 American College of Rheumatology guidelines for management of gout. Part 1: systematic non-pharmacologic and pharmacologic therapeutic approaches to hyperuricemia. *Arthritis Care Res* 2012;**64**(10):1431–46.

Paper 7.9: Mutations in *ANKH* cause chondrocalcinosis

Reference

Pendleton A, Johnson MD, Hughes A, et al. Mutations in *ANKH* cause chondrocalcinosis. *Am J Hum Genetics* 2002;71(4):933–40.

Purpose

CPPD is a common age-related phenomenon, and most cases are thought to occur sporadically. However, familial occurrence characterized by autosomal dominant inheritance, onset in the third and fourth decades, polyarticular involvement, and both attacks of acute CPP crystal arthritis and osteoarthritis with CPPD have been described [1, 2]. Recombinant mapping linked these familial forms to regions on chromosomes 5 (*CCAL2* MIM 118,600) and 8 (*CCAL1* MIM 600,688) [1–3]. In mice, a mutation in the progressive ankylosis gene *ank* behaves as an autosomal recessive trait and causes severe generalized arthritis resulting from calcium hydroxyapatite crystal arthritis. Progressive ankylosis is caused by a nonsense mutation in a multipass transmembrane protein which regulates levels of intra- and extracellular pyrophosphate and may act as a pyrophosphate transporter. The human equivalent of *ank*, named *ANKH* (MIM 605,145), maps to the region on Chromosome 5 previously linked to *CCAL2* in two families, one French and one British. Given the location and known role of the ANKH protein in pyrophosphate regulation and calcium crystal deposition, this paper explores the relationship of *ANKH* to CPPD in humans.

Study design

Blood-cell DNA was obtained from members of two families with *CCAL2*, 95 patients with sporadic CC diagnosed on plain radiographs, and 200 unaffected control subjects, and then used to amplify *ANKH* sequences. Gel electrophoresis was used to isolate and purify the amplification products prior to sequencing of the 12 exons (nucleotide sequences known to remain in the mature DNA) that make up *ANKH*.

The amplification products were sequenced using primers (specifically designed short sequences of approximately 20 base pairs each and which act as templates by which nucleotides can be added to an existing nucleotide sequence) by an automated process. All the heterogeneous base pair changes identified were then validated by independent resequencing or by cloning (where the fragment of interest is transferred to a new vector such as a bacterium in order to be further examined and resequenced) the amplification products and then resequencing individual subclones.

Changes identified in Exon 1 and Exon 12 were reproduced in 190 control chromosomes by amplification and direct sequencing using specific forward and reverse primers. The sequence from the French family differed from the others in that the mutation in it produced a restriction site, that is, a location at which a restriction enzyme will cut the sequence between two specific nucleotides, in Exon 2. Polymerase chain reaction (PCR) was used to amplify a 389 base pair (bp) segment spanning this mutation, using both a forward and reverse primer. This was followed by a second amplification using the same forward primer but a shorter nested reverse primer. Digestion of the product using a restriction enzyme resulted in the predicted band of 389 bp in unaffected family members and 107 controls, and additional smaller fragments (213 bp and 176 bp) in the affected patients carrying the missense mutation.

The effect of the mutations was then assessed by comparison with the wild-type sequence. First, both the wild-type sequence and the sequence containing the mutation identified in Exon 1 were subcloned, or moved from their existing vector into a specifically chosen alternative one, before amplification using primers with an upstream promoter (the region of DNA that initiates transcription of a particular gene) and downstream termination codons; then, the sizes of the proteins encoded were assessed and compared.

Each of the genes was then reconstructed in a previously described purpose built vector (pCMV-ANK) [4]. The French M48T mutation was generated using forward and reverse primers to produce a template including the particular sequence change of interest. Restriction enzymes were then used to separate and incorporate the fragment of interest into a new vector to ensure that experimental results were not influenced by other base pair changes incidentally present in the vector. The British −11CT mutation was generated by inserting 18 bp flanking the initiation codon of the mutant sequence into the pCMV-ANK vector by PCR. The E490del mutation was recreated in a similar way to the French M48T but using a vector containing the initiation codon for the wild-type human sequence.

The effect of these mutations on pyrophosphate levels was then tested by introducing fragments of DNA containing the identified mutant sequences into COS-7 cells (a simian fibroblast-like cell line often used to produce recombinant proteins in biology). Inorganic pyrophosphate concentration in these cells was measured 28–34 hours later by enzymatic assay, and the result compared to similar control experiments using wild-type DNA. The results of multiple experiments were compared using paired t-tests.

Results

All affected members of the French family were heterozygous for a thymine to cytosine base change at Exon 2 which led to a mutation in a transmembrane protein within the ANKH protein. All affected members of the British family were heterozygous for a cytosine to thymine base change at a location generating an initiation codon and which thus added four amino acids to the N-terminus of the ANKH protein. In both families, the mutation resided on the disease allele and segregated completely with CC. The mutations were not found in either unaffected family members or in 200 chromosomes from unaffected control individuals.

Of the 95 British patients with sporadic CC and in whom ANKH exons were sequenced, only one was shown to have a mutation. A 3 bp deletion in Exon 12 was identified in a patient with late-onset polyarticular CC and structural arthropathy of both knees. This deletion was not found in any of the control chromosomes. However, two other family members (the son and the sister of an index case) were also heterozygous for the same deletion. Neither had demonstrable CC and, although the sister had already undergone bilateral total knee replacement for 'osteoarthritis', her preoperative X-rays were not available for review, and X-rays of her pelvis and hands did not show any CC.

Overexpression of the wild-type full-length ANKH (the typical form for the species) was found to cause a significant reduction in intracellular pyrophosphate levels. The three mutations identified were also tested and shown to reduce intracellular pyrophosphate, by 148% (±33%) for the British family's mutation, 101% (±25%) for the French family's mutation, and 109% (±12%) for the deletion identified in the one sporadic CC patient, as compared with the reduction caused by the wild-type ANKH.

Critique of the paper

This study used a comparatively large sample for a study of its kind and used two separate families from different countries as well as unaffected control individuals in their investigation. Both families were European in origin, and comparison with patients of other ethnicities would have been useful in establishing the generalizability of this genetic variant; however, aside from this, the methodology was sound.

Significance of the paper

The identification of three different mutations (Figure 7.3) associated with onset of CC and associated arthropathy was an important step in explaining phenotypic differences that had been previously observed, even between families with primary hereditary CPPD, but not understood. In the UK family studied as part of this investigation, adult onset CC was preceded by repeated childhood seizures. The mutation identified in this family coded for an additional amino acid sequence, which may be expressed in neural cells (another known site of ANKH expression) possibly causing new or unusual activity resulting in these seizures.

Overexpression of *ank* in mice causes early and widespread deposition of calcium hydroxyapatite in cartilage and synovial fluid; in contrast, in humans, mutations in *ANKH* lead to slower, later-onset CPPD. These differences in crystal type and disease onset are likely to reflect different effects of the individual mutations on pyrophosphate levels. From their in vitro experiments, the authors were able to hypothesize that the mouse mutation truncates the ANK protein, significantly reducing its activity and thus causing a decrease in pyrophosphate levels outside cells. Since pyrophosphate levels are important in inhibition of hydroxyapatite formation, it is likely that this drop caused by the reduced activity of the truncated ANK protein in mice is what allows the widespread deposition of hydroxyapatite crystals in mice with this particular mutation. However, in humans, the mutations do not truncate the ANKH protein but rather cause small changes in amino acid sequences; in the experiments using COS cells, proteins carrying the replicated human mutations showed a higher level of activity than proteins carrying the mouse mutation but only a minor increase in activity level compared to the wild-type ANKH. However, the authors suggest that it is likely that these *ANKH* mutations are likely to lead to reciprocal increases in extracellular pyrophosphate, and that even a small increase in ANKH activity may be enough to lead to crystal formation in the longer term, since elevated pyrophosphate concentrations can trigger precipitation of calcium and pyrophosphate ions

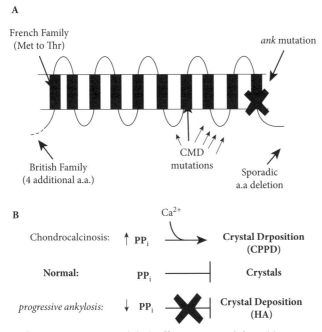

Fig. 7.3 Summary of *ANKH* mutations and their effects on crystal deposition.

and thus lead to CPPD. This is a plausible hypothesis, as metabolic conditions that raise extracellular pyrophosphate levels, such as hypomagnesaemia and hypophosphatasia, also predispose to CC [5].

The authors suggest that the human mutations are likely to cause increased activity of the ANKH transmembrane protein and thus lead to slow accumulation of pyrophosphate. A similar suggestion was made contemporaneously by Williams et al., who studied an Argentine family of northern Italian descent and with known autosomal dominant CPPD; the authors identified an mutation in the Chromosome 5p locus that was only found in those family members affected by the disease, with the exception of three who were much younger than the mean age of onset (29 years) and thus could not be reliably assessed for presence or absence of the disease. This mean age of onset is younger than the majority of patients found to have symptomatic CPPD and thus supports the theory that the presence of multiple mutations encoding differing mutations in the ANKH protein in humans results in multiple associated phenotypes [6].

The allele variants identified in this report provided the first evidence that CC and other forms of CPP deposition disease in humans are due to mutations in *ANKH*. It is suggested that these mutations result in increased activity of the ANKH protein, increasing transport of inorganic pyrophosphate into the extracellular compartment, where it is free to combine with calcium to form CPP crystals. The identification of these *ANKH* variants in humans with CC, and the mechanism by which they contribute to the formation of CPP crystals, raises the possibility of novel treatments targeted at the transmembrane protein encoded by *ANKH*.

References

1 **Baldwin CT, Farrer LA, Adair R, et al**. Linkage of early-onset osteoarthritis and chondrocalcinosis to human chromosome 8q. *Am J Hum Genet* 1995;**56**(3):692–7.

2 **Andrew LJ, Brancolini V, de la Pena LS, et al**. Refinement of the chromosome 5p locus for familial calcium pyrophosphate dehydrate deposition disease. *Am J Hum Genet* 1999;**64**(1):136–45.

3 **Hughes AE, McGibbon D, Woodward E, et al**. Localisation of a gene for chondrocalcinosis to chromosome 5p. *Hum Mol Genet* 1995;**4**(7):1225–8.

4 **Ho A, Johnson M, Kingsley DM**. Role of the mouse *ank* gene in tissue calcification and arthritis. *Science* 2000;**289**(5477):265–70.

5 **Jones AC, Chuck AJ, Arie EA, et al**. Diseases associated with calcium pyrophosphate deposition disease. *Semin Arthritis Rheum* 1992;**22**(3):188–202.

6 **Williams CJ, Zhang Y, Timms A, et al**. Autosomal dominant familial calcium pyrophosphate dihydrate deposition disease is caused by mutation in the transmembrane protein ANKH. *Am J Hum Genet* 2002;**71**(4):985–91.

Paper 7.10: Clinical and radiographic features of pyrophosphate arthropathy

Reference

Dieppe PA, Alexander GJM, Jones HE, et al. Pyrophosphate arthropathy: a clinical and radiological study of 105 cases. *Ann Rheum Dis* 1982;41(4):371–6.

Purpose

At the time of publication, several clinical syndromes were thought to result from the deposition of CPP crystals in articular cartilage. However, many patients with radiographic CC had been found to be asymptomatic, an observation resulting in uncertainty about the role played by crystal deposition in joint damage and arthropathy which had previously been attributed to their presence. This study aimed to survey a large cohort of unselected patients presenting to a rheumatologist with joint disease, for clinical and radiological evidence of CPPD and associated joint damage.

Patients

One-hundred and five consecutive patients presenting with joint disease and who had evidence of pyrophosphate deposition were studied. Inclusion criteria were the presence of radiological linear shadows of calcific density within hyaline or fibrocartilage, and the presence of positively birefringent crystals in synovial fluid or tissues samples.

Study design

A full medical history was obtained, including family history of arthritis, drug history, and any medical or surgical conditions that might predispose to CPPD. Number, site, and duration of acute attacks of arthritis (defined as episodes of severe joint pain, usually with swelling, lasting between 12 hours and 4 weeks) were recorded along with time of onset and site of chronic symptoms. Knees and hands were examined. Knees were scored on a scale of 0–3 (none, mild, moderate, and severe) for effusions, crepitus, and severity of involvement. Evidence of joint damage in the hands was scored on the same 0–3 scale. A modified Beighton score for hypermobility was recorded. X-rays of hands, wrists, the thoraco-lumbar spine, the pelvis, and any other clinically involved joints were examined for evidence of CC and joint disease. Synovial fluid was aspirated and examined under PLM for positively birefringent crystals. Both conventional histological examination and polarized light were used to examine tissue samples from five patients whose knees had been examined by arthroscopy.

Results

Pyrophosphate deposition as diagnosed on the basis of radiological features alone was present in 73 participants. Twenty-eight participants had both radiological features and synovial fluid or tissue crystals, three had only synovial fluid crystals but no radiographic

CC, and diagnosis was made on the basis of biopsy alone in one participant. Thus, only four participants had no radiological evidence of CC.

The majority of the 105 participants were women, with only 29 men included. Men were younger (mean age, 62 years) than women (mean age, 73 years). Of the 18 patients who presented under the age of 60, two-thirds were men.

The most commonly affected joints were the knee (men, 93%; women, 92%), shoulder (men, 36%; women, 48%), ankle (men, 32%; women, 35%), and hand (men, 32%; women, 41%). Spinal involvement was also common in women (49%). The first presentation was most commonly at the knee and involved the knee and ankle joints more frequently in men (82%) than in women (53%). Women were found to have a wider spectrum of both joint involvement and presenting symptoms, as well as a longer mean duration of joint symptoms (13 years) as compared to men (10 years).

Acute attacks of arthritis were experienced by 54% of men and 28% of women. The most commonly affected joint was the knee (men, 93%; women, 71%), followed by the wrist/hand (men, 13%; women, 62%), and ankle (men, 25%; women, 5%), with women more commonly experiencing upper limb and polyarticular acute involvement (three or more joints concurrently). Acute attacks only with no other joint symptoms were reported by 13 patients.

Of the 92 who experienced chronic joint symptoms, with or without acute attacks, the majority had polyarticular involvement, with the knee the most severely affected site. The spectrum of involved joints was wider in women, with clinical and radiological evidence of osteoarthritis also found at multiple sites in those with the longest duration of symptoms. Only 8% of participants had no knee involvement. Of those participants whose knees were affected, clinical findings of effusion and crepitus were found in 89% and 85%, respectively, with severe deformity or instability found in 30 participants, of whom 28 were women. The hands were affected in 76 participants; the pattern of hand joint involvement varied, although prevalence increased with age and was greater in women. The distal interphalangeal joint was most commonly affected (72%), followed by the proximal interphalangeal joint (54%), the first carpometacarpal joint (53%), and the metacarpophalangeal joints (43%).

By far the most commonly coexisting condition was generalized osteoarthritis, which was clinically diagnosed in 45 participants and was more common in women, particularly those with a longer duration of symptoms. A review of older X-rays from four of these patients revealed the presence of radiological evidence of the presence of osteoarthritis without CC. Rheumatoid arthritis, as defined by the American Rheumatism Association (ARA) criteria, was present in 8 participants, hypermobility in 13, and previous knee surgery prior to the onset of joint symptoms in 8, with CC only found in the operated knee in 3 of these. Previous treatment with steroids at a daily dose of 7.5 mg or more of prednisolone for five or more consecutive years was reported by 16 participants, for reasons including joint disease (n = 14), rheumatoid arthritis (n = 6), and presumed polymyalgia rheumatica (n = 8, one of whom had giant cell arteritis). Gout was the least common comorbidity, having been previously diagnosed in four participants but only having been confirmed by the presence of MSU crystals in synovial fluid in two of them. Clinically, there were no significant differences between those patients who had these associated conditions and those who did not, with the exception of those with rheumatoid arthritis and who thus had a younger mean age than the overall study population, and those who had received chronic steroid therapy and thus had experienced fewer acute attacks.

Radiological findings of linear and punctate calcification of hyaline and fibrocartilage were present in all except four participants (who showed other features typical of the arthropathy) and were usually bilateral. The knee meniscus was the site of the most densely calcified fibrocartilage; however, the triangular ligament of the wrist was also densely calcified, as was the pubic symphysis. Capsular calcification was seen in the metacarpophalangeal joints, metatarsophalangeal joints, shoulders, and hips, and periarticular soft tissue calcification was seen in tendons, particularly the Achilles, quadriceps, triceps, and supraspinatus. Features typical of degenerative joint disease were present in the majority of participants, including joint space narrowing, osteophytes, subchondral sclerosis, and cysts. The most severe damage was seen at the patella-femoral and radio-carpal joints. The knees, wrists, and metacarpophalangeal joints were the most frequently affected, followed by the elbow and glenohumeral joints.

Rapidly progressive destructive findings similar to Charcot joints were seen in 16 participants, resulting in 7 of these undergoing total hip replacement and 4 undergoing total knee replacement, with the remaining 5 with severe shoulder or elbow involvement.

Critique of the paper

This study used patients recruited from secondary care and potentially representing the more severe end of the disease spectrum. However, the study population was a large, unselected cohort and utilized both clinical and radiological examination to ensure accurate ascertainment of disease.

Significance of the paper

This study reported a clinical and radiological survey of 105 patients presenting to a rheumatologist with joint disease. This differed from the previous literature in that CPPD may be asymptomatic, and previous studies had included asymptomatic patients. However, this study also included patients with CC and a subsequent diagnosis of an alternative rheumatic disease, widening the spectrum of CC patients who were examined.

An important gender difference in the manifestation of CPPD deposition disease was uncovered by this study. The typical course of the disease in men began ten years earlier, had a shorter history of disease, and resulted in recurrent acute attacks in the joints of the lower limbs, whereas women tended to manifest a chronic polyarticular disease. Although the age/gender difference had been previously reported [1], the pattern of manifestation of the disease had not. Similarly the increased frequency of acute attacks in men had also previously been reported [2], but this study reported an equal gender incidence overall.

The coexistence of rheumatoid arthritis and osteoarthritis with CPPD strongly suggested joint damage as a risk factor for CC. This theory is supported by reports of patients who were only found to have CC in unstable or previously damaged joints [3–6] and by patients within this study who had CC only in joints which were the sites of previous surgery. Similarly, it was suggested that the previously reported associations between hypermobility, osteoarthritis, and CPPD might also be explained by chronic joint instability causing local mechanical damage and secondary crystal deposition [7].

Chronic steroid use was also suggested as a risk factor for crystal deposition, since steroids are known to adversely affect cartilage and bone. Sixteen of the 105 participants had been given long-term steroids, with 14 of the participants having been given steroids for diseases such as rheumatoid arthritis and polymyalgia rheumatica. The authors suggested that this could have been a coincidental finding, might have reflected arthropathy resulting from CPPD deposition mimicking polymyalgia rheumatica, or might have resulted from chronic steroid use predisposing to CC.

The authors also suggest that, in contrast to widely held opinion at the time, it is likely that CC is not a primary event but rather occurs following joint damage. However, once crystal deposition has occurred, it exerts a strong influence over the outcome, as destructive changes were seen frequently. This is also supported by findings that, in participants with a diagnosis of rheumatoid arthritis and coexisting pyrophosphate deposition, only three of the eight who met the ARA diagnostic criteria also had radiological findings which validated this diagnosis. These patients undoubtedly had rheumatoid arthritis, since they had a long history, typical joint deformities, nodules or vasculitis, and were strongly seropositive. The authors suggest that the CPPD appeared subsequently as a result of predisposing factors such as steroid therapy or pre-existing joint damage and modified the disease so that typical radiological signs were not seen.

The authors suggest hypothetical pathways linking predisposing factors with crystal deposition, and destructive arthropathies (Figure 7.4). Subsequent findings suggest that this pathway is likely to be common to other crystal arthropathies, since a similar predisposition to MSU crystal deposition has been shown in osteoarthritic joints [8].

Metabolic deposition of CPPD plays an important role in the pathway shown in Figure 7.5. In a companion paper, the authors report detailed findings of an investigation into the role that metabolic diseases play in predisposition to CC in this same cohort of 105 patients, matched with 105 age- and sex-matched patients admitted to the local hospital with acute medical conditions, and 48 unselected patients with uncomplicated clinical and radiological osteoarthritis [9]. After extensive biochemical, clinical, and radiological evaluation, they reported that, of the metabolic conditions previously linked with CPPD, only hypothyroidism and hyperparathyroidism were common. Chronic steroid use was also thought to be an important factor in CPPD, while hypertension, diabetes mellitus, hyperuricaemia, and mild uraemia were felt more likely to be related to age or drug therapy rather than the arthropathy itself. This companion paper also cited pre-existing joint damage as the most common cause of CPPD and found that metabolic associations were far less common in the patients studied. Furthermore, diagnosis of metabolic conditions in association with CPPD was made clinically, and thus extensive investigation in patients with CPPD for metabolic abnormalities was not felt to be appropriate.

HYPOTHESIS: CRYSTAL DEPOSITION ACTS AS AN"AMPLIFICATION
LOOP" IN CHRONIC DESTRUCTIVE ARTHROPATHIES

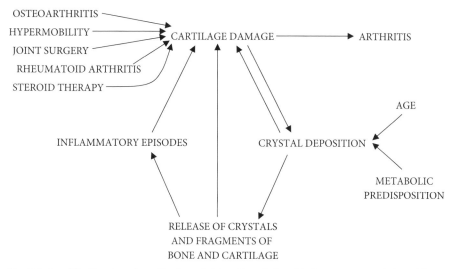

Fig. 7.4 Amplification loop hypothesis explaining the relationship between crystal deposition and joint damage.

Thus, pre-existing joint damage, for a variety of reasons, was felt to be the major cause of CPPD, and the mechanical and inflammatory damage which results from this deposition predisposes to further crystal deposition setting up a 'vicious cycle' that the authors describe as an 'amplification loop' in the pathogenesis of chronic arthritis.

This study is the first to survey a large cohort of unselected patients with joint disease for clinical and radiological evidence of CPPD and to hypothesize the role it plays in subsequent arthropathies. This led to the 'amplification' loop theory of pre-existing joint damage predisposing to CPPD, which in turn causes further cartilage damage, perpetuating the development of joint disease further. This study, along with its sister paper [9], also demonstrated that pre-existing joint damage is a far more common cause of CPPD than the metabolic associations previously described and that, of these, only hypothyroidism and hyperparathyroidism were common. As a result, the authors recommended that patients found to have CPPD should not be extensively investigated for underlying metabolic conditions.

References

1 **Atkins CJ, McIvor J, Smith PM, et al**. Chondrocalcinosis and arthropathy: studies in haemochromatosis and in idiopathic chondrocalcinosis. *QJMed* 1970;**39**(1):71–82.

2 **McCarty DJ**. Calcium pyrophosphate dihydrate crystal deposition disease: nomenclature and diagnostic criteria. *Ann Intern Med* 1977;**87**(2):241–2.

3 **Settas L, Doherty M, Dieppe P**. Localised chondrocalcinosis in unstable joints. *BMJ (Clin Res Ed)* 1982;**285**(6336):175–6.

4 **Doherty M, Watt I, Dieppe PA**. Localised chondrocalcinosis in post-meniscectomy knees. *Lancet* 1982;**319**(8283):1207–10.

5 **Ellman MH, Vazques LT, Brown NL, et al**. Calcium pyrophosphate dihydrate deposition in lumbar disc fibrocartilage. *J Rheumatol* 1981;**8**(6):955–8.

6 **de Lange EE, Keats TE**. Localized chondrocalcinosis in traumatized joints. *Skeletal Radiol* 1985;**14**(4):249–56.

7 **Bird HA, Tribe CR, Bacon PA**. Joint hypermobility leading to osteoarthrosis and chondrocalcinosis. *Ann Rheum Dis* 1978;**37**(3):203–11.

8 **Roddy E, Zhang W, Doherty M**. Are joints affected by gout also affected by osteoarthritis? *Ann Rheum Dis* 2007;**66**(10):1374–7.

9 **Alexander GM, Dieppe PA, Doherty M, et al**. Pyrophosphate arthropathy: a study of metabolic associations and laboratory data. *Ann Rheum Dis* 1982;**41**(4):377–81.

Chapter 8

Paediatric rheumatology

Nicola Ambrose, Despina Eleftheriou,
and John Ioannou

Introduction

This chapter aims to share with the reader a selection of paediatric rheumatology publications that we hope showcase this sub-speciality from its inception through to the
modern day.

The Ansell and Bywaters paper (Paper 8.1) was chosen because these authors are considered two of the founders of modern paediatric rheumatology. This seminal study set
the scene for randomized clinical trials undertaken to assess the efficacy of treatments in
juvenile arthritis patients.

'The treatment of Kawasaki syndrome with intravenous gamma globulin', a paper published by Newburger et al. (Paper 8.2), was chosen from a series of important papers that
Newburger published and which evaluated treatments for Kawasaki syndrome, a disease
that remains one of the most common vasculitides of childhood; this paper provides evidence for a treatment that may be life-saving in this condition.

The paper by Allen et al.—'Intraarticular triamcinolone hexacetonide in the management of chronic arthritis in children' (Paper 8.3)—was the first paper of its kind to attempt
to assess responses to steroid injections in a young population. Previously, children with
arthritis were treated as 'little adults' rather than being recognized as a distinct cohort.
The paper by Giannini et al., assessing the benefit of methotrexate with a double-blinded
randomized control trial (Paper 8.4), was a landmark paper in that it confirmed for the
first time anecdotal reports and provided evidence to support the use of methotrexate in
resistant juvenile arthritis, thus leading the way for this drug to be used first line in patients
failing to respond to non-steroidal anti-inflammatory drugs (NSAIDs); it remains the research upon which guidelines on methotrexate prescribing are based today.

One of the major obstacles to undertaking research in young patients with arthritis,
or in comparing published papers, was the lack of consistency in nomenclature and the
lack of definitions for disease improvement. We choose the 1977 paper by Giannini et al.
(Paper 8.5) and the 2004 paper by Petty et al. (Paper 8.8) to highlight these crucial developments, although Fink deserves special acknowledgement for having nine years earlier
undertaken the difficult task of establishing the first classification criteria for juvenile idiopathic arthritis.

Several of the papers highlight the evolution of modern treatments for juvenile idiopathic arthritis, with the first evidence for effectiveness of etanercept (Lovell et al.; Paper 8.7), evidence for the use of tocilizumab in systemic juvenile idiopathic arthritis (De Benedetti et al.; Paper 8.9), and the potential role for autologous haemopoietic stem-cell transplantation (Wulfrraat et al.; Paper 8.6) in resistant patients.

Finally, we choose a paper by Rettig and Atherya—'Adolescents with chronic disease. Transition to adult health care' (Paper 8.10). This was a landmark paper that helped shape the evolving specialty of adolescent rheumatology. Important work in this field was also undertaken by several others such as Janet McDonagh, and today adolescent and young adult rheumatology and the important role of transition is being acknowledged as an important part of a rheumatology service that bridges paediatric and adult care.

For each paper that was chosen for this chapter, there were numerous other papers that we would have liked to have also included, and some of these are referenced. Our hope is that this chapter provides the reader with a flavour of the history of paediatric rheumatology, and an appetite to read more.

Paper 8.1: Comparison of cortisone and aspirin in treatment of juvenile rheumatoid arthritis

Reference

Ansell BM, Bywaters EG, Isdale IC. Comparison of cortisone and aspirin in treatment of juvenile rheumatoid arthritis. *BMJ*. 1956;1(4975):1075–7.

Purpose

To compare the efficacy of cortisone vs aspirin therapy in juvenile rheumatoid arthritis patients.

Patients

Patients were diagnosed on clinical grounds as having 'rheumatoid type' polyarthritis involving two or more joints and with onset before the age of 16. Joint biopsies confirmed the diagnosis in seven cases. All the patients had active disease. Twenty-five patients were recruited, of whom 13 were assigned to the cortisone arm and 12 to the aspirin arm. The mean age was 9.3 years in the cortisone arm, and 9.4 years in the aspirin arm. There were four males in each arm. Baseline characteristics such as the disease activity and erythrocyte sedimentation rate (ESR) were similar in both groups.

Study design

This was a randomized, controlled, unblinded trial.

Treatment

Therapy was given for 12 weeks, following which patients had 1 week without treatment. They were then retreated if necessary, initially with another 12-week course, thereafter by continuous treatment. The cortisone group initially received 300 mg daily, 200 mg daily, and then five days of 100 mg of oral cortisone, following which the dose was adjusted to the individual (between 25 mg and 200 mg oral cortisone daily). The dosage of aspirin for older children started at 6 g daily for the first week, 2 g daily for the second week, and thereafter individually adjusted at between 3 g and 6 g daily. Smaller children were given proportionately less, down to an initial starting dose of 1.3 g at the age of 2.

Trial end points measured

Assessments included the patient's functional capacity in five grades; the disease activity (none, mild, severe); grip strength; a timing test (either using pegs or walking, depending on joint involvement); joint tenderness; and range of movement. The sedimentation rate and haemoglobin was measured and X-rays of the affected joints were undertaken before treatment and at one year and graded by blinded assessors.

Follow-up

Patients were assessed at intervals up to the period of one year from the start of treatment. Most outcome measures reported pertained to the 13-week and one-year time points.

Results

Results at 13 weeks and 1 year showed no significant differences between the two treatment arms. Overall, both treatment groups improved clinically and functionally to a similar extent. X-ray films showed an increase in the number of erosions (the number roughly doubling) in both groups. Timing of tasks was not found to be a useful outcome measure. For most outcomes assessed, the mean result at one year was slightly better in the aspirin group, with the exception of the haemoglobin, but differences were not significant. One patient in the cortisone group developed haemolytic anaemia and agranulocytosis and died at one year. The cause was not ascertained but was not attributed to the cortisone. Five of the 13 patients in the cortisone group were in complete remission and off all medication at one year, and 6 of the 12 aspirin patients were also disease and drug free at one year.

Critique of the paper

The paper includes 25 patients, which is a small number when assessing multiple output measures. It was unlikely to have had the power to show statistical differences for small changes between the groups. No attempt was made to blind the assessors of clinical disease activity, although those assessing radiographs were blinded. The paper predates the development of validated scoring systems for arthritis but despite this demonstrated efficacy of these two medications and was the first randomized trial undertaken in this population. It is interesting to note that the number of erosions doubled in both groups, highlighting that both treatments were suboptimal.

Significance and importance of the paper

This seminal study, undertaken by Barbara Ansell and Eric Bywaters, set the scene for undertaking randomized clinical trials to assess the efficacy of treatments in juvenile arthritis patients. In 1954 a similar trial had been undertaken in adult rheumatoid arthritis patients but until this point treatment in children was empiric rather than evidence-based.

Barbara Ansell and Eric Bywaters are two of the founders of modern paediatric rheumatology. The first book on paediatrics published in the English language was written by Thomas Phaer, who lived in a remote part of Wales. His book ('The Boke of Chyldren') devotes a section to 'the sytffnesse of the lymmes', which he describes as being produced by leaving children out in the frost, the cure being gentle thawing. In the following centuries, tuberculosis was recognized to involve joints, but non-tuberculous arthritis in children did not emerge until Cornil described a case in 1864. The first children's hospital in Great Britain was founded by Charles West in 1852 and had ten beds in Richard Mead's house in Great Ormond Street. West published several paediatric books but even in later editions

(1881) only allocated four paragraphs to childhood arthritis. Internationally, physicians Adams, Bouchet, and Marfan described case series of chronic rheumatism.

George Frederic Still joined Great Ormond Street, where in 1896 he described 19 cases of juvenile chronic polyarthritis, cases given to him by his superiors to review. He thought that chronic polyarthritis in childhood included a number of different conditions. He was inclined to view 'that the disease was infectious in nature' and noted that 'the synovial membrane showed active proliferation and fibrosis spreading to cartilage'. Still's article is famous because it was the first series of cases big enough to separate out subgroups on a clinical basis. Still was the first of the paediatricians to confine his work solely to children, and therefore he is better remembered as the founder of paediatrics in Great Britain rather than the founder of rheumatology, as the remainder of his career following residency was not devoted to any further rheumatology. For the first half of the twentieth century, little further advance occurred. Between the wars, Group A β-haemolytic streptococcus was identified as the causative organism of rheumatic fever and, simultaneously, pharmaceutical advances lead to the development of rheumatic fever treatments and prophylaxis.

In 1947 Eric Bywater set up a 100-bed rheumatism research unit at Taplow. This was an era when rheumatic fever was still one of the biggest problems in rheumatology. Initially, 96 beds were occupied by rheumatic fever and only 4 with polyarthritis but, due to improving public health conditions, the problem rapidly declined and rheumatoid arthritis became the point of interest.

Barbara Ansell came to work with Bywaters at Taplow in 1952. She later moved to become the head of the Division of Rheumatology at the Clinical Research Centre at Northwick Park Hospital in 1976. She was awarded a CBE in 1982 for her work in juvenile arthritis. Not only did she have a huge amount of clinical experience treating patients with juvenile chronic polyarthritis but, more importantly, she studied them thoroughly. Together with Eric Bywaters, they devised a follow-up scheme to enable them to keep track of almost all of their 1,000 patients. Their research interests included characterizing accurate subtypes of arthritis and running drug trials including the use of steroids in arthritis; they described the first large case series of 65 patients undergoing treatment with gold; they assessed the usefulness of outcome measures; they described diagnostic criteria for Still's disease; and they set the scene for modern-day paediatric rheumatology. [1–3]

References

1 **Ansell BM, Bywaters EG**. Rheumatoid arthritis (Still's disease). *Pediatr Clin North Am* 1963;**10**:921–39.

2 **Bywaters EG**. The history of pediatric rheumatology. *Arthritis Rheum* 1977;**20**(2 Suppl):145–52.

3 **Bywaters EG, Ansell BM**. Monoarticular arthritis in children. *Ann Rheum Dis* 1965;**24**(2):116–22.

Paper 8.2: The treatment of Kawasaki syndrome with intravenous gamma globulin

Reference

Newburger JW, Takahashi M, Burns JC, et al. The treatment of Kawasaki syndrome with intravenous gamma globulin. *N Engl J Med* 1986;315(6):341–7.

Purpose

To compare the efficacy of intravenous gamma globulin (IVIG) plus aspirin therapy vs aspirin alone in reducing the frequency of coronary artery abnormalities in children with acute Kawasaki syndrome.

Patients

Patients were recruited from six centres across the US. They were diagnosed on clinical grounds requiring the presence of five of the following six criteria: (1) fever; (2) non-exudative conjunctivitis; (3) changes in the oropharynx (mucosal erythema; dry fissured lips or strawberry tongue); (4) changes in the extremities (erythema of the palms/soles/oedema of the hands and feet, or periungueal desquamation in the subacute phase of the disease); (5) rash; and (6) cervical lymphadenopathy. Patients were recruited within ten days of the onset of the fever. One hundred and sixty eight patients were recruited, of whom 84 were randomized to each treatment arm. The mean age was 2.3 years in the aspirin arm and 2.7 years in the IVIG arm. Both arms had 41 females. Demographics between the two groups were similar. Patients in both groups were on average 6.4 days into their illness at the time of recruitment. Clinical and laboratory features were comparable.

Study design

This was a multicentre, randomized, unblinded trial.

Treatment

Patients in both treatments groups received aspirin, 100 mg/kg per day administered every six hours through to day 14 of the illness. Salicylate levels were measured five days after enrolment. On day 15 of the illness, the aspirin dose was reduced to 3–5 mg kg^{-1} day^{-1}, administered as a single daily dose. In children with normal echocardiographs, aspirin therapy was discontinued at seven weeks. Patients randomly assigned to the gamma globulin group received IVIG 400 mg kg^{-1} day^{-1} given over two hours on four consecutive days in addition to aspirin. The first infusion was administered on the day of enrolment.

Trial end points measured

The primary end point was the prevalence of coronary artery involvement at seven weeks in the two groups.

Follow-up

Echocardiograms (ECHOs) and blood tests were obtained at weeks 0, 2, and 7. ECHOs were interpreted blindly and independently by two paediatric echocardiographers.

Results

Six children by enrolment (day 7+) had abnormalities in one or more coronary arteries (four in the aspirin group, two in the IVIG group) and by seven weeks this had resolved completely in one of these patients in each group. The incidence of coronary aneurysms peaked at the two-week scan and had declined by seven weeks in both groups. At two weeks, 23% of the aspirin group and 8% of the IVIG group had detectable lesions (P = 0.01). By seven weeks, lesions were detected in 14% of the aspirin group vs 2.6% of the IVIG group (P = 0.01). It was estimated that the intervention reduced risk to a third of the risk for two weeks and one-fifth the risk by seven weeks. The age of the patient was not found to be a contributing factor regarding the impact of the treatments (Breslow–Day test for homogeneity). The group detected abnormalities most often in the left main and left anterior descending coronary arteries and least often in the circumflex. Children in the aspirin group tended to have a larger number of affected vessels after both intervals but this difference did not reach statistical significance. The majority of children treated with IVIG became afebrile after the first infusion, which was not the case in the aspirin group. Laboratory markers of inflammation also had a more rapid resolution in the IVIG group (white cells; absolute granulocyte counts, platelet counts, and serum alpha 1 antitrypsin in the first two days). These results were comparable between the groups by two and seven weeks. Of the five IVIG failures, these children had a greater rise in platelet count and a smaller decline in white cell counts. No child had a serious adverse effect to IVIG. Mild congestive failure developed in three children (4%) after the first infusion but in each case the child tolerated subsequent infusions without difficulty. A comparable number of children in the aspirin group had congestive heart failure. Children underwent hepatitis B and HIV screening and these remained negative in all cases at seven weeks post treatment.

Critique of the paper

Patients, their families, and the physicians were aware of the treatment assignment in this study. The authors argued that the likelihood of bias was low given the fact that those interpreting ECHOs and laboratory findings were blinded. The numbers were too small to comment on the potential impact IVIG may have had on existing aneurysms. Lastly, this trial did not find the optimum dosage of IVIG or the optimum number of days that children should be treated.

Significance and importance of the paper

Kawasaki syndrome remains one of the most common vasculitides of childhood. It is typically a self-limited condition with fever and manifestations of acute inflammation lasting for an average of 12 days without therapy. However, cardiovascular complications, particularly coronary artery aneurysms, can lead to significant morbidity and mortality.

This multicentre randomized trial demonstrated that high-dose IVIG administered early in the course of KS was effective in reducing the prevalence of coronary artery abnormalities. They also found that IVIG significantly reduced fever and laboratory indications of the acute phase response, suggesting a rapid generalized anti-inflammatory effect. Two earlier Japanese studies had asked the same question. In one a low dose of IVIG was used ($100 \text{ mg kg}^{-1} \text{ day}^{-1}$) and had shown no significant difference. The other study used the $400 \text{ mg kg}^{-1} \text{ day}^{-1}$ dose and had similar results to this trial but had been strongly criticized for the fact that echocardiographers were not blinded and that extensive protocol exclusions had applied. [1]

In 1991 a multicentre randomized controlled trial involving 549 children with acute KS was undertaken, to compare a single IVIG infusion (2 g/kg over ten hours) to four infusions (400 mg/kg over four consecutive days). Both treatment groups received aspirin. The relative prevalence of coronary abnormalities among patients treated with the four-day regimen, as compared to the one-day arm, was 1.94 two weeks after enrolment and 1.84 at seven weeks after enrolment. Children in the one-day arm also had lower mean temperatures while hospitalized, shorter mean duration of fever, and a more rapidly normalizing acute phase response. The two groups had similar rates of adverse events. This trial led to the adoption of a one-day regimen. [2]

In 1995, a meta-analysis was published assessing the efficacy of aspirin and IVIG treatment in the prevention of coronary artery aneurysms in KS. They found that the incidence of aneurysms was lowest in the high-IVIG, and lower especially in the single-dose IVIG group. There was no apparent difference whether aspirin was low or high dose. [3]

In 2004, guidelines by the American Heart Association and the American Academy of Pediatrics were developed. They recommended initial therapy with IVIG 2 g/kg administered as a single infusion over 8–12 hours, and aspirin.

Interestingly, recent clinical trials and meta-analyses have demonstrated that the addition of corticosteroids to IVIG is beneficial for the prevention of coronary artery aneurysms in severe cases with highest risk of IVIG resistance. [4–6] Outside of Japan, however, clinical scores to predict IVIG resistance perform suboptimally. Other therapies, including anti-TNFα [7], could also have a role for IVIG-resistant KD or as a first-line therapy to rapidly reduce the ongoing inflammatory responses and improve outcome.

References

1 Furusho K, Nakano H, Shinomiya K, et al. High-dose intravenous immunoglobulin for Kawasaki Disease. *Lancet* 1984;**2**(8411):1055–8.

2 Newburger JW, Sleeper LA, McCrindle BW, et al. A single intravenous infusion of gamma globulin as compared with four infusions in the treatment of acute Kawasaki syndrome. *N Engl J Med* 1991;**324**(23):1633–9.

3 **Durongpisitkul K, Gururaj VJ, Park JM, et al**. The prevention of coronary artery aneurysm in Kawasaki disease: a meta-analysis on the efficacy of aspirin and immunoglobulin treatment. *Pediatrics* 1995;**96**(6):1057–61.

4 **Inoue Y, Okada Y, Shinohara M, et al**. A multicenter prospective randomized trial of corticosteroids in primary therapy for Kawasaki disease: clinical course and coronary artery outcome. *J Pediatr* 2006;**149**(3):336–41.

5 **Chen S, Dong Y, Yin Y, et al**. Intravenous immunoglobulin plus corticosteroid to prevent coronary artery abnormalities in Kawasaki disease: a meta-analysis. *Heart* 2013;**99**(2):76–82.

6 **Kobayashi T, Saji T, Otani T, et al**. Efficacy of immunoglobulin plus prednisolone for prevention of coronary artery abnormalities in severe Kawasaki disease (RAISE study): a randomised, open-label, blinded-endpoints trial. *Lancet* 2012;**379**(9826):1613–20.

7 **Burns JC, Best BM, Mejias A, et al**. Infliximab treatment of intravenous immunoglobulin-resistant Kawasaki disease. *J Pediatr* 2008;**153**(6):833–8.

Paper 8.3: Intra-articular triamcinolone hexacetonide in the management of chronic arthritis in children

Reference

Allen RC, Gross KR, Laxer RM, et al. Intraarticular triamcinolone hexacetonide in the management of chronic arthritis in children. *Arthritis Rheum* 1986;29(8):997–1001.

Purpose

To investigate the use of intra-articular triamcinolone hexacetonide in the management of persistent knee arthritis that is unresponsive to nonsteroidal anti-inflammatories, in children.

Patients

All patients were under 16 years old at the onset of chronic arthritis. Forty children were recruited. Twenty-nine fulfilled the American Rheumatism Association criteria, four had seronegative enthesopathy-related arthropathy, six had psoriatic arthritis, and one had juvenile ankylosing spondylitis. All patients had arthritis in more than four joints at the time of study. All had active arthritis for >4 months, all had received >3 months acetylsalicylic acid for inflammation, and approximately a fifth had received other NSAIDS.

Study design

This was a prospective, unblinded, uncontrolled study.

Treatment

Fifty-three knees from 40 patients were injected at least once. Following cleansing of the skin and local anaesthetic, fluid was drained from the knee; then, 20–40 mg of triamcinolone hexacetonide was injected.

Trial end points measured

A good response was defined as complete resolution of the signs and symptoms of active inflammation (joint effusion, heat, and tenderness), with or without complete correction of deformity. A relapse was defined as a sustained re-accumulation of joint effusion, with or without heat, tenderness, or loss of range of motion. The time of relapse was taken as the point at which the attending physician believed the signs of inflammation had recurred.

Follow-up

The effects of the injections were evaluated at 6, 12, and 24 months. All patients were followed for at least three months, 49 knees were followed for six months, 40 knees for one year, and 31 knees for two years.

Results

Of 49 knees that were injected and followed for six months, all knees responded well to injection initially. The procedure was well tolerated. One patient developed a small area of subcutaneous atrophy at the injection site.

By six months, 63.3% of knees were still in remission: 67.6% of the juvenile rheumatoid arthritis vs 50% of the knees of children from other groups. In the juvenile rheumatoid arthritis group, a good response was associated with male sex. The mean age was higher in the relapse group (14.39 years old) than in the persistent responders group (8.75 years old; P < 0.005) In addition, the duration of arthritis at the time of injection differed in the two groups, with a mean duration of 3.5 years in the juvenile rheumatoid arthritis response group vs 8.6 years in the relapse group (P < 0.005). There were no significant differences among human leukocyte antigen (HLA) allele groups or between the presence and absence of antinuclear antibodies. Of patients who had both knees injected, a concordant response was observed in only 8 of 12.

At one year, 50% of the juvenile rheumatoid arthritis group continued to have a good response, vs 30% in the other groups. There were no differences between the groups with respect to sex or dose. The good responders were younger than the relapsers and had a shorter disease duration. At two years, of the 31 knees still being followed, 16.1% remained in the good response group. Of the eight knees that were re-injected following a relapse, five achieved remission that lasted for at least six months.

Critique of the paper

The paper includes 40 patients, which is a small number when assessing multiple outcomes at multiple time points. The non-juvenile rheumatoid arthritis groups were very small. The study claims that there is no association between response and HLA antigen type or the presence of antinuclear antibodies but it is unlikely that it had sufficient power for this to be a convincing negative. There is no control group undergoing a sham procedure or being followed prospectively with no procedure. No comparison was made using other steroids, and no explanation was given as to why some patients received 20 mg and others 40 mg triamcinolone hexacetonide.

Significance and importance of the paper

The importance of this paper is that it was the first of its kind to attempt to assess responses to steroid injections in a young population. Previously, physicians treated children with arthritis as 'little adults' rather than recognizing that these patients represent a distinct cohort. Steroid injections were given empirically rather than because of any evidence to support their use. Despite the lack of a sham-control, this paper demonstrates that intra-articular steroid injections were effective for juvenile arthritis, particularly juvenile rheumatoid arthritis.

Intra-articular corticosteroid injections are still utilized for active arthritis, usually when there are a small number of active joints. They are used most commonly in oligoarticular

JIA but may also be used in other subtypes of JIA when a few joints remain inflamed despite systemic therapy. Following on from this paper, studies were next undertaken to assess the duration of sustained benefit after injections but these had widely varying results. [1–4] The injections are generally considered to be effective for six weeks to three months. Later it was shown that the concomitant use of methotrexate leads to longer periods of remission. An important paper demonstrated a superior efficacy of triamcinolone hexacetonide over triamcinolone acetonide. [5] More recently, a larger study studied 95 joints (37 patients) that had received a total number of 125 injections [6]. Remission of the joint inflammation, lasting at least 6 months, was obtained in 62 of 95 injections (65%), which is about equivalent to the findings reported by Allen and colleagues. Treatment of joint contractures was successful in 35 of 51 joints (69%). In patients with oligoarticular arthritis, 21 of 26 injected joints (81%) were in full remission at six months. The six-month remission was significantly lower in the other subtypes of JIA, again supporting the observations by Allen et al. These studies in combination have demonstrated that steroid injections are an effective and safe treatment for inflammatory joints in JIA, particularly in the oligoarticular form. Injections have also been shown to be effective in correcting joint contractures and deformities. Current best practise is to administer steroid injections for mono/oligoarthritis in JIA and for some cases of polyarticular JIA.

References

1 **Eberhard BA, Sison MC, Gottlieb BS, et al**. Comparison of the intraarticular effectiveness of triamcinolone hexacetonide and triamcinolone acetonide in treatment of juvenile rheumatoid arthritis. *J Rheumatol* 2004; **3**(12):2507–12.

2 **Beukelman T, Guevara JP, Albert DA**. Optimal treatment of knee monoarthritis in juvenile idiopathic arthritis: a decision analysis. *Arthritis Rheum* 2008;**59**(11):1580–8.

3 **Beukelman T, Guevara JP, Albert DA, et al**. Variation in the initial treatment of knee monoarthritis in juvenile idiopathic arthritis: a survey of pediatric rheumatologists in the United States and Canada. *J Rheumatol* 2007;**34**(9):1918–24.

4 **Padeh S, Passwell JH**. Intraarticular corticosteroid injection in the management of children with chronic arthritis. *Arthritis Rheum* 1998;**41**(7):1210–4.

5 **Zulian F, Martini G, Gobber D, et al**. Triamcinolone acetonide and hexacetonide intra-articular treatment of symmetrical joints in juvenile idiopathic arthritis: a double-blind trial. *Rheumatology* 2004;**43**(10):1288–91.

6 **Unsal E, Makay B**. Intraarticular triamcinolone in juvenile idiopathic arthritis. *Indian Pediatr* 2008;**45**(12):995–7.

Paper 8.4: A USA-USSR double-blind, placebo-controlled trial on methotrexate in resistant juvenile rheumatoid arthritis

Reference

Giannini EH, Brewer EJ, Kuzmina N, et al. Methotrexate in resistant juvenile rheumatoid arthritis. Results of the U.S.A.-U.S.S.R. double-blind, placebo-controlled trial. *N Engl J Med* 1992;326:(16)1043–9.

Purpose

To compare the efficacy of two different doses of oral methotrexate vs placebo therapy in resistant juvenile rheumatoid arthritis patients.

Patients

Patients were diagnosed on clinical grounds as having juvenile rheumatoid arthritis by using the American College of Rheumatology (ACR) criteria. Patients between 18 months and 18 years and who had disease that was not adequately controlled by NSAIDs or second-line agents were recruited. Patients who had received other disease-modifying antirheumatic drugs (DMARDs) or intra-articular or intramuscular long-acting steroids within the preceding three months were excluded, as were patients who had previously received methotrexate. Of the 127 patients who took part, 31 were boys. Sixty-six subjects were recruited in the USA, and 61 in the former USSR. The average age was 10.1 years old and the average disease duration was 5.1 years. Twenty-five per cent of participants had systemic disease. For patients to be included, they had to be 100% compliant with medication use for at least 80% of the six-month study. In total, 108 (85%) of the patients completed the full six months.

Study design

This was a double-blind, parallel, randomized, placebo-controlled trial undertaken in the USA and the former USSR. One hundred and twenty-seven children took part.

Treatment

Methotrexate was prescribed orally at either 10 mg/m^2 body surface (low dose) or 5 mg/m^2 (very low dose), or a placebo was given. The maximum dose was 15 mg/week. Patients were allowed to take up to two NSAIDs, as well as prednisolone not exceeding 0.5 mg/kg (max 10 mg per day), concurrently with the study medication, and the dose of these had to be stable for one month before and for the duration of the trial.

Trial end points measured

Assessments included the patient's disease activity measured as follows: joint swelling (none, mild, moderate, or severe); pain on motion; joint tenderness; and limitation of motion. The number of joints deemed to be active and the duration of morning stiffness was noted. These formed a composite score, and a positive result was counted if there was more than a 25% improvement in this score. As well as this composite score, other primary outcomes included the physician's global assessment of response and the articular severity score. Secondary outcomes included number of joints with swelling, pain on motion, tenderness and limitation of motion, duration of morning stiffness, and blood markers of inflammation (haemoglobin and sedimentation rate). X-rays were not deemed to be useful because of the short duration of the trial and were not undertaken.

Follow-up

The primary end point was at six months. Patients were assessed at seven visits over a seven-month period. At each assessment, arthritis was clinically assessed and bloods were taken.

Results

Efficacy was demonstrated for the low-dose methotrexate but not the very-low-dose, compared with placebo. A reduction in the articular severity score of more than 25% was one of the primary outcome measures. Using this score, 63% of patients in the low-dose group were classified as improved, compared to 32% of the very-low-dose, and 36% of the placebo group. This difference between low-dose methotrexate and the other groups was significant (P = 0.013). The physician's global assessment, another primary end point, showed that a significantly higher proportion of patients improved in the low-dose group than in the placebo group (P = 0.023) but no difference was found with the very-low-dose vs placebo. The secondary outcomes, which together formed the composite score, all showed better values in the low-dose methotrexate group vs the other two groups; however, for most of these scores, results were not statistically significant. The one that did reach significance even with correction for multiple testing was the number of joints with limitation of motion. The medication was well tolerated, with 12% of low-dose, 20% of very-low-dose, and 12% of placebo patients reporting clinical side effects mostly related to gastrointestinal complaints, which were deemed to be possibly related to the medication by blinded assessors. No patient had pulmonary symptoms. Regarding laboratory outcomes, 15 patients in the low- and very-low-dose vs only 5 of the placebo patients had abnormalities deemed to be likely to be secondary to medications. The most frequent abnormalities were elevation of aminotransferase levels and anaemia.

Critique of the paper

This study had a short follow-up of only six months, which was too short to assess outcomes such as progression of erosive disease or long-term safety. It reached its primary end points successfully but did not reach its secondary end points, probably because there were too few patients to detect small differences between subgroups once corrections were made for multiple comparisons. Over 40% of the placebo group—a high percentage—reached the primary end point of greater than 25% improvement of the composite score.

The fact that patients were allowed take steroids and two NSAIDS during the trial probably accounts for this result and made it difficult to show improvement in the very-low-dose methotrexate group. Patients had to be 100% compliant for 80% of the six-month study, had to have not received intra-articular/intramuscular steroids, and could not have previously taken methotrexate therapy; these conditions may have skewed the population being tested away from the normal outpatient population. Finally, the paper does not tell us about the breakdown of the juvenile arthritis subtypes, other than stating that 25% were systemic. It also does not tell us if patients with spinal symptoms showed any response to treatment.

Significance and importance of the paper

The efficacy of the antimetabolite methotrexate had already been shown in placebo-controlled trials in adults with rheumatoid arthritis. However, supporting data in children had come from uncontrolled trials. For the first time, this trial confirmed anecdotal reports and provided evidence to support the use of methotrexate in resistant juvenile arthritis, leading the way for this drug to be used first line in patients failing to respond to NSAIDs. This trial heralded the beginning of randomized controlled trials to assess the efficacy of DMARDs in the paediatric arthritis population.

This study remains the research upon which guidelines on methotrexate prescribing are based today. Empiric escalation of the dose of methotrexate in less responsive patients has occurred as experience with methotrexate in juvenile idiopathic arthritis has increased. Small trials and, non-controlled descriptive reports advocated the use of higher doses of methotrexate in patients with juvenile idiopathic arthritis unresponsive to initial standard doses, [1] until in 2010 a retrospective cohort study compared children in whom methotrexate >0.5 mg kg^{-1} week^{-1} ('high-dose') had been started, to children in whom methotrexate ≤ 0.5 mg kg^{-1} week^{-1} ('low-dose') had been prescribed. [2] Of the 220 children identified, at six months, the high-dose group was more likely to have an elevated aspartate aminotransferase or alanine aminotransferase (adjusted OR 3.89; 95% CI, 1.82–8.29; P < 0.0001). Subjects receiving both methotrexate and NSAIDs had no significant difference between groups in change of active joint count, while subjects in the high-dose group but not taking NSAIDs had more active joints (P = 0.036) at six months compared to the low-dose group. Initial high-dose methotrexate was associated with an increased risk of at least one liver enzyme abnormality, with no significant improvement in active joint count. This suggests that there was no apparent benefit, while the potential for liver toxicity was increased, when using higher doses of methotrexate at treatment inception in patients with juvenile idiopathic arthritis.

In 2010 a prospective, open, multicentre medication-withdrawal randomized clinical trial was published, assessing the likelihood of relapse if methotrexate was withdrawn in patients in remission for 6 or 12 months. [3] At 24 months approximately 55% of patients in both groups had flared. This study found that in juvenile idiopathic arthritis in remission, a 12-month vs a 6-month withdrawal of methotrexate did not reduce the relapse rate.

Other DMARDs were also studied over the coming years. In 1998 a 24-week randomized, placebo-controlled, double-blind, multicentre study of patients with active juvenile idiopathic arthritis was undertaken to assess the efficacy, tolerability, and safety of sulphasalazine. Of the 69 patients enrolled, 52 (75%) completed the trial. Six patients (18%) withdrew from the placebo group, and 11 (31%) withdrew from the sulphasalazine group (P = 0.18). There was a significant difference in the articular severity score (P = 0.02), all global assessments (P = 0.01), and the laboratory parameters (P < 0.001) with the sulphasalazine group performing better. Adverse events occurred more frequently in the sulphasalazine group. [4] The results demonstrated that sulphasalazine was effective and safe in the treatment of children with oligoarticular- and polyarticular-onset juvenile idiopathic arthritis, although it was not well tolerated in one-third of the patients.

In 2005 Silverman et al. undertook a multinational, multicentre, randomized, controlled trial to compare leflunomide and methotrexate in children with juvenile idiopathic arthritis. [5] Of 94 patients randomized, 86 completed 16 weeks of treatment, 70 of whom entered into the 32-week extension study. At week 16, more patients in the methotrexate group than in the leflunomide group had an ACR Pediatric (Pedi) 30 response (89% vs 68%; P = 0.02), whereas the values for the Percent Improvement Index did not differ significantly (−52.87% vs −44.41%; P = 0.18). In both groups, the improvements achieved at week 16 were maintained at week 48. Aminotransferase elevations were more frequent with methotrexate than with leflunomide during the initial study and the extension study.

These studies together provided evidence to support the use of DMARDs in juvenile idiopathic arthritis which had until this point been treated empirically. Furthermore, together they support the use of methotrexate as first line after NSAIDs but also show efficacy of sulphasalazine and leflunomide.

References

1 **Ruperto N, Murray KJ, Gerloni V, et al**. A randomized trial of parenteral methotrexate comparing an intermediate dose with a higher dose in children with juvenile idiopathic arthritis who failed to respond to standard doses of methotrexate. *Arthritis Rheum* 2004;**50**(7):2191–201.

2 **Becker ML, Rose CD, Cron RQ, et al**. Effectiveness and toxicity of methotrexate in juvenile idiopathic arthritis: comparison of 2 initial dosing regimens. *J Rheumatol* 2010;**37**(4): 870–5.

3 **Foell D, Wulffraat N, Wedderburn LR, et al**. Methotrexate withdrawal at 6 vs 12 months in juvenile idiopathic arthritis in remission: a randomized clinical trial. *JAMA* 2010;**303**(13):1266–73.

4 **Van Rossum MA, Fiselier TJ, Franssen MJ, et al**. Sulfasalazine in the treatment of juvenile chronic arthritis: a randomized, double-blind, placebo-controlled, multicenter study. *Arthritis Rheum* 1998;**41**(5):808–16.

5 **Silverman E, Mouy R, Spiegel L, et al**. Leflunomide or methotrexate for juvenile rheumatoid arthritis. *N Engl J Med* 2005;**352**(16):1655–66.

Paper 8.5: Preliminary definition of improvement in juvenile arthritis

Reference

Giannini EH, Ruperto N, Ravelli A, et al. Preliminary definition of improvement in juvenile arthritis. *Arthritis Rheum* 1997;40(7):1202–9.

Purpose

To identify a core set of outcome variables for the assessment of children with juvenile arthritis in order to use this core set to develop a definition of improvement of juvenile arthritis. The rationale was to have consensus measures to use in determining whether individual patients demonstrate clinically important improvement and to promote this definition as a single efficacy measure in future juvenile arthritis clinical trials.

Methods

Identification of a core set of outcome variables

A multistep process was involved in searching for, defining, and validating a set of core outcome variables. Initially, a 16-member advisory council was formed consisting of members of the rheumatology section of the American Academy of Pediatrics, the paediatric section of the ACR and the Arthritis Foundation, OMERACT (an outcome measures in rheumatology network) members, and private and academic practitioners. The council first completed a questionnaire ranking the usefulness of 25 variables. They were also asked to suggest other variables they felt were important. They then met in Florida and developed a core set of response variables. This included (1) the physician's global assessment of overall disease activity VAS, (2) the parent/patient global assessment of overall well-being VAS, (3) functional ability, (4) the number of joints with active arthritis, (5) the number of joints with limited range of motion, and (6) ESR. A follow-up questionnaire was then sent to a larger international cohort (198 sent; 140 completed and returned) of practitioners to obtain their reaction to the core set and its proposed use. This survey validated the Florida findings, as the core six variables chosen in Florida also scored highest in the larger survey. Further questions revealed that participants felt that the number of core variables that were needed to improve to demonstrate improvement was 3, and the number of variables worsening that could be ignored if they worsened was 2. The task force then put each of these variables through several previously conducted trials and found that they correlated well with each other (i.e. they changed in the same direction) but were not redundant (each added useful information).

Development and selection of a definition of improvement

Once the core variables had been established, the group next developed multiple definitions of improvement based on the core variables and set out to decide on the best combination. A second conference took place in Pavia, Italy, in 1996 and was attended by 21 paediatric rheumatologists from 14 countries. First, they reviewed 72 patient profiles from a published trial that had documented each of the six core outcome measures of interest. They reviewed profiles from patients who were near the threshold level of improvement (i.e. patients with 100% improvement were excluded). Each participant was asked to say whether they thought a patient had improved, and patients where a consensus of 80% was reached were further evaluated to calculate the false-positive and the false-negative rates for each definition of improvement. Their specificity, sensitivity, and hence validity were then established.

Results

Final definition of improvement

The final definition of improvement with the highest final score was as follows: at least 30% improvement from baseline in three of any six core variables, with no more than one of the remaining variables worsening by >30%. The second-highest scoring definition was closely related to the first, thus indicating convergent validity of the process used.

Critique of the paper

The majority of expert participants were from North America and Europe, and the patient cohort used for defining improvement was an Italian population. Other ethnic populations were not considered. The lack of a valid, widely available laboratory marker of inflammation in children with arthritis is the other limitation, and this group chose ESR as the marker of disease activity. However, some children with active disease may have a normal ESR, and the authors proposed that ESR be replaced as soon as a more reliable laboratory biomarker of disease activity became available. The authors chose not to attempt to create different definitions of improvement for the various subtypes of JRA and instead focused on the central features of arthritis, function, and well-being. These core outcomes may also under-represent arthritis in joints where swelling cannot be clinically appreciated, such as the hips or axial spine. Finally, improvement as per this definition is a categorical outcome, being either present or absent. It may be useful to have a scale to grade improvement, similar to the ACR 20/50/70 response used in adults.

Significance and importance of the paper

Prior to this paper, no consensus definition of improvement existed for juvenile arthritis, and thus it was difficult to combine study outcomes for meta-analysis or to compare treatments assessed in different trials. The establishment of core variables and the consensus definition of improvement was a huge advancement, allowing a more rigorous approach to clinical research and drug trials.

Hand in hand with this paper was the equally important development two years earlier of a classification criteria published by Fink et al. for idiopathic arthritis of childhood. [1] It had long been recognized that juvenile arthritis was not a homogenous disease. However, several classification systems were being used around the world that varied enough that comparisons between trials were difficult to undertake. The Pediatric Standing Committee of the International League of Associations for Rheumatology (ILAR) was established in 1993 with Chester Fink as chairman and it was decided that the first priority was to develop a classification criteria. Similar to the process used by Giannini to develop a definition of improvement, this process was complicated and required establishment of international task forces, several meetings, and layers of consensus seeking and validation. The committee eventually decided on the following groups: (1) systemic arthritis; (2) polyarthritis, rheumatoid factor negative; (3) polyarthritis, rheumatoid factor positive; (4) Oligoarthritis (up to four joints during the first six months of the disease, and no more than five joints after this point); (5) extended oligoarthritis (four joints up to the first six months, and five or more joints after this point); (6) enthesitis-related arthritis, and (7) psoriatic arthritis. One of the principles underlying these classifications was that there should be no overlap between the seven diseases. Therefore, patients with criteria for more than one classification were left unclassified but were to be given ongoing consideration as part of a continuing study.

The result of these two major undertakings to establish an international consensus for both the classification of juvenile arthritis and a definition of improvement allowed for the development of more robust, reproducible, and comparable trials over the coming years.

Reference

1 **Fink CW**. Proposal for the development of classification criteria for idiopathic arthritides of childhood. *J Rheumatol* 1995;**22**(8):1566–9.

Paper 8.6: Autologous haemopoietic stem-cell transplantation in refractory juvenile chronic arthritis

Reference

Wulffraat N, Van Royen A, Bierings M, et al. Autologous haemopoietic stem-cell transplantation in four patients with refractory juvenile chronic arthritis. *Lancet* 1999;353(9152):550–3.

Purpose

To report on the first four children with juvenile idiopathic arthritis to undergo autologous haemopoietic stem-cell transplantation.

Patients

Patients were diagnosed on clinical grounds as having systemic (n = 3) or polyarticular (n = 1) juvenile arthritis with onset before the age of 16 years. All had active disease. The systemic patients were 6 (n = 1) and 11 (n = 2) years old, respectively. Two were girls. The patient with polyarticular juvenile idiopathic arthritis was a 7-year-old girl. All had severe resistant disease, raised inflammatory markers, and significant growth delays.

Study

This was a case series of four patients.

Treatment

Bone marrow aspiration was performed to obtain haemopoietic stem cells without priming. The graft was purged via two cycles of T-cell depletion with CD2 and CD3 antibodies, and the suspension was then stored in liquid nitrogen.

The patient conditioning regimen included two days of antithymocyte globulin at 5 mg/kg daily from day −9 to day −6; cyclosporin at 50 mg/kg daily from day −5 to day −2, and low-dose (4 Gy) single-fraction total body irradiation on day −1. At day 0 the frozen stem-cell suspension was thawed and infused. DMARDs had been previously stopped. NSAIDs were continued. Prednisolone was tapered over two months.

Trial end points measured

Clinical markers of disease activity improvement (based on factors described by Giannini et al.) were assessed. Patients were monitored to assess reconstitution of blood profiles and normalization of inflammatory markers.

Follow-up

Follow-up ranged from 6 months to 18 months.

Results

The conditioning was well tolerated in all four patients and there was substantial resolution of signs and symptoms of active disease by two weeks with normalization of ESR and C-reactive protein. Haemoglobin returned to normal by eight weeks. Two patients developed varicella zoster virus eruptions, which were treated with acyclovir. One patient was platelet transfusion dependent for 28 days. All patients remained well over follow-up. Owing to existing erosive damage, some markers of pain and function did not improve but all patients came off DMARD medications. Two patients developed mild joint swelling at four months and which subsided without treatment. All had an increase in their growth velocity over the follow-up period.

Critique of the paper

The paper reports on a series of four juvenile arthritis patients who successfully underwent autologous bone marrow transplantation. This was not a trial, and the patient numbers were small. The bone marrow aspirate was T-cell depleted and there is no evidence to say if this was or was not critical. Likewise, the addition of the low-dose body irradiation regimen used requires more investigation. Long-term consequences cannot be ascertained due to the short follow-up period but the authors comment that no long-term effects of 4 Gy single-dose therapy have been observed in patients undergoing this treatment for aplastic anaemia. In contrast, high-dose irradiation therapy has been associated with the development of solid tumours in later life. Longer follow-up would be needed to ascertain if the remission would be long-lasting. The usefulness of this treatment for other forms of juvenile arthritis cannot be ascertained from this paper. The centre did not mobilize bone marrow progenitor cells with cyclophosphamide and granulocyte colony stimulating factor because the latter had been associated with reactivation of rheumatoid arthritis and the development of leukocytoclastic vasculitis.

Significance and importance of the paper

This seminal paper by Wulfrraat et al. published in 1999 was the first to demonstrate the efficacy of autologous bone marrow transplantation in the treatment of juvenile arthritis. This study offered a new mechanism of treatment for those patients who fail to respond or lose their response to DMARDs and biologic monoclonal antibody treatments or in whom long-term steroid toxicity is pronounced. In particular, growth retardation, obesity, osteoporosis, and cataracts are some of the many major disadvantages associated with prolonged use of steroids.

The mechanism of action of autologous haematopoietic stem-cell transplantation in autoimmune disease is stringent immunosuppression with chemotherapy followed by autologous stem-cell rescue from which the immune repertoire can be rebuilt. The goal is to reset the immune system. Long-term data were published by the same group in 2004 and showed a 40%–50% long-term rate of relapse in juvenile arthritis (both in polyarticular and systemic), and a 10%–15% mortality risk. [1] Results were similar in a UK cohort followed from 2000–2007 [2]. There is an increased incidence of macrophage activation syndrome in patients with systemic juvenile idiopathic arthritis, along with opportunistic and viral infections. While steroids, DMARDs, and biologics remain the standard of care, patients with juvenile idiopathic arthritis refractory to all these treatments may be considered for autologous haematopoietic stem-cell transplantation in the setting of severe resistant disease. Current protocols are based on the University Medical Centre Utrecht autologous transplantation protocol. This involves mobilizing stem cells after a cyclophosphamide pulse with granulocyte colony stimulating factor. Apheresis is performed approximately four weeks prior to infusion. Peripheral blood stem cells are collected. At approximately two weeks the patient receives anti-thymocyte treatment, cyclophosphamide, and fludarabine, followed by reinfusion of the thawed autologous graft.

A more recent development is the use of mesenchymal stromal cells (MSCs). These cells are an adherent subset of the non-haematopoietic stem cells that can be easily cultured and expanded from the bone marrow and adipose tissue. They are poorly immunogenic so treatment with allogeneic MSCs does not require conditioning therapy. MSCs were first used as second-line therapy for the treatment of steroid refractory acute graft vs host disease after allogeneic haematopoietic stem-cell transplantation. In a study which included children, they offered a valuable treatment option with higher overall survival (from 10% to 53%) for patients with acute graft vs host disease. More recently, MSCs have been used instead of haematopoietic stem-cell transplantation in some settings. The first patient to receive MSCs for an autoimmune disease was a patient with systemic sclerosis and the treatment was deemed to be successful. Wulfrraat's group is currently conducting a pilot study on efficacy and safety of local administration of allogeneic bone marrow-MSCs for therapy in refractory juvenile idiopathic arthritis patients.

The use of allogeneic haematopoietic stem-cell transplantation is felt by those in the transplant field to offer the highest chance of cure for severe AIDS, [3] but in humans no head-to-head study has yet been undertaken and most current data come from patients treated with allogeneic haematopoietic stem-cell transplantation for other haematological diseases. Other future considerations will be changes to the chemotherapy regimens, and protocols combining allogeneic haematopoietic stem-cell transplantation with MSC infusions. Hand in hand with these advancements will have to be methods to better identify patients who will benefit from these therapies, before these patients have accumulated huge damage and while they are at lower risk for the procedure.

References

1 De Kleer IM, Brinkman DM, Ferster A, et al. Autologous stem cell transplantation for refractory juvenile idiopathic arthritis: analysis of clinical effects, mortality, and transplant related morbidity. *Ann Rheum Dis* 2004;**63**(10):1318–26.

2 Abinun M, Flood TJ, Cant AJ, et al. Autologous T cell depleted haematopoietic stem cell transplantation in children with severe juvenile idiopathic arthritis in the UK (2000–7). *Mol Immunol* 2009;**47**(1):46–51.

3 Daikeler T, Hügle T, Farge D, et al. Allogeneic hematopoietic HSCT for patients with autoimmune diseases. *Bone Marrow Transplant* 2009;**44**(1):27–33.

Paper 8.7: Etanercept in children with polyarticular juvenile rheumatoid arthritis

Reference

Lovell DJ, Giannini EH, Reiff A, et al. Etanercept in children with polyarticular rheumatoid arthritis. *N Engl J Med* 2000;342(11):763–9.

Purpose

To evaluate the safety and efficacy of etanercept therapy in juvenile rheumatoid arthritis patients.

Patients

Patients were diagnosed on clinical grounds as having active polyarticular juvenile arthritis. This required that at least five joints be swollen, and three or more joints have limitation in movement, pain, or tenderness. Patients could have initially presented with oligoarticular or systemic disease. Patients were 4 to 17 years old. They had failed methotrexate therapy or had not tolerated it. They were required to have stopped DMARDs two to four weeks before commencement of etanercept and were required to be on stable doses or any other medications such as NSAIDs or low-dose prednisolone. Patients with significant co-morbidities were excluded, as were those who had received a recent intra-articular cortisone injection.

Study design

This was a randomized, controlled, multicentre blinded trial of 69 patients. The study had two phases. In the first phase, all patients received etanercept. In the second phase, patients who had responded to etanercept were randomized to receive etanercept or placebo. The second phase was double-blinded.

Treatment

Etanercept was prescribed at 0.4 mg/kg subcutaneously for up to three months in the open-label part of the trial. Patients who responded (as per the Gianinni criteria, with improvement of 30% or more in at least three of six indicators, or no more than one indicator worsening by more than 30%) were then entered into the double-blind study and were randomly assigned to receive for four months either etanercept or placebo.

Trial end points measured

The trial end point was either four months after enrolment into the double-blind trial, or when the disease flared, whichever was earlier. Following this, patients were allowed continue etanercept in an open-label manner. Efficacy was assessed according to the number of patients with disease flare after receipt of placebo or etanercept, and the time to relapse of those patients. The core outcome variables and definition of improvement were those proposed by Giannini et al. The primary end point evaluated in the double-blind study was the number of patients with disease flare. This was based on the change in the core set of response variables from the beginning of the double-blind study; patients who met these criteria had worsening of 30% or more in three of the six variables and a minimum of two active joints. They also could have improvement of 30% or more in no more than one of the six variables.

Follow-up

Patients were assessed initially at day 1 and day 15; after that, they were assessed at the end of each month during the study. Final safety assessments were made 30 days after the discontinuation of the study drug, for patients who withdrew, or at the patient's next scheduled visit. The final assessment was seven months after the commencement of etanercept (three months open-label followed by four months blind study).

Results

At the end of the open-label study, 74% of patients had responded to etanercept. Of the 51 patients who entered the double-blind study, 81% of patients who received placebo withdrew because of disease flare vs only 21% of the etanercept patients (P = 0.003). The median time to flare was 28 days in the placebo group, vs 116 days in those treated with etanercept (P < 0.001). There was no significant difference between the two treatment groups in terms of the frequency of adverse events.

Critique of the paper

No patients were maintained on methotrexate; therefore, no information could be ascertained about whether it was preferable to use etanercept as monotherapy or in combination with methotrexate. There was a difference in the age and ethnicity of the patient groups: the placebo group was slightly older than the etanercept group, with a mean age of 12.2 years vs 8.9 years, respectively, more of the placebo group were white (88% vs 56%), and more of the etanercept group were Hispanic (8% vs 24%). The study was relatively small and there was no long-term follow-up to assess outcomes such as progression of erosive disease and growth. The end point in the study was flare of the disease, which is a composite measure that includes subjective assessments by both patient and physician. In the absence of X-ray data or surrogate markers such as plasma cytokine levels, it is difficult to gauge the biologic effects of etanercept in these patients—specifically, whether it alters the course of the disease, including the development of deformity. Psoriatic or enthesitis-related juvenile arthritis were not included in the study.

Significance and importance of the paper

This was the first placebo-controlled trial to assess the use of biological therapies in children with arthritis. The efficacy of these therapies had been firmly established in the adult population several years earlier. This paper confirmed that blockade of tumour necrosis factor (TNF) was a valid therapeutic intervention in the paediatric cohort with severe polyarticular arthritis and who did not tolerate or have an adequate response to methotrexate.

Clinical trials involving children with juvenile rheumatoid arthritis pose obstacles not encountered with adults, including the limited number of potential subjects, difficulties in ascertaining symptoms in young patients, and difficulties with the physical examination. Because of ethical issues, standard study designs may also need modification in trials of treatment for serious childhood illness. In the study by Lovell et al., all patients who entered the trial initially received etanercept in an open-label fashion and then were randomly assigned to either continued therapy with etanercept or placebo according to a double-blind design. The rates of disease flare in the second, double-blind part of the study were used to assess the efficacy of etanercept. This ethically acceptable model of study design was used subsequently in a number of landmark studies.

Eight years after this randomized controlled trial, Lovell et al. published long-term follow-up data. [1] Of the 69 patients originally enrolled, 58 (84%) participated in the follow-up, for a total of 318 patient-years of etanercept exposure. The overall rate of serious adverse effects (0.12 per patient-year) did not increase with long-term exposure to etanercept. The rate of medication-induced infections (0.03 per patient-year) remained low. No cases of tuberculosis, opportunistic infections, malignancies, lymphomas, lupus, demyelinating disorders, or deaths were reported. An ACR Pedi 70 response or higher was achieved by 100% of patients (n = 11) with eight years of data. These data suggested that the acceptable safety profile of etanercept therapy is maintained for up to eight years in this population of juvenile idiopathic arthritis patients. Improvements in the signs and symptoms of juvenile idiopathic arthritis were also maintained for up to eight years. Studies by other groups highlighted the positive impact of etanercept on growth rate in juvenile idiopathic arthritis. [2]

In 2008 Lovell et al. published results of a randomized, placebo-controlled, double-blind trial of the use of adalimumab with or without methotrexate in the *New England Journal of Medicine*. [3] This study had the same structure as the etanercept trial. The authors found adalimumab monotherapy to be safe and effective. The addition of methotrexate led to a higher proportion of patients having an ACR Pedi 30, 50, or 70 response, although the authors commented that the trial was not designed to compare monotherapy with combination therapy. Follow-up was for two years.

Recent trial data also show efficacy of infliximab for juvenile idiopathic arthritis as well as evidence to support the use of TNF blockade in juvenile onset ankylosing spondylitis [4]. One retrospective study has suggested that TNF blockade may be less efficacious in patients with enthesitis-related arthritis [5]. Wallace et al. evaluated the use of early aggressive treatment with etanercept plus methotrexate plus prednisolone (Arm 1) vs methotrexate alone (Arm 2) in patients with juvenile idiopathic arthritis. [6]. This study failed to show statistical differences. By six months, clinical inactive disease had been achieved in 17 (40%) of 42 patients in Arm 1, and 10 (23%) of 43 patients in Arm 2 (P = 0.088). After 12 months, clinical remission on medication was achieved in nine patients in Arm 1, and three patients in Arm 2 (P = 0.053). However, despite the lack of a statistical difference, early aggressive therapy in this cohort of children with recent-onset polyarticular juvenile idiopathic arthritis resulted in clinical inactive disease by 6 months, and clinical remission on medication within 12 months of treatment in substantial proportions of patients in both arms. Further studies may provide more evidence for the early use of biologics in this population.

References

1 Lovell DJ, Reiff A, Ilowite NT, et al. Safety and efficacy of up to eight years of continuous etanercept therapy in patients with juvenile rheumatoid arthritis. *Arthritis Rheum* 2008;**58**(5):1496–504.

2 Tynjälä P, Lahdenne P, Vähäsalo P, et al. Impact of anti-TNF treatment on growth in severe juvenile idiopathic arthritis. *Ann Rheum Dis* 2006;**65**(8):1044–9.

3 Lovell DJ, Ruperto N, Goodman S, et al. Adalimumab with or without methotrexate in juvenile rheumatoid arthritis. *N Engl J Med* 2008;**359**(8):810–20.

4 Horneff G, Fitter S, Foeldvari I, et al. Double-blind, placebo-controlled randomized trial with adalimumab for treatment of juvenile onset ankylosing spondylitis (JoAS): significant short term improvement. *Arthritis Res Ther* 2012;**14**(5):R230.

5 Visvanathan S, Wagner C, Marini JC, et al. The effect of infliximab plus methotrexate on the modulation of inflammatory disease markers in juvenile idiopathic arthritis: analyses from a randomized, placebo-controlled trial. *Pediatr Rheumatol Online J* 2010;**8**:24.

6 Wallace CA, Giannini EH, Spalding SJ, et al. Trial of early aggressive therapy in polyarticular juvenile idiopathic arthritis. *Arthritis Rheum* 2012;**64**(6):2012–21.

Paper 8.8: Classification of juvenile idiopathic arthritis: second revision, Edmonton, 2001

Reference

Petty RE, Southwood TR, Manners P, et al. International League of Associations for Rheumatology classification of juvenile idiopathic arthritis: second revision, Edmonton, 2001. *J Rheumatol* 2004;31(2):390–2.

Purpose

To delineate, for research purposes, relatively homogenous, mutually exclusive categories of idiopathic childhood arthritis based on predominant clinical and laboratory features.

Participants

The ILAR taskforce met in Edmonton in 2001 to discuss modifications of the proposed juvenile idiopathic arthritis classification. The aim was twofold: to outline modifications to the revised classification proposed as a result of the Edmonton meeting and to correct misconceptions highlighted by the published studies concerning the clinical use of the classification.

The Edmonton revision

The changes made to the classification criteria previously published were as follows:

1 Clarification of the definitions of each category.

2 Improvement in the congruity between inclusion and exclusion criteria.

3 Removal of the requirement that a dermatologist makes the diagnosis of psoriasis.

4 Removal of the requirement that there be medical confirmation of HLA-B27-associated disease in a relative.

5 Reduction in the age for Criterion 3 of enthesitis-related arthritis and Exclusion b from 8 years to 6 years of age.

6 Improvement in the consistency of structure.

Results

The new classification criteria defined juvenile idiopathic arthritis as arthritis of unknown aetiology beginning before the sixteenth birthday and persisting for at least six weeks, other known conditions having been excluded. Categories include systemic arthritis, oligoarthritis, polyarthritis (rheumatoid factor negative), polyarthritis (rheumatoid factor positive), psoriatic arthritis, enthesitis-related arthritis, and undifferentiated arthritis.

Significance and importance of the paper

In 1995 Fink et al. had undertaken the difficult task of establishing a classification criterion for juvenile idiopathic arthritis. This had occurred around the time that Giannini et al. had defined core outcome variables for assessment of disease activity and had proposed a definition of improvement.

These two publications revolutionized clinical research in juvenile arthritis, by allowing meta-analytical evaluation of studies and enabling the undertaking of reliable and reproducible research in large multicentre, multinational collaborations.

Ten years later when this Edmonton revision was undertaken, there was both an acknowledgement of the great work done but also a recognition of the need for research tools such as classification criteria and criteria to define improvement to be updated to reflect experience over the preceding decade. There had been major clinical advances during this time, including a shift towards early aggressive treatment and the development of new therapeutic strategies. This paper improved the existing classification criteria to allow it to be more useful to clinicians undertaking research.

The Giannini definition of response to treatment had been defined as a 30% improvement in at least three of six core outcome variables, and over time this became known as the ACR Pedi 30 criteria. It remains a useful scoring system. Although not prospectively evaluated, the ACR Pedi 20, Pedi 50, Pedi 70, and Pedi 90 measures are now also used as outcome measures in clinical trials and offer the advantage of a providing graded rather than purely categorical information. Definitions of disease flare had also been developed. [1] Although the development of the ACR paediatric response measures was a significant advance for paediatric rheumatology, the utility of these measures was limited because they assess the relative response (i.e. the change in disease status relative to a baseline clinic visit or other prior clinic visit) and do not provide an absolute measure of the disease state. Recent trials for biologics in juvenile idiopathic arthritis have added data on systemic symptoms, including recording tympanic temperatures and the presence of rash.

The use of a specific composite disease activity score for juvenile idiopathic arthritis, the juvenile arthritis disease activity score (JADAS), was developed, and in validation analyses it was found to have be a useful and reliable test. [2, 3] It is computed by assessing variables including (1) the physician global rating of overall disease activity VAS, (2) Parent/child ratings of well-being and pain VAS, (3) the number of active joints, assessed in 71, 27, or 10 joints (JADAS 71/27/10), and (4) ESR normalized on a 1–10 point scale.

Given the advances in aggressive treatments, more effective treatments, and improving outcomes, there was now a need to define remission, minimal disease activity, and acceptable symptoms state in juvenile idiopathic arthritis. In 2012 Consoloaro et al. published an article defining these outcomes based on the JADAS. [4, 5] With all versions of the JADAS, the cut-off score for classifying a patient as having inactive disease was 1, whereas the cut-off for classification of minimal disease activity was 2 for oligoarticular juvenile idiopathic arthritis and 3.8 for polyarticular juvenile idiopathic arthritis. Cut-offs for physicians', parents', and children's subjective rating of remission ranged from 2 to 2.3. Cut-offs for acceptable symptom state ranged from 3.2 to 5.4 for parents and from 3 to 4.5 for children. Results of cross-validation analyses strongly supported the selected cut-off values.

The other major advance during these years was the increasing use of ultrasound and MRI, in addition to plain X-rays, in the evaluation of disease activity. As scoring systems become more reliable and refined, these also offer an additional tool in clinical research. [6]

Together, these pieces of work allow for more efficient and reliable clinical trials to be undertaken and enable researchers to extract useful information from studies.

References

1 **Brunner HI, Lovell DJ, Finck BK, et al**. Preliminary definition of disease flare in juvenile rheumatoid arthritis. *J Rheumatol* 2002;**29**(5):1058–64.

2 **van der Heijde DM, van 't Hof M, van Riel PL, et al**. Development of a disease activity score based on judgment in clinical practice by rheumatologists. *J Rheumatol* 1993;**20**(3):579–81.

3 **Ringold S, Chon Y, Singer NG**. Associations between the American College of Rheumatology pediatric response measures and the continuous measures of disease activity used in adult rheumatoid arthritis: a secondary analysis of clinical trial data from children with polyarticular-course juvenile idiopathic arthritis. *Arthritis Rheum* 2009;**60**(12):3776–83.

4 **Wallace CA, Ruperto N, Giannini E, et al**. Preliminary criteria for clinical remission for select categories of juvenile idiopathic arthritis. *J Rheumatol* 2004;**31**(11):2290–4.

5 **Consolaro A, Bracciolini G, Ruperto N, et al**. Remission, minimal disease activity, and acceptable symptom state in juvenile idiopathic arthritis: defining criteria based on the juvenile arthritis disease activity score. *Arthritis Rheum* 2012;**64**(7):2366–74.

6 **Malattia C, Consolaro A, Pederzoli S, et al**. MRI versus conventional measures of disease activity and structural damage in evaluating treatment efficacy in juvenile idiopathic arthritis. *Ann Rheum Dis* 2013;**72**(3):363–8.

Paper 8.9: Randomized trial of tocilizumab in systemic juvenile idiopathic arthritis

Reference

De Benedetti F, Brunner HI, Ruperto N, et al. Randomized trial of tocilizumab in systemic juvenile idiopathic arthritis. *N Engl J Med* 2012;367(25):2385–95.

Purpose

To evaluate the safety and efficacy of the addition of tocilizumab vs placebo in patients with systemic juvenile idiopathic arthritis.

Patients

Patients were diagnosed on clinical grounds using ILAR criteria as having systemic juvenile idiopathic arthritis. Patients were between 2 and 17 years old. They had persistently active joint disease (>6 months) or fevers (of >38 degrees for 5 days during the 14-day screening period) with an inadequate response to conventional therapy and on stable doses of NSAIDs, oral glucocorticoids (max of 0.5 mg kg^{-1} day^{-1}) and methotrexate (<20 mg/m^2 for >8 weeks before baseline). Other DMARDs or biologics were not permitted. One hundred and twelve patients participated.

Study design

This was a two-phase study. The first phase was a 12-week, randomized, placebo-controlled, double-blinded, multicentred international trial. Patients were randomly assigned in a 2:1 ratio to receive tocilizumab or placebo. During the second phase, all participants received tocilizumab. If patients flared during the first 12 weeks they were also switched to open-label tocilizumab. Glucocorticoid tapering was permitted from week 6 according to pre-defined rules.

Treatment

Therapy was given for 12 weeks during the first phase of the trial. Patients received placebo or tocilizumab biweekly. Children >30 kg received 8 mg/kg, and those <30 kg received 12 mg/kg. After 12 weeks, all children received tocilizumab.

Trial end points measured

Biweekly clinical assessment were undertaken, which included the six core variables of the ACR core set for juvenile idiopathic arthritis (the number of joints with active arthritis, the number of joints with limited range of motion, the physicians global assessment of disease active, the parent/patient's global assessment of overall well-being, physical function (CHAQ-QI), and the ESR). Fevers were recorded at least twice daily. The primary outcome was the proportion of patients who had a juvenile idiopathic arthritis ACR 30 (improvement in three of six core outcome variables, with no more than one variable worsening by more than 30%, and an absence of fever). The juvenile idiopathic arthritis ACR 50/70 and 90 responses were also assessed. Flare, inactive disease, and adherence to the glucocorticoid tapering guidelines were determined by independent evaluators.

Follow-up

Patients were assessed biweekly throughout the study. The first phase was a 12-week study, and the second phase followed patients out to 52 weeks.

Results

The study met the primary end point with significantly more patients in the tocilizumab group than the placebo group having an ACR 30 response (85% vs 24%; P < 0.001). At 52 weeks, 80% of the patients who had received tocilizumab had at least a 70% improvement, with no fever, and 59% had an ACR 90 response. Fifty-two per cent had discontinued glucocorticoids. There was a higher proportion of patients in the tocilizumab group with serious adverse events (serious infections in 18 patients during the 52 weeks, neutropenia in 19 patients, transaminitis in 21 patients, and macrophage activation syndrome in 3). Opportunistic infections and tuberculosis were not reported. Three deaths occurred during tocilizumab treatment (pneumothorax, road accident, and sepsis) and three deaths occurred in patients who had received tocilizumab but had later withdrawn from the study (two pulmonary hypertension and one macrophage activation syndrome occurred at >6 months after tocilizumab; two were, by then, on other biological agents). Anti-tocilizumab antibodies developed in two patients. Patients treated with tocilizumab appeared to have a 25% risk of a serious adverse event and an 11% risk of a serious infection per year of treatment.

Critique of the paper

The paper only includes patients with persistent systemic features and arthritis resistant to conventional DMARD therapy, while the response of systemic juvenile idiopathic arthritis with a polyarticular course was not assessed. The trial was relatively large for a paediatric study. It was a placebo-controlled, randomized, multinational trial. The overall death rate was high, probably reflecting the severity of disease in this population more than the drug being studied. The safety profile of tocilizumab is difficult to assess, given the severe underlying disease of the study participants and the high percentage of patients with previous exposure to biologic agents. Lipid profiles were not reported, despite lipid abnormalities being reported in adult populations.

Significance and importance of the paper

This study was one of a series of studies published from 2008, assessing the next generation of biological agents in robust double-blind, randomized, placebo-controlled trials. For patients with severe resistant systemic juvenile idiopathic arthritis, this opened up the treatment options. Previously, there were no effective therapies for children and young adults with systemic juvenile idiopathic arthritis, particularly those with severe disease, despite successful management of other types of juvenile idiopathic arthritis with methotrexate and TNFα inhibitors. In 2008 Yokota et al. had published a smaller (n = 56) withdrawal trial in a Japanese cohort which had similar findings. [1] In 2011 the UK's National Institute for Health and Care Excellence recommended the use of tocilizumab in severe systemic juvenile idiopathic arthritis based on the data of this randomized controlled trial, even though not in full publication at that stage.

In 2008 a multicentre randomized controlled trial reported efficacy of abatacept in patients with juvenile idiopathic arthritis. [2] This study enrolled 190 patients, of whom 143 (75.3%) responded in the lead-in phase. Responders were then randomized to continue receiving abatacept (10 mg/kg every 28 days) or switch to placebo for six months. The primary end point was time to flare. Flares occurred in 53% of the placebo group and only 20% of the treatment group (P = 0.0003). Median time to flare was six months for the placebo arm but insufficient flares had occurred in the treatment arm for assessment to occur. This study included all subtypes of juvenile idiopathic arthritis; the highest proportion were patients with polyarthritis (negative for rheumatoid factor). The authors did not find differences in the response between subtypes of juvenile idiopathic arthritis, although the study was not designed to assess for differences.

Canakinumab is a fully human anti–IL1β monoclonal antibody that had been shown to be very effective in autoinflammatory illnesses. [3] Therefore, there was a strong rationale to investigate its potential use in systemic juvenile idiopathic arthritis. In 2012 the results of two randomized controlled trials assessing the use of canakinumab in systemic juvenile idiopathic arthritis were reported together. [4] In the first trial, patients with active systemic juvenile idiopathic arthritis were assigned to receive either canakinumab (4 mg/kg every 28 days) or placebo. The second trial was a withdrawal trial. In the first trial, patients in the treatment arm were significantly more likely to have an ACR Pedi 30 response (84% vs 10%). In the second trial, 75% of patients switched from canakinumab to placebo flared, vs only 26% of patients maintained on treatment.

Together, these well-run trials have significantly contributed to the evidence base available to clinicians when deciding on biologic treatment options for severe or resistant systemic juvenile idiopathic arthritis. The successful design and performance of the trials of these agents is commendable, given the severity and rarity of systemic juvenile idiopathic arthritis and the ethical challenges of placebo-controlled paediatric studies. The therapeutic benefits of these biologic agents will need to be weighed against the apparent risks of infection, neutropenia, and liver dysfunction. Macrophage activation syndrome developed in a small number of patients in both the placebo and active-treatment groups in these trials but an understanding of the overall effect of the agents on the macrophage activation syndrome will require additional investigation.

References

1 **Yokota S, Imagawa T, Mori M, et al**. Efficacy and safety of tocilizumab in patients with systemic-onset juvenile idiopathic arthritis: a randomised, double-blind, placebo-controlled, withdrawal phase III trial. *Lancet* 2008;**371**(9617):998–1006.

2 **Ruperto N, Lovell DJ, Quartier P, et al**. Abatacept in children with juvenile idiopathic arthritis: a randomised, double-blind, placebo-controlled withdrawal trial. *Lancet* 2008;**372**(9636):383–91.

3 **Lachmann HJ, Kone-Paut I, Kuemmerle-Deschner JB, et al**. Use of canakinumab in the cryopyrin-associated periodic syndrome. *N Engl J Med* 2009;**360**(23):2416–25.

4 **Ruperto N, Brunner HI, Quartier P, et al**. Two randomized trials of canakinumab in systemic juvenile idiopathic arthritis. *N Engl J Med* 2012;**367**(25):2396–406.

Paper 8.10: Adolescents with chronic disease: transition to adult health care

Reference

Rettig P, Athreya BH. Adolescents with chronic disease. Transition to adult health care. *Arthritis Care Res* 1991;4(4):174–80.

Purpose

To describe the experience of a US paediatric rheumatology centre in transitioning patients from a paediatric clinic to an adult clinic. The authors undertake a review of the literature, describe the pitfalls of transition, and make a set of recommendations to transition patients to adult services.

Justification for a structures system of formally transitioning patients

The authors initially undertake a review of the literature in other specialties and comment on the following points: (1) more children with chronic disease are now surviving into adulthood; (2) paediatric teams take a more holistic approach to patient care which assures good care but may increase dependency of the patient and family on the team; (3) adult internists expect their adult patients to take care of their own needs and liaise less with multidisciplinary teams; and (4) some adult internists may not be familiar with diseases of childhood and may not feel comfortable treating these patients.

Goals of a transition programme

The authors propose five goals for transition programmes: (1) to promote continuity of care; (2) to promote independence in the young adult; (3) to assess the impact of the disease on the patient's ability to achieve optimal vocational and educational goals, and to intervene accordingly; (4) to promote optimal adolescent development by addressing issues regarding sexuality, psychosocial, and future planning concerns; and (5) to provide emotional support to the members of the family during transition.

Obstacles to transition

The authors outline many obstacles in the way of successful transition to adult services. These include patient-related obstacles (e.g. dependent behaviour, immaturity, and trust); family-related obstacles (e.g. need for control, emotional dependency, and trust); paediatrician obstacles (e.g. emotional bonds with patient and family, and distrust of adult caregiver), and internist concerns (e.g. lack of understanding of childhood disease, and heightened perception of care demands).

Proposal of recommendations for a transition programme

The authors proposed recommendations for a successful transition. They advocated the involvement of a multidisciplinary team including doctors, nurse specialists, social workers, physical therapists, and occupational therapists. They defined a pre-transitional phase where the paediatric team would prepare the patient and family for transfer. Transition should happen ideally while disease is under good control. They advocate the use of questionnaires to assess the readiness of the patient for transfer, and the involvement of social workers and nurses in the process. The transition phase involves being seen by an adult rheumatologist in a specific transition clinic in conjunction with the paediatrician. Questions relating to issues such as alcohol and sexual risks and implications regarding medications should be addressed by members of the team as appropriate. Having a transition clinic facilitates these conversations between internist and patient.

Results

The authors report that in the three years of their transition programme, they transitioned 36 patients to adult services. Only two had been lost to follow-up.

Critique of the paper

This publication is not an evidence-based trial. There is no control group, and few specific details of the patients transitioned are provided. This is simply a discursive article relating the experience of a centre, allowing for a review of available literature and general recommendations based on experience rather than being based strictly on evidence. The two authors did not collaborate with other similar centres when creating the set of recommendations.

Significance and importance of the paper

This was an important paper that helped mould the evolving specialty of adolescent rheumatology. Adolescents (11–19 years old) represent a large cohort of patients who have, traditionally, received very little attention. Up to 60% of patients with juvenile idiopathic arthritis have ongoing joint inflammation or disability into adulthood. [1, 2] Though with the universal use of biologics this figure may now be less, this still represents a significant burden of morbidity during a period of what is supposed to be peak physical health. They present unique challenges with regard to their growth and sexual development, risk-taking behaviour, vocational planning, mental health, adherence, and attendance. Treating patients effectively during this period of change and enabling them to transition confidently into the adult health-care system empowers them to reach their potential with regard to their health and employment potential, with resultant benefits both to patients as well as to the health service (i.e. employment vs long-term disability). [3–5] This paper created a discussion that influenced future evidence-based trials.

In 2007 McDonagh and colleagues published a study to determine whether the quality of life of adolescents with juvenile idiopathic arthritis could be improved by a co-ordinated, evidence-based programme of transitional care. [6] Adolescents with juvenile idiopathic arthritis aged 11, 14, and 17 years, and their parents, were recruited from ten rheumatology centres in the UK. Data were collected at baseline, 6 months, and 12 months, including core outcome variables. The primary outcome measure was health-related quality of life

(HRQL) as determined by the Juvenile Arthritis Quality of Life Questionnaire (JAQQ). Secondary outcome measures included knowledge, satisfaction, independent health behaviours, and pre-vocational experience. Of the 359 families invited to participate, 308 (86%) adolescents and 303 (84%) parents accepted. A fifth of them had persistent oligoarthritis. Median disease duration was 5.7 (0–16) years. Compared with baseline values, significant improvements in JAQQ scores were reported for adolescent and parent ratings at 6 months and 12 months, and for most secondary outcome measures, with no significant deteriorations, between 6 and 12 months. Continuous improvement was observed for both adolescent and parent knowledge, with significantly greater improvement in the younger age groups at 12 months (P = 0.002). This study provided the first objective evaluation of an evidence-based transitional care programme and demonstrated that such care could potentially improve adolescents' HRQL.

The importance of transitional health care is now fully established and embedded in formal standards of care. Important issues still to be addressed pertain to rolling the system out so that all adolescents with chronic disease benefit from a planned and individualized transition plan. Furthermore, it is also important to ensure this population is included in research, to ensure continuing access to clinical trials, guide management decisions such as choice of DMARDs and biologics, and define long-term outcomes and early predictors of disease and response to treatment.

References

1 **Minden K.** Adult outcomes of patients with juvenile idiopathic arthritis. *Horm Res* 2009;**72**(Suppl 1): 20–5.

2 **Scott DL, Symmons DP, Coulton BL, et al.** Long-term outcome of treating rheumatoid arthritis: results after 20 years. *Lancet* 1987;**1**(8542):1108–11.

3 **Shaw KL, Southwood TR, McDonagh JE, et al.** Developing a programme of transitional care for adolescents with juvenile idiopathic arthritis: results of a postal survey. *Rheumatology* 2004;**43**(2):211–19.

4 **Klostermann BK, Slap GB, Nebrig DM, et al.** Earning trust and losing it: adolescents' views on trusting physicians. *J Fam Pract* 2005;**54**(8):679–87.

5 **McDonagh JE, Shaw KL, Southwood TR.** Growing up and moving on in rheumatology: development and preliminary evaluation of a transitional care programme for a multicentre cohort of adolescents with juvenile idiopathic arthritis. *J Child Health Care* 2006;**10**(1):22–42.

6 **McDonagh JE, Shaw KL, Southwood TR.** The impact of a coordinated transitional care programme on adolescents with juvenile idiopathic arthritis. Rheumatology 2007;**46**(1):161–8.

Chapter 9

Metabolic bone disease

Ashok Bhalla and Tehseen Ahmed

Introduction

The term 'metabolic bone disease' covers a wide variety of disorders that can ultimately lead to alteration in bone strength. The disorders can be both inherited and acquired. Abnormalities of calcium, phosphate, and/or vitamin D are commonly seen. However, the most common metabolic bone disorder is osteoporosis, in which the density and quality of bone architecture is adversely affected.

Osteoporosis is a major health problem, with one in two women and one in five men over the age of 50 expected to sustain a fragility fracture in their remaining lifetime. As one might expect, this leads to significant morbidity and excess mortality. We can expect osteoporosis to represent an increasing burden on health resources as life expectancy continues to increase.

In this chapter, we have chosen eight landmark papers that cover various aspects of metabolic bone disease but with a primary focus on osteoporosis.

Paper 9.1 addresses the issue of fracture risk in osteoporosis. Since the publication of this paper, fracture risk assessment has become an increasingly important topic and continues to evolve with time. This presents a real shift in clinical practice with a move away from relying on absolute bone density as the only risk factor of significance. A comprehensive assessment of fracture risk now underpins many national guidelines on the management of osteoporosis.

Papers 9.2, 9.3, and 9.4 examine the evidence for some of the most commonly used treatments in osteoporosis. Paper 9.2 looks at the issue of calcium and vitamin D supplementation in patients at increased risk of fragility fractures. This was the first large-scale study to show beneficial effects of calcium and vitamin D supplementation on fracture risk in a well-defined population. The results of this study continue to influence our management of patients to this day, although controversies remain as to which populations may benefit most from this intervention.

Paper 9.3 looks at the role of alendronate therapy in reducing fracture risk. It was the first large-scale study to demonstrate a reduction in clinical fractures. The evidence provided by this and allied studies has had a huge impact on osteoporosis management, with alendronate remaining the most widely prescribed of the bisphosphonates in current practice.

Paper 9.4 provides another landmark moment in the management of osteoporosis, describing the use of anabolic therapy and demonstrating evidence of significant reductions in vertebral and non-vertebral fractures. Parathyroid hormone remains one of the most effective treatments to date and it is possible that further research may lead to novel indications for its use.

Papers 9.5 and 9.6 continue the story of osteoporosis and its management but concentrate on the potential adverse effects of bisphosphonate therapy. These potential adverse effects (atypical femoral fractures and osteonecrosis of the jaw) have been making headlines in recent years and there is increasing physician and patient awareness of these issues, highlighting the need for continuing education, accumulation of evidence, and debate. Papers 9.5 and 9.6 help to summarize current thinking on the pathophysiology and management of these rare, but significant, problems.

Paget's disease of bone, depending on geographical location and ethnic make-up, is the second most common metabolic bone disease. Paper 9.7 looks at the early pharmacological therapy of Paget's disease and is significant in that it introduced concepts of management that still hold true in current clinical practice.

Finally, Paper 9.8 looks at the issue of hypercalcaemia in patients with sarcoidosis. This work has helped to enhance our understanding of calcium metabolism. This study led to the realization that hypercalcaemia could occur as a result of increased levels of activated vitamin D that were independent of renal 1α-hydroxylase and parathyroid hormone activity. Subsequent work has proven the existence of extra-renal 1α-hydroxylase activity in tissues such as lymph nodes and skin.

Paper 9.1: Epidemiology of osteoporotic fracture

Reference

Kanis JA, Johnell O, Oden A, et al. Ten-year probabilities of osteoporotic fractures according to BMD and diagnostic thresholds. *Osteoporosis Int* 2001;12(12):989–95.

Purpose

To estimate ten-year probabilities of osteoporotic fractures in men and women according to age and bone mineral density (BMD) at the femoral neck.

Patients

Combined data on incidence of first fracture of the hip, forearm, proximal humerus, and clinical vertebral fracture from the population of Malmo, Sweden, was utilized in association with fracture and mortality hazards to calculate ten-year probabilities as applied to the mean population size of Sweden in 1994.

Study design

This was an observational, data-based study.

Treatment

This study did not address treatment.

Trial end points measured

The trial end points comprised average ten-year probabilities of forearm, proximal humerus, hip, and vertebral fractures in men and women over the age of 45.

Follow-up

There was no follow-up in this study.

Results

The ten-year probabilities of fracture at all sites, for men and women, increased with worsening T-score for a given age. For a given T-score, forearm fracture probability in men remained relatively stable with advancing age. For all other fracture types in men and women, fracture risk increased with age up to 80 years. Thereafter, fracture risk plateaued or decreased secondary to the rising risk of mortality. Fracture risk was higher in women than in men at given ages. Age is an independent risk factor for fracture.

Critique of the paper

This was an observational study to calculate fracture probabilities based on data of a limited number of risk factors for fracture; therefore, the fracture probabilities calculated could be further refined by taking account of other risk factors. An assumption has been made that fracture risk increases with worsening BMD with the same order of magnitude in men as is the case in women. The calculated probabilities may not be applicable to patients from other geographical locations or ethnic backgrounds.

Significance and importance of the paper

Diagnostic criteria for osteoporosis and low bone mass were proposed in 1994 based on T-scores [1, 2]. These criteria have been widely accepted and continue to influence many clinicians' decisions on treatment. Historically, national bodies have used BMD and T-scores to guide intervention thresholds [3, 4]. However, T-scores have limitations in their use as a clinical diagnostic test. There are discrepancies in T-scores within individuals at different anatomic sites. There are also differences between dual-energy X-ray absorptiometry machines from different manufacturers. But most importantly, it is difficult to contextualize a T-score as an absolute risk of fracture. For example, a T-score of −2.5 signifies osteoporosis in an 80-year old patient as well as in a 50-year old patient but the risk of fracture is markedly increased in the 80-year old as compared to the 50-year old. This is not to say that this method of estimating fracture risk is perfect; for example, it does not take account of rates of bone turnover, although these also influence the risk of fracture [5].

The goal of trying to better characterize fracture risk has led to the development of fracture risk calculators. The most widely used of these calculators is FRAX®. It was developed by the World Health Organization Collaborating Centre for Metabolic Bone Diseases and has been available for use since 2008 [6, 7]. It takes in to account many risk factors, beyond age and BMD, and can be used to calculate ten-year fracture probabilities for major osteoporotic and hip fracture, both with and without femoral neck BMD measurement. Data from many different population cohorts has allowed the FRAX® model to provide more accurate fracture risk assessments for many different countries around the world, as it can be calibrated to take account of local epidemiology of fractures and death. Like any predictive tool, there are limitations to its use. For example, it does not take account of the number of prior fractures sustained nor type of fracture sustained, there is no adjustment for current or prior treatment, nor does it take account of the magnitude of alcohol consumed or cigarettes smoked. It has, however, been updated to take some account of the dose of glucocorticoids that a patient has been receiving [8]. Guidance has also been issued to take account of situations when there is a large discrepancy in T-scores at the femoral neck and lumbar spine within the same individual [9].

FRAX® is not the only fracture risk calculator available. In the UK, QFracture has been validated on large primary care populations [10]. It allows for computation of multiple risk factors, including falls, but is not designed to incorporate BMD measurements. It can provide estimates of fracture incidence over time periods shorter than ten years and thus may be of more use in the very elderly population, where short-term fracture risk may be of more value in view of shorter life expectancy.

Assessing fracture risk necessitates consideration of intervention thresholds. In the UK, the National Osteoporosis Guideline Group (NOGG) have produced decision management guidance that links to FRAX® [11]. The intervention threshold is set at the age-specific fracture probability equivalent to women with a prior fragility fracture. There is no such intervention guidance that links to QFracture. The NOGG guidance is only applicable in the UK; other countries have outlined intervention thresholds of their own, but this needs to be done at a national level to take account of local epidemiology and availability of health resources.

Paper 9.1 was the first to introduce the concept of absolute fracture risk. It also helped to imbed the concepts that risk factors other than BMD contribute to fracture risk (in this case, age) and that the use of a T-score alone is an unsatisfactory measure on which to base intervention thresholds. These concepts have been crucial to the development of the now widely used fracture risk calculators and the development of intervention thresholds based on fracture risk estimates and health economic analyses. Fracture risk assessment and intervention thresholds will need to be continually refined over time to ensure that precious resources are targeted effectively.

References

1 **World Health Organization**. Assessment of fracture risk and its application to screening for postmenopausal osteoporosis. WHO technical report series 843. Geneva: WHO; 1994.

2 **Kanis JA, Melton LJ, Christiansen C, et al**. The diagnosis of osteoporosis. *J Bone Miner Res* 1994;**9**(8):1137–41.

3 **Royal College of Physicians**. Osteoporosis: clinical guidelines for prevention and treatment. London: RCP; 1999.

4 **National Osteoporosis Foundation**. Osteoporosis: review of the evidence for prevention, diagnosis and treatment and cost-effectiveness analysis. *Osteoporos Int* 1998;**8**(Suppl 4):1–88.

5 **Kanis JA, Johnell O, Oden A, et al**. Prediction of fracture from low bone mineral density measurements overestimates risk. *Bone* 2000;**26**(4):387–91.

6 **Kanis JA, on behalf of the World Health Organization Scientific Group (2007)**. Assessment of osteoporosis at the primary health-care level. Technical Report. World Health Organization Collaborating Centre for Metabolic Bone Diseases, University of Sheffield, UK. 2007.

7 **Kanis JA, Johnell O, Oden A, et al**. FRAX™ and the assessment of fracture probability in men and women from the UK. *Osteoporos Int* 2008;**19**(4):385–97.

8 **Kanis JA, Johansson H, Oden A, et al**. Guidance for the adjustment of FRAX according to the dose of glucocorticoids. *Osteoporos Int* 2011;**22**(3):809–16.

9 **Leslie WD, Lix LM, Johansson H, et al**. Spine–hip discordance and fracture risk assessment: a physician-friendly FRAX enhancement. *Osteoporos Int* 2011;**22**(3):839–47.

10 **Collins GS, Mallett S, Altman DG**. Predicting risk of osteoporotic and hip fracture in the United Kingdom: prospective independent and external validation of QFractureScores. *BMJ* 2011;342:d3651. doi:10.1136/bmj.d3651.

11 **Kanis JA, McCloskey EV, Johansson H, et al**. Case finding for the management of osteoporosis with FRAX®—assessment and intervention thresholds for the UK. *Osteoporos Int* 2008;**19**(10):1395–1408; erratum in 2009 *Osteoporos Int* 20(3):499–502.

Paper 9.2: Calcium and vitamin D in the prevention of fractures

Reference

Chapuy MC, Arlot ME, Duboeuf F, et al. Vitamin D3 and calcium to prevent hip fractures in elderly women. *N Engl J Med* 1992;327(23):1637–42.

Purpose

To assess whether calcium and vitamin D_3 supplements reduce the risk of non-vertebral fractures, particularly fractures of the femoral neck, among ambulatory elderly women living in nursing homes.

Patients

Ambulatory female nursing/residential home residents aged 69–106 (mean 84 ± 6 years) without serious medical conditions. Patients were excluded if they had been treated with sodium fluoride for more than 3 months, had received drugs that alter bone metabolism in the previous 12 months, or received calcium and vitamin D in the previous 6 months (or for more than 1 year in the previous 5 years). Women with previous fractures were eligible.

Study design

This study described a randomized, double-blind, placebo-controlled trial involving 3,270 women.

Treatment

Treatment comprised daily placebo (n = 1,636) or daily tricalcium phosphate (containing 1.2 g elemental calcium) and 20 μg vitamin D_3 (800 IU) (n = 1,634) for 18 months.

Trial end points measured

The trial end points comprised new non-vertebral fractures, serial serum parathyroid hormone and 25-hydroxyvitamin D levels in a subgroup of patients (n = 142), and femoral BMD measurements in a subgroup of patients (n = 56).

Follow-up

Follow-up was 18 months.

Results

There was a 43% reduction of hip fractures and a 32% reduction in the total number of non-vertebral fractures in patients treated with calcium and vitamin D_3 supplements as compared to placebo (P < 0.05). There was a 44% reduction in mean serum parathyroid hormone levels and a 162% increase in serum 25-hydroxyvitamin D levels as compared to baseline (P < 0.001) in patients treated with calcium and vitamin D_3 supplements. The bone density of the proximal femur increased 2.7% in the calcium and vitamin D_3 cohort and decreased 4.7% in the placebo cohort (P < 0.001).

Critique of the paper

The results are only applicable to a very specific population (elderly, Caucasian nursing-home residents). In addition, there were high dropout rates and there was no analysis of the intervention on risk of falls.

Significance and importance of the paper

This landmark study was the first to show that calcium and vitamin D_3 supplementation can reduce the risk of non-vertebral fragility fractures in a specific elderly population. This was an important finding, as this was a relatively simple and low-cost intervention in a population at high risk of fractures.

Previous studies have shown that there is a reduction in 25-hydroxyvitamin D levels and increase in parathyroid hormone levels in elderly patients [1, 2]. This leads to increased bone resorption. Supplementation with calcium and vitamin D_2 acts to reduce biochemical indices of secondary hyperparathyroidism [1, 2]. In Paper 9.2, Chapuy et al. postulated that supplementation with calcium and vitamin D_3 would act to lower serum parathyroid hormone levels, which in turn would have a beneficial effect on BMD and fracture risk.

The two cohorts of patients in this study had similar baseline characteristics with regard to age, weight, height, dietary calcium intake, and percentage of 'fallers' (defined as at least one fall in the three months prior to recruitment). Of the 3,270 patients originally enrolled in the study, 1,765 were treated and followed for the 18 months. Forty-six per cent of patients in each group dropped out of the study. Reasons for dropout included death, non-compliance, inability to walk during the study, loss to follow-up, intercurrent illness, and adverse effects. There was no significant difference between the groups in this regard.

Among the patients who completed the study, there were 21 hip fractures and 66 non-vertebral fractures in the calcium and vitamin D_3 group versus 37 hip fractures and 97 non-vertebral fractures in the placebo group. This represents relative risks of 0.57 and 0.68 for hip fractures and non-vertebral fractures, respectively. The result of the intention to treat analysis was similar.

The results of this study are not necessarily applicable to all patients at an increased risk of fracture, and not even applicable to all elderly patients. This study shows the value of calcium and vitamin D_3 supplementation in elderly, Caucasian nursing-home residents with relatively low calcium intake, low serum 25-hydroxyvitamin D levels, and good adherence to supplementation.

Subsequent to this study, numerous randomized controlled trials have looked at the effects of calcium and/or vitamin D supplementation on fracture risk. The trials varied in the populations studied as well as the doses of calcium and/or vitamin D administered to participants. There have also been a number of meta-analyses of these studies. Unfortunately, the studies and meta-analyses have reached differing conclusions regarding the effect on fracture risk, adding to the uncertainties that practising clinicians face.

However, a few key points can be taken from the conclusions drawn. Calcium supplementation, in isolation, does not appear to reduce fracture risk [3]. Vitamin D in combination with calcium supplementation appears to be most effective in reducing the risk of fractures [4, 5]. The effects of vitamin D appear to be dose dependent. A meta-analysis showed that received doses (product of administered dose and percentage adherence to therapy) >400 IU per day significantly reduced non-vertebral and hip fractures with relative risks of 0.80(0.72–0.89) and 0.82 (0.69–0.97), respectively [4]. Received doses of vitamin D <400 IU per day did not result in a reduction in fracture risk [6]. Thus, as would be expected, the value of the intervention depends to a large extent on adherence to therapy. Finally, it is likely that calcium and vitamin D supplementation is of most benefit in those populations with low dietary calcium intake and low 25-hydroxyvitamin D levels, as seen in this landmark study.

There remains a need for further research in a number of areas. These include the potential benefits of calcium and vitamin D supplementation in populations at lower risk of fracture, in childhood/young adulthood, and in the offspring of mothers supplemented during pregnancy. The benefit of calcium and vitamin D supplementation on health outcomes other than bone health remains unclear. In addition, it is just as important to continue to assess the potential harms of therapy, especially in light of the uncertainty surrounding an association with risk of cardiovascular disease [7].

References

1 **Chapuy MC, Durr F, Chapuy P**. Age-related changes in parathyroid hormone and 25 hydroxycholecalciferol levels. *J Gerontol* 1983;**38**(1):19–22.
2 **Chapuy MC, Chapuy P, Meunier PJ**. Calcium and vitamin D supplements: effects on calcium metabolism in elderly people. *Am J Clin Nutr* 1987;**46**(2):324–8.
3 **Bischoff-Ferrari HA, Dawson-Hughes B, Baron JA, et al**. Calcium intake and hip fracture risk in men and women: a meta-analysis of prospective cohort studies and randomized controlled trials. *Am J Clin Nutr* 2007;**86**(6):1780–90.
4 **Tang BM, Eslick GD, Nowson C, et al**. Use of calcium or calcium in combination with vitamin D supplementation to prevent fractures and bone loss in people aged 50 years and older: a meta-analysis. *Lancet* 2007;**370**(9588):657–66.
5 **Boonen S, Lips P, Bouillon R, et al**. Need for additional calcium to reduce the risk of hip fracture with vitamin D supplementation: evidence from a comparative meta-analysis of randomized controlled trials. *J Clin Endocrinol Metab* 2007;**92**(4):1415–23.
6 **Bischoff-Ferrari HA, Willett WC, Wong JB, et al**. Prevention of nonvertebral fractures with oral vitamin D and dose dependency: a meta-analysis of randomized controlled trials. *Arch Intern Med* 2009;**169**(6):551–61.
7 **Bolland MJ, Avenell A, Baron JA, et al**. Effect of calcium supplements on risk of myocardial and cardiovascular events: Meta-analysis. *BMJ* 2010;**341**:c369.

Paper 9.3: Alendronate and reduction of clinical vertebral fractures

Reference

Black DM, Cummings SR, Karpf DB, et al. Randomised trial of effect of alendronate on risk of fracture in women with existing vertebral fractures. *Lancet* 1996;348(9041):1535–41.

Purpose

To investigate the effect of alendronate on the risk of morphometric as well as clinically evident fractures in postmenopausal women with low bone mass and prevalent vertebral fracture.

Patients

The patients in this study were postmenopausal women aged 55–81 with low femoral-neck BMD and the presence of an existing vertebral fracture.

Study design

This was a randomized, double-blind, placebo-controlled trial involving 2,027 women.

Treatment

Treatment comprised placebo (n = 1,005) or daily alendronate (n = 1,022) at a dose of 5 mg daily (increased to 10 mg daily after 24 months).

Trial end points measured

The trial end points comprised new vertebral fractures—morphometric and clinical—and non-spine clinical fractures.

Follow-up

Follow-up was 36 months.

Results

Eight per cent of participants in the alendronate group sustained one or more new morphometric vertebral fractures, as compared with 15% in the placebo group (relative risk 0.53). In addition, 2.3% of women in the alendronate group sustained one or more clinically apparent vertebral fractures, as compared with 5% in the placebo group (relative risk 0.45). The relative risk of any clinical fracture was significantly lower in the alendronate group, with a relative risk of 0.72. The effects were independent of baseline BMD. The relative risks for hip and wrist fractures in the alendronate group versus placebo were 0.49 and 0.52, respectively. There was no significant difference between the groups for adverse events.

Critique of the paper

The dose of alendronate was altered during the period of study. The study design precluded analysis of the efficacy of the different doses. In addition, the results are not necessarily generalizable to all ethnic groups, as the vast majority of the study subjects were Caucasian.

Significance and importance of the paper

Bisphosphonates, an anti-resorptive class of drugs, have been used to treat osteoporosis since the 1970s. They work by inhibiting the activity, and inducing apoptosis, of osteoclasts.

Previous studies have shown that intermittent cyclical sodium etidronate (EHDP) can improve BMD and reduce the incidence of morphometric (radiographically defined) vertebral fractures [1, 2]. Liberman et al. showed that 10 mg of daily alendronate treatment resulted in improved BMD versus placebo (8.8% at the lumbar spine, 5.9% at the femoral neck) [3]. The 10 mg dose was more effective than a 5 mg dose of daily alendronate and as effective as a 20 mg dose of daily alendronate. They were also able to show a 48% reduction in morphometric vertebral fractures (absolute rate of 3.2% vs 6.2% in the placebo group) when data for all the alendronate arms (5 mg, 10 mg, and 20 mg) was pooled. Post hoc analysis showed a trend towards reduction in non-vertebral fractures but this did not reach statistical significance.

Black's landmark study formed the first part of the Fracture Intervention Trial (FIT) and looked to assess the effect of alendronate in postmenopausal women with low bone density and prior vertebral fracture. The study showed that treatment with daily alendronate could reduce the incidence of clinical as well as morphometric vertebral fractures. The study commenced with participants in the alendronate arm receiving a dose of 5 mg daily. This was increased to 10 mg daily after 24 months in light of the findings by Liberman et al. [3]. Black's study was a pivotal trial, as a reduction in clinical vertebral fractures had not been shown previously. Given the complicated administration regime and lack of clinical benefit apparent to patients for what is essentially a preventative treatment, it comes as no surprise that adherence to bisphosphonate therapy is notoriously poor in routine clinical practice. Evidence such as that provided by Black et al. can be useful to educate patients about the very real benefits of bisphosphonate therapy.

Black's study was closely followed in 1998 by the publication of the second part of the FIT by Cummings et al. [4]; in this part, 2,218 women were randomized to placebo and 2,214 to alendronate. The women in the alendronate arm received 5 mg daily for the first 24 months before the dose was increased to 10 mg daily, as per Black's study. Results at 4 years showed significant increases in BMD compared to placebo (6.6% at the lumbar spine, and 4.6% at the femoral neck) that were independent of baseline BMD. There was a 44% reduction in morphometric vertebral fractures in the alendronate cohort. A statistically significant reduction in clinical fractures was demonstrated in the subset of patients with a femoral-neck T-score <−2.5; that is, the beneficial effect of alendronate on clinical fractures was dependent on baseline BMD.

Subsequent pooling of the data from the two FIT studies produced a cohort of 3,658 patients with femoral-neck T-scores <−2.5 and/or prevalent vertebral fracture [5]. Analysis of this data showed a 48% reduction in morphometric vertebral fracture, a 45% reduction in clinical vertebral fracture, and a 27% reduction in non-vertebral fracture in patients treated with alendronate. In addition, a 53% reduction in hip fracture and 30% reduction in wrist fracture were observed.

Large-scale studies have confirmed fracture risk reduction with other oral bisphosphonates, including risedronate and ibandronate [6, 7]. Concerns around adherence to daily bisphosphonates led to the development of once-weekly formulations of alendronate and risedronate, and a once-monthly preparation of oral ibandronate. These new formulations have gone some way to improving adherence to therapy. Subsequent development of effective parenteral bisphosphonates has provided clinicians with a broader choice of treatments for patients who cannot tolerate oral bisphosphonates secondary to gastro-intestinal side effects and for those who are unable to comply with the special instructions for administration.

It remains unclear for how long patients at increased risk of fracture should be treated with bisphosphonates. However, an extension of the FIT trials has provided some further data on this subject [8]. Patients who had completed five years of therapy with alendronate were randomized to placebo, 5 mg of daily alendronate, or 10 mg of daily alendronate. They were then followed for a further five years. The results showed a reduced incidence of clinical vertebral fractures in the groups randomized to alendronate (2%) versus placebo (5%). Rates of non-vertebral fractures and hip fractures were similar in the alendronate and placebo arms.

The potential long-term adverse effects of bisphosphonate therapy have garnered increasing attention, particularly with regard to associations with atypical femoral fractures and osteonecrosis of the jaw (see Papers 9.5 and 9.6). However, a causal relationship has not been demonstrated to date.

Black's work was a landmark study in terms of its size and design. It was the first study to assess the effect of treatment on fracture incidence as a primary end point and provided excellent quality fracture data. Its clinical impact is such that alendronate remains the most widely prescribed medication for the treatment of osteoporosis in the western world. Issues that still require clarification include differences between bisphosphonates in clinical efficacy, optimal duration of use, long-term adverse events, and the potential utility of combination therapy with other agents.

References

1 **Storm T, Thamsborg G, Steiniche T, et al**. Effect of intermittent cyclical etidronate therapy on bone mass and fracture rate in women with postmenopausal osteoporosis. *N Engl J Med* 1990;**322**(18):1265–71.

2 **Watts NB, Harris ST, Genant HK, et al**. Intermittent cyclical etidronate treatment of postmenopausal osteoporosis. *N Engl J Med* 1990;**323**(2):73–9.

3 **Liberman UA, Weiss SR, Broll J, et al**. Effect of oral alendronate on bone mineral density and the incidence of fractures in postmenopausal osteoporosis. *N Engl J Med* 1995;**333**(22):1437–43.

4 **Cummings SR, Black DM, Thompson DE, et al**. Effect of alendronate on risk of fracture in women with low bone density but without vertebral fractures. *JAMA* 1998;**280**(24):2077–82.

5 **Black DM, Thompson DE, Bauer DC, et al**. Fracture risk reduction in women with osteoporosis: the Fracture Intervention Trial. *J Clin Endocrinol Metab* 2000;**85**(11):4118–24.

6 **Harris ST, Watts NB, Genant HK, et al**. Effects of risedronate treatment on vertebral and nonvertebral fractures in women with postmenopausal osteoporosis: a randomized controlled trial. *JAMA* 1999;**282**(14):1344–52.

7 **Chesnut CH, Ettinger MP, Miller PD, et al**. Effects of oral ibandronate administered daily or intermittently on fracture risk in postmenopausal osteoporosis. *J Bone Miner Res* 2004;**19**(8):1241–9.

8 **Black DM, Schwartz AV, Ensrud KE, et al**. Effects of continuing or stopping alendronate after 5 years of treatment. The Fracture Intervention Trial Long-term Extension (FLEX): a randomized trial. *JAMA* 2006;**296**(24):2927–38.

Paper 9.4: Anabolic therapy in the treatment of osteoporosis

Reference

Neer RM, Arnaud CD, Zanchetta JR, et al. Effect of parathyroid hormone (1–34) on fractures and bone mineral density in postmenopausal women with osteoporosis. *N Engl J Med* 2001;344(19):1434–41.

Purpose

Treatment with parathyroid hormone may provide protection against fractures in humans.

Patients

The patients in this study were postmenopausal women with a history of prior vertebral fractures.

Study design

This was a randomized, placebo-controlled trial involving 1,637 postmenopausal women.

Treatment

Treatment comprised placebo or 20 µg or 40 µg of recombinant human parathyroid hormone (1–34) in a regimen of daily, self-administered injections.

Trial end points measured

The trial end points comprised occurrence of new vertebral and non-vertebral fractures, and percentage change in BMD.

Follow-up

The median duration of observation was 21 months.

Results

Treatment with parathyroid hormone at doses of 20 µg or 40 µg daily resulted in relative risks of vertebral fractures of 0.35 and 0.31, respectively, as compared to placebo. The relative risks of non-vertebral fractures were 0.47 and 0.46, respectively. Compared with placebo, 20 and 40 µg doses of parathyroid hormone increased bone density in the lumbar spine by 9 and 13 more percentage points, respectively, and in the femoral neck by 3 and 6 more percentage points, respectively.

Critique of the paper

Patients received variable strengths of vitamin D supplements. No attempt was made to analyse worsening of pre-existing vertebral deformities. In addition, only a low proportion of participants had previously received treatment to reduce fracture risk.

Significance and importance of the paper

Parathyroid hormone, produced by the parathyroid glands, is involved in calcium homeostasis. This was first conclusively demonstrated in 1925 by Collip [1]. Parathyroid hormone deficiency leads to hypocalcaemia, hyperphosphataemia, and tetany, while parathyroid hormone excess can lead to hypercalcaemia, hypophosphataemia, bone pain, pathological fractures, and renal calculi.

The synthesis of human parathyroid hormone in 1974 helped to drive research into the biological actions of the hormone [2]. Intuitively, exogenous administration of parathyroid hormone should result in net bone loss, as is the case in patients with hyperparathyroidism. However, paradoxically, intermittent administration of parathyroid hormone produces an anabolic response in bone with stimulation of osteoblast activity. This finding led the way to parathyroid hormone becoming the first anabolic agent to be studied for the treatment of osteoporosis.

Early work by Reeve et al. showed that once-daily subcutaneous administration of parathyroid hormone (1–34) in human subjects with osteoporosis, given for 6–24 months, substantially increased iliac trabecular bone volume by a mean of 70% [3]. They hypothesized that parathyroid hormone may prove useful in treating patients with vertebral fractures. Lane et al. conducted a randomized clinical trial of parathyroid hormone (1–34) in postmenopausal women with osteoporosis who were taking corticosteroids and receiving hormone replacement therapy (HRT) [4]. The authors were able to show significant improvements in bone density at the lumbar spine in the group receiving parathyroid hormone as compared to the group receiving HRT. Within the first three months of treatment, markers of bone formation increased approximately 150% whereas markers of bone resorption increased 100%, suggesting early uncoupling of bone turnover in favour of bone formation. Lindsay et al. conducted a three-year randomized controlled trial of parathyroid hormone (1–34) in postmenopausal women with osteoporosis and taking HRT [5]. The primary outcome was BMD of the lumbar spine. The authors showed significant increases in BMD at the lumbar spine (13%) and total body (8%) in patients taking parathyroid hormone. There was also a reduction in vertebral fractures in patients taking parathyroid hormone when compared to those receiving HRT, although the number of patients in each cohort was small (n = 17).

The above studies provided the background for Neer and colleagues' landmark piece of work. This study was, and remains, the largest trial of parathyroid hormone to date, involving 1,637 women with postmenopausal osteoporosis. It demonstrated dramatic reductions in vertebral and non-vertebral fracture risk and large improvements in lumbar spine BMD. The magnitude of fracture risk reduction was greater than that seen with other available therapies for osteoporosis at the time of publication. This study was pivotal in the subsequent licensing and establishment of parathyroid hormone as a treatment for individuals at high risk of fracture, particularly vertebral fracture. Just as importantly, Neer's study led to parathyroid hormone becoming the first available anabolic treatment for osteoporosis. It remains one of the most effective treatments to date, although other agents (zoledronate and denosumab) have subsequently shown a similar magnitude of vertebral fracture risk reduction, as well as significant reductions in hip fracture incidence [6, 7].

Of note, Neer's study was terminated early by the sponsors after the finding that osteosarcoma developed in rats receiving high-dose parathyroid hormone [8]. However, there appears to be no evidence of an increased risk of osteosarcoma in human subjects receiving parathyroid hormone. In addition, there is no evidence to suggest an increased risk of osteosarcoma in patients with hyperparathyroidism. Parathyroid hormone treatment is associated with side effects including dizziness, leg cramps, irritation at injection sites, headache, nausea, hypercalcaemia, and arthralgias/myalgias. Neer's study showed that adverse effects were more common in patients receiving the 40 µg dose of parathyroid hormone. This group also had the greatest dropout rate (11% vs 6% in the 20 µg and placebo arms).

In summary, parathyroid hormone remains the only truly anabolic agent available in the routine clinical care of patients at high risk of fractures. It improves bone mass and architecture and reduces fracture risk. However, the high cost of treatment and method of administration somewhat limit its utility. Neer's landmark study has undoubtedly contributed to the ongoing quest to produce new anabolic agents.

References

1 **Collip JB**. The extraction of a parathyroid hormone which will prevent or control parathyroid tetany and which regulates the level of blood calcium. *J Biol Chem* 1925;**63**(2):395–438.

2 **Tregear GW, van Rietschoten J, Greene E, et al**. Solid-phase synthesis of the biologically active N-terminal 1–34 peptide human parathyroid hormone. *Hoppe Seylers Z Physiol Chem* 1974;**355**(1):415–21.

3 **Reeve J, Meunier PJ, Parsons JA, et al**. Anabolic effect of human parathyroid hormone fragment on trabecular bone in involutional osteoporosis: a multicentre trial. *BMJ* 1980;**280**(6228):1340–4.

4 **Lane NE, Sanchez S, Modlin GW, et al**. Parathyroid hormone treatment can reverse corticosteroid-induced osteoporosis. Results of a randomized controlled clinical trial. *J Clin Invest* 1998;**102**(8):1627–33.

5 **Lindsay R, Nieves J, Formica C, et al**. Randomised controlled study of effect of parathyroid hormone on vertebral-bone mass and fracture incidence among postmenopausal women on oestrogen with osteoporosis. *Lancet* 1997;**350**(9077):550–5.

6 **Black DM, Delmas PD, Eastell R, et al**. Once-yearly zoledronic acid for treatment of postmenopausal osteoporosis. *N Engl J Med* 2007;**356**(18):1809–22.

7 **Cummings SR, San Martin J, McClung MR, et al**. Denosumab for prevention of fractures in postmenopausal women with osteoporosis. *N Engl J Med* 2009;**361**(8):756–65.

8 **Vahle JL, Sato M, Long GG, et al**. Skeletal changes in rats given daily subcutaneous injections of recombinant human parathyroid hormone (1–34) for 2 years and relevance to human safety. *Toxicol Pathol* 2002;**30**(3):312–21.

Paper 9.5: Atypical femoral fractures

Reference

Goh SK, Yang KY, Koh JSB, et al. Subtrochanteric insufficiency fractures in patients on alendronate therapy: a caution. *J Bone Joint Surg Br* 2007;89(3):349–53.

Purpose

This is a retrospective chart review over ten months of patients who presented with low-energy subtrochanteric fractures after the authors became aware of an apparent rise in numbers of such fractures in women aged between 50 and 70 years and occurring after minimal or no trauma.

Patients

This study examined patients who had been treated surgically for subtrochanteric fracture of the femur.

Study design

Between 1 May 2005 and 28 February 2006, a retrospective review of operating records of all orthopaedic surgeons from two hospitals were examined to identify patients who had been treated surgically for subtrochanteric fracture of the femur. Subtrochanteric fracture was defined as one in the region of the femur which extended from the lesser trochanter to the junction of the proximal and middle third of the femoral shaft. Only fractures sustained in low-energy trauma were included. The details collected were patient demographics, the classification of the subtrochanteric fracture, co-morbidities, the results of bone density measurement and medication, the presence or absence of prodromal pain before the fracture, and the histological findings of bone from the site of fracture when available.

Results

Thirteen women with subtrochanteric fractures sustained by low-energy trauma were identified, of whom nine had been taking alendronate. The patients in the alendronate group were younger, with a mean age of 66.9 years (55–82 years) versus 80.3 years (64–92 years).

Four patients in the alendronate group reported that the fracture had occurred in the absence of a fall, and each recorded experience of sharp pain or hearing a snapping sound at the moment of the fracture.

In the alendronate group, five patients reported that prodromal symptoms of pain or discomfort had occurred in the fractured limb 2–6 months before the injury. One patient localized the prodromal pain in the groin on the fracture site, whereas the remainder localized the pain at the lateral aspect of the thigh. None of the patients in the non-alendronate group had prodromal symptoms.

Of the 13 patients, 9 were taking alendronate and oral calcium for the treatment of osteoporosis either at the time of or within a year before the injury. Four patients were not taking alendronate; of these, two were taking oral calcium supplements.

BMD results were available in only five patients: four had osteopenia, and one had osteoporosis. The duration of alendronate treatment in the nine patients was 2.5–5 years.

In the alendronate group, eight of the patients had an AO type-A fracture occurring at the metaphyseal–diaphyseal junction, while the ninth had a type-B fracture. In six, cortical hypertrophy was observed on the lateral side of the subtrochanteric region of the femur. In three, a similar hypertrophic cortex was observed in the contralateral subtrochanteric region.

Three patients in the non-alendronate group had AO type-B fractures, and one had a type-C fracture. As judged by plain radiographs, the bones of these patients appeared to be extremely osteoporotic, with loss of the trabecular pattern.

In five patients in the alendronate group, bone biopsies were sent for histological analyses. All were found to be benign.

Critique of the paper

It is known that the subtrochanteric region of the femur is subjected to maximal bending movement and is one of the strongest parts of the femur; it is unlikely to fail in low-energy trauma unless extreme osteoporosis is present. The authors noted that the literature indicated that only 10%–34% of all fractures of the hip are in the subtrochanteric region.

The authors noted that the alendronate group had been on medication for a mean of 4.2 years, that the trauma was minimal in nine patients, that a few had experienced prodromal symptoms in the months preceding the fracture, and that most were in the early stages of the menopause and had led relatively active lifestyles at the time of injury.

The authors noted that bisphosphonates have been proven to reduce fractures in patients with osteopenia/osteoporosis and made reference to the FIT. The mechanism by which alendronate acts is through inhibition of bone resorption by suppressing activity of the osteoclast and inducing apoptosis. The authors speculated that a reduction in bone turnover could lead to an accumulation of skeletal microdamage and an increased risk of insufficiency fractures.

The authors noted the fractures in the alendronate group had radiologically good cortical bone stock and contrasted with the presence of extreme osteoporosis in the non-alendronate group. They speculated that the observations of thickening in the lateral femoral cortex in six of the alendronate patients, in three of whom the cortical thickening was bilateral, together with a history of prodromal pain, support the hypothesis that the fractures in these patients were insufficiency fracture resulting from altered bone metabolism. The authors observed this was the first report of a series of fractures in the subtrochanteric region of the femur in patients who had received alendronate for a long period. They agreed that the study did not establish a cause and effect relationship but suggested a potential, as yet unrecognized, side effect of prolonged pharmacological suppression of bone turnover.

Significance and importance of the paper

This initial publication was followed by many case reports and case series on atypical femoral fractures (AFFs). In 2010 the American Society for Bone and Mineral Research (ASBMR) Task Force reported on AFFs and concluded that the incidence of AFFs associated with bisphosphonate therapy for osteoporosis was very low when compared to other fractures that are prevented by bisphosphonates and noted that a causal association between bisphosphonates and AFFs had not been established [1].

A Swedish study, using a national dataset but being constrained by having access to less than three years of medication history, suggested a rapid, reversible, and an important increase in AFFs among bisphosphonate users [2]. They found an atypical fracture rate of 0.9/100,000 person-years in Sweden among those who had not used bisphosphonates, compared to 55/100,000 person-years among bisphosphonate users, with a relative risk of 47.3 among every user. There was a tenfold increase in risk within two years of treatment and a 124-fold increased risk in the first five years. In this study the researchers were unable to assess trends in atypical fractures. This was analysed in a publication by Feldstein et al., who undertook a retrospective medical record and radiographic review among women over the age of 50 years and men over the age of 65 from January 1996 to 2009 in the United States [3]. The authors reviewed the radiographs and suggested that the definition of atypical fractures, as proposed by the task force report of the ASBMR in 2010 [1], may need to be modified. The AFFs were divided into those with major features only, a group who were older with lower BMD, and those with additional one or more minor criteria. It was only the latter subtype of fractures that showed an increasing time trend and an association with bisphosphonate use. There were no such fractures in the years 1996 to 1999, after which there was a slow increase.

Since the publication of this report, numerous epidemiological studies have examined the relationship of such fractures to bisphosphonate therapy and other risk factors for AFFs. As a result, and because concerns were raised about the limitation of the ASBMR case definition, the ASBMR task force was reconvened in 2012 and subsequently reported their findings [4]. In the second task force report, a revised case definition for AFFs was suggested (Box 9.1).

After examining studies with radiographic evaluation, the task force concluded that a causal relation between bisphosphonates and AFFs had not been established but that evidence for an association continues to accumulate.

The task force suggested, as they did in 2010, that patients with stress reactions/stress fracture or incomplete or complete subtrochanteric or femoral shaft fracture should have anti-resorptive therapy discontinued. They should receive adequate dietary calcium and vitamin D, supplemented if necessary. Prophylactic reconstruction nail fixation was recommended for incomplete fractures accompanied by pain. For those in minimal pain, a conservative trial of limited weight bearing through crutches could be considered. Prophylactic nail fixation should be considered if there is no symptomatic or radiographic improvement after two to three months. In those with incomplete fractures and no pain, or

Box 9.1 American Society for Bone and Mineral Research Task Force 2013 revised case definition of atypical femoral fractures*

To satisfy the case definition of atypical femur fracture (AFF), the fracture must be located along the femoral diaphysis from just distal to the lesser trochanter to just proximal to the supracondylar flare.

In addition, at least four to five major features must be present. None of the minor features is required but have sometimes been associated with those fractures.

Major features[†]

- The fracture is associated with minimal or no trauma, as in a fall from a standing height or less.

- **The fracture line originates at the lateral cortex and is substantially transverse in its orientation, although it may become oblique as it progresses medially across the femur.**

- Complete fractures extend through both cortices and may be associated with a medial spike; incomplete fractures involve only the lateral cortex.

- The fracture is noncomminuted **or minimally comminuted.**

- **Localized periosteal or endosteal thickening of the lateral cortex is present at the fracture site ('beaking' or 'flaring').**

Minor features

- Generalized increase in cortical thickness of the **femoral diaphysis.**

- Unilateral or bilateral prodromal symptoms such as dull or aching pain in the groin or thigh.

- Bilateral incomplete or complete femoral diaphysis fractures.

- Delayed **fracture** healing.

* Changes made to the original definition are in bold.
[†] **Excludes** fractures of the femoral neck, intertrochanteric fractures with spinal subtrochanteric extension, periprosthetic fractures, and pathological fractures associated with primary or metastatic bone tumours and miscellaneous bone diseases (e.g. Paget's disease, fibrous dysplasia).

those with periosteal thickening but no cortical lucency, reduced weight bearing should be continued with avoidance of strenuous activity until there is no evidence of bone oedema on MRI. The task force also considered anecdotal reports of various medical therapies, although they concluded that, in the absence of a randomized, placebo-controlled trial, no definite conclusion could be reached regarding the efficacy of teriparatide in the treatments of AFFs.

References

1 **Shane E, Burr D, Ebeling PR, et al**. Atypical subtrochanteric and diaphyseal femoral fractures: report of a task force of the American Society for Bone and Mineral Research. *J Bone Miner Res* 2010;**25**(11):2267–94.

2 **Schilcher J, Michaëlsson K, Aspenberg P**. Bisphosphonate use and atypical fractures of the femoral shaft. *N Engl J Med* 2011; **364**(18):1728–37.

3 **Feldstein AC, Black D, Perrin N, et al**. Incidence and dermography of femur fractures with and without atypical features. *J Bone Miner Res* 2012; **27**(5):977–86.

4 **Shane E, Burr D, Abraham B, et al**. Atypical subtrochanteric and diaphyseal femoral fractures: second report of a task force of the American Society for Bone and Mineral Research. *J Bone Miner Res* 2014;**29**(1):1–23.

Paper 9.6: Bisphosphonates and osteonecrosis of the jaw

Reference

Marx RE. Pamidronate (Aredia) and zoledronate (Zometa) induced avascular necrosis of the jaws: a growing epidemic. *J Oral Maxillofacsurg* 2003;61(9):1115–17.

Purpose

Bisphosphonates, either orally or intravenously, are licensed for use in osteoporosis, hypercalcaemia caused by malignancy, Paget's disease of the bone, and metastatic bone disease of multiple myeloma, breast, lung, and prostatic cancer. This paper and another one by Migliorati were the first reports of an association of bisphosphonates with osteonecrosis of the jaw (ONJ) [1].

Patients

This study examined patients receiving bisphosphonates and presenting with painful exposed avascular bone in the mandible or maxilla.

Study design

This was an observational study. Thirty-six patients were described, of whom 24 had received intravenous pamidronate, 6 had received pamidronate previously but had been switched to zoledronate intravenously, and 6 had received only zoledronate.

In 18 patients, the indication for using a bisphosphonate was hypercalcaemia related to multiple myeloma, in 17 patients the indication was hypercalcaemia related to metastatic breast cancer, and in 1 patient the indication was osteoporosis. Although patients were taking other medications, only pamidronate or zoledronate was the single class of drug in all 36 cases. Twenty-two (61%) of patients were also receiving dexamethasone, 24 (67%) were receiving maintenance chemotherapy, and 4 (11%) had received radiotherapy in the past.

Results

Twenty-nine (80.5%) of the patients presented with painful exposed avascular bone in the mandible, and 14% in the maxilla, with 5.5% at both sites. The presentation simulated dental abscesses, 'toothache', denture sore spots, and osteomyelitis. Removal of painful teeth was often the initiator of the exposed non-healing bone, as noted in 28 (77.7%) patients, with the remaining 8 patients developing exposed bone spontaneously.

Critique of the paper

Although written as a letter to the editor, the authors noted that there were no reports of ONJ with EDHP and speculated that the problem may have been with nitrogen-containing bisphosphonates such as pamidronate and zoledronate.

The authors observed jaws are the only bones in the skeleton exposed to the external environment through the presence of teeth, with frequent occurrence of periodontal inflammation, dental abscesses, and other pathologies that may lead to an increase in bone turnover. They observed that 77.7% of their patients had ONJ initiated by tooth-removal surgery. For the rest, they speculated that thinning of the oral mucosa of the posterior mandible may be a factor and observed the occurrence of this in two other conditions associated with non-healing avascular exposed bone: osteoradionecrosis and osteopetrosis.

The authors suggested that most patients will be unresponsive or worsen with major debridement surgery, which should be avoided if at all possible. They suggested controlling and limiting progression with long-term or intermittent courses of antibiotics, mouthwashes, and periodic minor debridement of soft-textured sequestrated bone and wound irrigation.

Significance and importance of the paper

Since this report and that by Migliorati [1], over a thousand cases of ONJ have been reported in the literature. In understanding the relationship of the condition to bisphosphonate therapy, it is worth noting that osteomyelitis of the jaw was observed in the eighteenth century in factory workers who made phosphorous-containing matches; at this time, the condition was termed 'phossy jaw'. The first medical report of this, following the availability of the yellow phosphorous matchsticks in 1832, was in 1858 and led to a ban of these matches in 1906 [2]. In the US, a patient was admitted to the Massachusetts General Hospital in July 1895 with a diagnosis of 'necrosis of the jaw in a phosphorous worker'. Sixty-one years later, after a collection of 150 cases, legislation was passed in Congress prohibiting the use of white phosphorous in match manufacturing [3]. ONJ remains a rare adverse event in the UK, with an estimated incidence of 620 cases per year [4]; it has been observed with both intravenous and oral bisphosphonates, although the frequency is higher with intravenous bisphosphonates. The estimated rate of ONJ due to oral bisphosphonates for the treatment of osteoporosis ranges from 1.04 to 69 per 100,000 patient-years. [5].

Definition of ONJ

The American Association of Oral and Maxillofacial Surgeons have recently updated their definition of medication-related ONJ to (1) current or previous treatment with antiresorptive or antiangiogenic agents; (2) exposed bone or bone that can be probed through an intraoral or extraoral fistula (e) in the maxillofacial region that has persisted for more than 8 weeks; and (3) no history of radiation therapy to the jaws or metastatic disease to the jaw (6). The International Task force on Osteonecrosis of the Jaw defines ONJ as: (1) exposed bone in the maxillofacial region that does not heal within 8 weeks after identification; (2) exposure to an antiresorptive agent; (3) no history of radiation therapy to the craniofacial region.

Although most observers accept an association between bisphosphonate exposure and development of ONJ, there is controversy about the epidemiology, pathophysiology, and management of ONJ. Several risk factors for ONJ have been identified. One of the most striking is the consistent use of nitrogen-containing bisphosphonates, particularly zoledronic acid. This drug, rather than pamidronate, is the preferred bisphosphonate for treating multiple myeloma and metastatic cancers. It is estimated that patients with cancer and who are on zoledronic acid have 9.1–15 times the risk of developing ONJ as compared to 1.6–4 times the risk when pamidronate is followed by the use of zoledronic acid. Other risk factors include the duration of exposure to the medication. Most cancer patients who are exposed to zoledronic acid develop ONJ within 9–13 months of treatment, with most cases occurring after three months [7]. Other risk factors identified include age, smoking, glucocorticoid therapy, diabetes, cancer, anti-cancer treatment, pre-existing dental disease, dental extraction, and thin dental mucosa where there is a risk of non-surgical trauma.

Osteonecrosis of the jaw has also been reported with the RANKL inhibitor denosumab.

Unlike in patients with cancer, the median time of development of ONJ in patients with osteoporosis is 3.5 years [8].

Clinical presentation

The exposed, yellowish to white, necrotic bone varies in size from a few millimetres to several centimetres. The edges of the exposed bone may be rough and sharp or smooth. The mandible is more frequently affected than the maxilla in the ratio of 2:1, and lesions are more common in areas with a thin mucosa overlying bone prominence, such as mandibular and maxillary tori, bone exostoses, and the mylohyoid ridge. The lesions may develop at sites of previous dental extraction. The bone may become loose and fragmented in the process of sequestration, causing pain and irritation. The adjacent teeth may become progressively mobile and symptomatic and may fall out. Sixty per cent of cases present initially with pain but many remain asymptomatic for a long time. The necrotic bone may be colonized by dental plaque, forming a biofilm [7]. Infection of the bone may cause pain, suppuration, and osteomyelitis, sometimes associated with a sinus causing a purulent discharge.

Management

The goal of management includes education and reassurance, pain control, infection control, and limiting the progression of the disease [7]. A staging system has been advocated (Table 9.1) [6, 7]. In this the disease is staged according to the clinical extent of involvement. In stage one, treatment aims to control and limit the process with antibacterial mouth rinse with limited debridement to eliminate sharp edges or lose bone. In Stage 2 disease, often the result of infection, oral therapy with broad spectrum antibiotics is used as well as limited debridement of exposed bone. In stage three of the disease additional therapy includes surgery to remove necrotic infected bone.

ONJ does not resolve completely once it has developed. Even where there is complete epithelization and normalization of the mucosa, the defect of the underlying bone may persist for many years.

When ONJ develops, bisphosphonates should be discontinued, although there is no evidence this makes any difference to the outcome. Since the major defect for the development of ONJ is osteoclast suppression, case reports have suggested that the anabolic agent teriparatide may be useful [5, 9].

Table 9.1 The American Association of Oral and Maxillofacial Surgeons Clinic staging system for bisphosphonate-associated osteonecrosis of the jaw

Stage 0	Stage 1	Stage 2	Stage 3
no clinical evidence of necrotic bone but nonspecific clinical findings, radiographic changes, and symptoms	1—exposed and necrotic bone or fistulas that probes to bone in patients who are asymptomatic and have no evidence of infection	exposed and necrotic bone or fistulas that probes to bone associated with infection as evidenced by pain and erythema in the region of exposed bone with or without purulent drainage	exposed and necrotic bone or a fistula that probes to bone in patients with pain, infection, and ≥1 of the following: exposed and necrotic bone extending beyond the region of alveolar bone (i.e., inferior border and ramus in mandible, maxillary sinus, and zygoma in maxilla) resulting in pathologic fracture, extraoral fistula, oral antral or oral nasal communication, or osteolysis extending to inferior border of the mandible or sinus floor

Source data Ruggiero SL, Dodson TB, Fantasia J et al et al. American Association of Oral and Maxillofacial Surgeons position paper on medication-related osteonecrosis of the jaws—2014update. *J Oral Maxillofac Surg* 2014;72(10): 1938–56 and 7. Mawardi HH, Treister NS, Woo S-B. Bisphosphonate-associated osteonecrosis of the jaws. Rosen CJ (ed). Primer on the metabolic bone diseases and disorders of mineral metabolism. 8th Edition. Wiley-Blackwell 2013 pp. 929–40.

References

1 **Migliorati CA**. Bisphosphonates and oral cavity avascular bone necrosis. *J Clin Oncol* 2003;**21**(22):4253–8.

2 **Miles AE**. Phosphorus necrosis of the jaw: 'phossy jaw'. *Br Dent J* 1972;**133**(5):203–6.

3 **Cannon IM, Hum D**. The meaning of the patient to the hospital. *N Engl J Med* 1947;**236**(13):457–60.

4 **Faculty of General Dental Practice**. National study on avascular necrosis of the jaws including bisphosphonate-related necrosis. Dec 2012; <http://www.fgdp.org.uk/_assets/pdf/research/final%20 report-27.11.12.pdf>, accessed 2 February 2015.

5 **Khan AA, Morrison A, Hanley DA, et al**. Diagnosis and Management of the Jaw; A Systematic Review and International Consensus. J Bone Mineral Res 2015;**30**(1): 3–23.

6 **Ruggiero SL, Dodson TB, Fantasia J et al**. American Association of Oral and Maxillofacial Surgeons position paper on medication-related osteonecrosis of the jaws—2014 update. *J Oral Maxillofac Surg* 2014;**72**(10):1938–56.

7 **Mawardi HH, Treister NS, Woo S-B**. 'Bisphosphonate-associated osteonecrosis of the jaws' in Primer on the metabolic bone diseases and disorders of mineral metabolism, 8th edn (Rosen CJ, ed.); Ames, IA: Wiley-Blackwell; 2013; pp. 929–40.

8 **Lo JC, O'Ryan FS, Gordon NP, et al**. Prevalence of osteoporosis of the jaw in patients with oral bisphosphonate exposure. *J Oral Maxillofac Surg* 2010;**68**(2):243–53.

9 **Lau AN, Adachi JD**. Resolution of osteonecrosis of the jaw after teriparatide [recombinant human PTH-(1–34)] therapy. *J Rheumatol* 2009;**36**(8):1835–7.

Paper 9.7: Treatment of Paget's disease of bone

Reference

Khairi MR, Altman RD, DeRosa GP, et al. Sodium etidronate in the treatment of Paget's disease of bone. A study of long-term results. *Ann Intern Med* 1977;87(6):656–63.

Purpose

To assess the effect of longer-term treatment with EHDP in Paget's disease of bone, to assess factors influencing relapse after a course of therapy with EHDP, to assess the effect of retreatment with EHDP, to identify long-term side effects, and to identify the optimal dose of EHDP with respect to risks and benefits of treatment.

Patients

Patients with Paget's disease of bone as evidenced by radiologic examination, pain at one or more sites of pagetic bone involvement, and serum alkaline phosphatase or urinary hydroxyproline levels more than 1.5 times the normal upper limits.

Study design

This was an open-label, unblinded, observational study of 109 patients (a follow-on study from a previous one-year double-blind crossover study [1]).

Treatment

Treatment consisted of 5 mg, 10 mg, or 20 mg of EHDP kg^{-1}day^{-1} for 6–24 months.

Trial end points measured

The trial end points were percentage change in serum alkaline phosphatase and urinary hydroxyproline levels, clinical observations (primarily subjective improvement in pain), and bone histology.

Follow-up

There was open-label follow-up for up to 24 months after the cessation of EHDP therapy.

Results

Significant decreases in serum alkaline phosphatase and urinary hydroxyproline were noted after six months of therapy; no significant further improvement resulted after prolonged therapy. Some patients maintained biochemical remission after withdrawal of EHDP but others showed a relapse, related primarily to the pretreatment severity of the disease. Clinical improvement was noted in 61% of the patients. Similar findings were seen after a second course of EHDP. No side effects were noted in patients treated with 5 mg EHDP kg^{-1}day^{-1}. In patients treated with 10 mg EHDP kg^{-1}day^{-1} or 20 mg EHDP kg^{-1}day^{-1}, severe diarrhoea, bone pain, and non-traumatic fractures were noted in 3, 13, and 12 patients, respectively. Quantitative histomorphometry showed mineralization delay in patients receiving 10 mg EHDP kg^{-1}day^{-1} or 20 mg EHDP kg^{-1}day^{-1} but not in those receiving 5 mg EHDP kg^{-1}day^{-1}; 5 mg EHDP kg^{-1}day^{-1} was effective and appeared to be safer than the higher doses.

Critique of the paper

There was no placebo arm running throughout the course of the study. Patients and investigators were not blinded to the treatments. In addition, there was no clear validated scoring system to define clinical improvement.

Significance and importance of the paper

Paget's disease of bone is characterized by a dramatic increase in bone turnover. It has long been recognized that efforts to slow bone turnover, particularly suppressing activity of osteoclasts, may help to treat the condition. Various therapies have been utilized over the years to try and suppress the bone remodelling process, including antibiotics, radiotherapy, calcitonin, and fluoride. These were followed by the diphosphonates.

The therapeutic role of EHDP in the treatment of Paget's disease of bone had been established in prior studies [1–3]. However, this study was pivotal in exploring longer-term outcomes of therapy in a larger number of subjects and attempting to identify an optimal treatment regimen.

This study highlighted the adverse effects of higher doses of EHDP (diarrhoea, bone pain, non-traumatic fractures, and inhibition of bone mineralization) and suggested an optimal dose regimen of 5 mg EHDP kg^{-1}day^{-1} for six months as having the lowest risk–benefit ratio.

EHDP was the first bisphosphonate approved in the US for the treatment of Paget's disease of bone and continues to be licensed for this indication. The usual recommended dose regime remains 5 mg EHDP kg^{-1}day^{-1} for six months.

Other bisphosphonates (tiludronate and clodronate) have been utilized in the treatment of Paget's disease and, together with EHDP, have been shown to decrease alkaline phosphatase levels. However, despite these reductions, these treatments only normalize alkaline phosphatase levels in a minority of patients. The relative success of the early bisphosphonates, but noted deficiencies of treatment, laid the foundation for the subsequent trials of the newer generation of more potent nitrogen-containing bisphosphonates (pamidronate, alendronate, risedronate, and zoledronate).

Both oral alendronate and risedronate have been shown to be superior to EHDP in terms of improvement in alkaline phosphatase levels and, in the case of risedronate, improvement in pain [4, 5]. However, intravenous zoledronate (the most potent of the bisphosphonates) can justifiably lay claim to being the current 'gold standard' treatment, with approximately nine of ten treated patients showing normalization of alkaline phosphatase levels after a single infusion [6, 7]. In addition, it appears to be the most effective treatment to date in producing a sustained response. Head-to head studies show superiority over oral risedronate and intravenous pamidronate [6, 7].

The concepts of 'courses of treatment' and sustained response following therapy can trace their roots back to the landmark paper that is the subject of this review. Khairi's study helped to show that prolonging therapy beyond a six-month course of treatment did not result in further biochemical or clinical improvement and that subjects could remain in remission for some time after cessation of therapy. It also identified that retreatment at the time of clinical or biochemical relapse resulted in similar improvements to the first treatment course. These findings continue to influence our use of the nitrogen-containing bisphosphonates in current practice.

References

1 **Khairi MRA, Johnston CC Jr, Altman RD, et al**. Treatment of Paget's disease of bone (osteitis deformans): results of a one-year study with sodium etidronate. *JAMA* 1974; **230**(4):562–7.

2 **Altman RD, Johnston CC Jr, Khairi MRA, et al**. Influence of sodium etidronate on clinical and laboratory manifestations of Paget's disease of bone (osteitis deformans). *N Engl J Med* 1973;**289**(26):1379–84.

3 **Russell RGG, Smith R, Preston C, et al**. Diphosphonates in Paget's disease. Lancet 1974; **303**(7863):894–8.

4 **Siris E, Weinstein RS, Altman R, et al**. Comparative study of alendronate versus etidronate for the treatment of Paget's disease of bone. *J Clin Endocrinol Metab* 1996;**81**(3):961–7.

5 **Miller PD, Brown JP, Siris ES, et al**. A randomized, double-blind comparison of risedronate and etidronate in the treatment of Paget's disease of bone. *Am J Med* 1999;**106**(5):513–20.

6 **Reid IR, Miller P, Lyles K, et al**. Comparison of a single infusion of zoledronic acid with risedronate for Paget's disease. *N Engl J Med* 2005;**353**(9):898–908.

7 **Merlotti D, Gennari L, Martini G, et al**. Comparison of different intravenous bisphosphonate regimens for Paget's disease of bone. *J Bone Miner Res* 2007; **22**(10):1510.

Paper 9.8: Mechanisms of altered calcium homeostasis in sarcoidosis

Reference

Barbour GL, Coburn JW, Slatopolsky E, et al. Hypercalcaemia in an anephric patient with sarcoidosis: evidence for extrarenal generation of 1,25-dihydroxyvitamin D. *N Engl J Med* 1981;305(8):440–3.

Background

Mild-to-severe hypercalcaemia is present in 10% of patients with sarcoidosis, and up to 50% of patients will at some time during the course of the illness become hypercalciuric [1].

Briefly, exposure to solar ultraviolet B radiation converts 7-dehydroxycholesterol in the skin to pre-vitamin D_3, which is immediately converted to vitamin D_3. Vitamin D, bound to vitamin D-binding protein, is transported to the liver to undergo conversion by vitamin D-25-hydroxylase to 25-hydroxyvitamin D (25-(OH)D), the major circulating form of vitamin D used clinically to assess an individual's vitamin D status. 25-(OH)D is converted in the kidneys to the biologically active form 1,25-dihydroxyvitamin D (1,25(OH)$_2$D) through the action of the renal 1α-hydroxylase. This active metabolite is the natural ligand for the vitamin D receptor. The conversion of 25-(OH)D to 1,25(OH)$_2$D is primarily controlled at the level of the kidney, where low serum phosphorous, low serum calcium, low FGF23 and high parathyroid hormone levels favour the production of 1,25(OH)$_2$D [2].

In the active phase of sarcoidosis, increased absorption of calcium from the intestine leads to hypercalciuria and occasionally hypercalcaemia. In these patients, unlike normal individuals, a small-to-moderate increase of circulating 25-(OH)D causes significant increases in serum 1,25(OH)$_2$D. Additionally, hypercalcaemic patients have higher or inappropriately elevated 1,25(OH)$_2$D concentrations, even though parathyroid hormone levels are suppressed and serum phosphorous elevated. Furthermore, the increased production of 1,25(OH)$_2$D, is unusually amenable to inhibition by glucocorticoids which normally do not affect the renal 1α-hydroxylase enzyme. The finding of elevated circulating levels of 1,25(OH)$_2$D in hypercalcaemic patients with sarcoidosis suggests the increased endogenous levels of 1,25(OH)$_2$D from the precursor is either due to an altered production or degradation of 1,25(OH)$_2$D [3].

Under normal circumstances, the endogenous production of 1,25(OH)$_2$D occurs only in the kidney, thus explaining why there is a deficiency of 1,25(OH)$_2$D in patients with advanced renal failure and which contributes to the development of renal osteodystrophy.

Patient

Barbour et al. described a patient with asymptomatic hilar lymphadenopathy due to sarcoidosis and who developed IgA (Henoch–Schönlein) glomerulonephritis and nephrotic syndrome. The patient's renal disease and arthralgias were managed by prednisolone but renal function continued to decline, leading to peritoneal dialysis. The patient developed hypercalcaemia, which responded to prednisolone, and subsequently underwent bilateral nephrectomy and splenectomy in preparation for a cadaveric renal transplant.

Following this, attempts to reduce the prednisolone led to recurrences of hypercalcaemia.

Methods

Serum samples were collected at intervals and analysed for parathyroid hormone and vitamin D sterols.

Results

During episodes of hypercalcaemia, levels of $1,25(OH)_2D$ were elevated, with suppression of immunoreactive parathyroid hormone (iPTH). With prednisolone, the serum levels of $1,25(OH)_2D$ and calcium lowered, with a reciprocal rise in iPTH. This relationship was seen both before and after nephrectomy.

On chromatography of lipid extract of serum samples, the serum contained material that co-migrated with authentic $1,25(OH)_2D_3$ and competed with authentic $1,25(OH)_2D_3$ in a competitive binding assay.

Critique of the paper

At the time of this report, it was thought that there were only two sources of 1α-hydroxylase: the renal cortex and the placenta. It was assumed that the renal enzyme was responsible for the production of $1,25(OH)_2D$. The findings in this patient suggested that there was an extrarenal source of $1,25(OH)_2D$ production but where this occurred was unknown.

Significance and importance of the paper

This publication provided good evidence that the endogenous production of $1,25(OH)_2D$ in sarcoidosis with hypercalcaemia was not from the kidney. In 1985 Adams et al. showed that primary cultures of pulmonary alveolar macrophages from two patients with biopsy-proven sarcoidosis and with recent abnormalities of calcium metabolism were able to synthesize in vitro from $25-(OH)D_3$ a metabolite that resembled $1,25(OH)_2D_3$ [4]. The reason for the expression of 1α-hydroxylase in macrophages remains unknown. Although the enzyme has similar substrate specificity and enzyme kinetics as the renal enzyme, there are important differences in how the macrophage 1α-hydroxylase regulates the synthesis of $1,25(OH)_2D_3$ [5]. The macrophage 1α-hydroxylase is not induced by parathyroid hormone but is sensitive to stimulation by immunoactivators such as interferon-γ and tumour necrosis factor-α. Unlike the renal 1α-hydroxylase, the macrophage enzyme is refractory to negative feedback regulation by $1,25(OH)_2D$ but is sensitive to inhibition by glucocorticoids [6].

Hypercalcaemia has been associated with a number of granulomatous diseases, including TB and lymphoma. In B-cell lymphoma, the source of the elevated $1,25(OH)_2D$ is not the tumour itself but the adjacent macrophages. The syndrome of hypercalcaemia in granulomatous disease is reversed with glucocorticoids or the treatment of the underlying disorder as well as by lowering dietary intake of vitamin D and calcium. Since the main source of vitamin D is sunlight, sun exposure should be minimized.

References

1 **Studdy RR, Bird R, Neville E, et al**. Biochemical findings in sarcoidosis. *J Clin Pathol* 1980; **33**(6):528–33.

2 **Holick MF**. Vitamin D deficiency. *N Engl J Med* 2007;**357**(3):266–81.

3 **Papapoulos SE, Clemens TL, Fraher LF, et al**. 1,25-Dihydroxycholecalciferol in the pathogenesis of hypercalcaemic in sarcoidosis. *Lancet* 1979;**313**(8117):627–30.

4 **Adams JD, Singer FR, Gacad MA, et al**. Isolation and structural identification of 1,25-dihydroxyvitamin D_3 production by cultured alveolar macrophage in sarcoidosis. *J Clin Endocrinol Metab* 1985;**60**(5):960–6.

5 **Reichel H, Koeffler HP, Bishop JE, et al**. 25-Hydroxyvitamin D_3 metabolism by lipopolysaccharide—stimulated normal human macrophages. *J Clin Endocrinol Metab* 1987; **64**(1):1–9.

6 **Adams JS, Gacad MA**. Characterisation of 1α-hydroxylation of vitamin D_3 sterols by cultured alveolar macrophage from patients with sarcoidosis. *J Exp Med* 1985;**161**(4):755–65.

Chapter 10

Ehlers–Danlos syndrome and Marfan syndrome

Alan Hakim and Asma Fikree

Introduction

Hereditary disorders of connective tissue (HDCT) comprise a varied group of conditions that arise from abnormalities of collagen, fibrillin, elastin, and other matrix proteins, and as a consequence of genetic and molecular aberrations. There are a number of rare HDCTs. However, three disorders are relatively common, namely, Ehlers–Danlos syndrome, Marfan syndrome, and osteogenesis imperfecta.

This chapter focuses on Ehlers–Danlos syndrome and Marfan syndrome: the early observations of inheritance in Ehlers–Danlos syndrome, the classification of subgroups in Ehlers–Danlos syndrome, and specific examples of advances in molecular genetics in Ehlers–Danlos syndrome; and the recognition of the association of Marfan syndrome with life-threatening cardiac complications, surgical intervention to correct aortic root pathology in Marfan syndrome, and the identification and therapeutic implications of transforming growth factor ß in the pathogenesis of Marfan syndrome. For both Ehlers–Danlos syndrome and Marfan syndrome, there is a wealth of historical landmarks over a short period of time. A chronology of the different discoveries is outlined on a timeline for each condition (Box 10.1 and Box 10.2).

Box 10.1 A timeline of landmarks in Ehlers–Danlos syndrome

400 BC	Hippocrates description of Ehlers–Danlos syndrome
1657	Van Meek'ren: first description of disorder
1883	Wile: case presentation of Ehlers–Danlos syndrome
1892	Tschernogobow: case presentation of Ehlers–Danlos syndrome
1897	Gould and Pye: case presentation of Ehlers–Danlos syndrome
1901	Danish physician Edvard Ehlers publishes detailed description of disorder
1908	French physician Henri-Alexandre Danlos publishes detailed description of disorder
1916	Finkelstein describes the familial/congenital nature of joint 'hypotonia'
1927	Key describes a father and sons who have joint hypermobility and early osteoarthritis, recognizing the familial nature of joint hypermobility
1936	The term 'Ehlers–Danlos syndrome' is coined by Frederick Parkes-Weber
1937	Stuart: description of individuals (mother and two children) affected with Ehlers–Danlos syndrome within the same family
1938	Goldsmith: description of individuals (girl and uncle) affected with Ehlers–Danlos syndrome within the same family
1949	Johnson and Falls: the first comprehensive description of Ehlers–Danlos syndrome as an inherited trait, drawing on data from large pedigrees involving six generations
1955	Jansen publishes his 'collagen wickerwork' theory to account for abnormalities in Ehlers–Danlos syndrome: abnormal collagen fibres lead to abnormal/weak collagen fibrils, which lead to the Ehlers–Danlos syndrome phenotype
1956	McKusick coins the term 'hereditary disorders of connective tissue' to include Ehlers–Danlos syndrome, osteogenesis imperfecta, pseudoxanthoma elasticum, and Hurler syndrome
1967	Barabas: first clinical and histological characterization of Ehlers–Danlos syndrome into three groups: classical, varicose, and arterial
1969	Beighton: revised classification of Ehlers–Danlos syndrome into five groups: gravis, mitis, benign hypermobile, ecchymotic, and X-linked
1971	Miller: recognition of different subtypes of collagen in different tissues

Box 10.1 A timeline of landmarks in Ehlers–Danlos syndrome *(continued)*

1972	Pinnell: first molecular defect of collagen is discovered; lysyl hydroxylase deficiency is associated with recessive form of Ehlers–Danlos syndrome VII
1975	Pope: collagen III is absent in tissue from patients with Ehlers–Danlos syndrome IV (vascular)
1977	Pope: determined that Ehlers–Danlos syndrome IV is inherited as an autosomal recessive disorder
1982–1983	Junien, Herre, Henderson, Solomon: *COLIA2* linked to Chromosome 7
1984	Strom: *COL2A1* linked to Chromosome 12
1985	Emmanuel: *COL3A1* and *COL5A2* linked to Chromosome 2
1986	Tsipouras: linkage of *COL3A1* defect to Ehlers–Danlos syndrome IV
1987	Wirtz: first account of linking a genetic defect in *COL1A2* to Ehlers–Danlos syndrome VII
1991	Weil, Vasan, Nicholls, Chiodo, Watson: different genetic mutations in *COL1A2* discovered in patients with Ehlers–Danlos syndrome VII
1992	Greenspan: *COL5A1* linked to Chromosome 9
1995	Loughlin: *COL5A1* mutations are linked to Ehlers–Danlos syndrome II
1996	Kadler: biochemistry of collagen
1996	Toriello, Nicholls, Wenstrup, Richards, Michalickova: different genetic mutations in *COL5A1* and *COL5A2* discovered in patients with Ehlers–Danlos syndrome I/II
1997	The Villefranche classification for Ehlers–Danlos syndrome is published
1998	The revised (Brighton) classification for the joint hypermobility syndrome is published
2000	Schalkwijk: deficiency of tenascin X is associated with recessive form of classical Ehlers–Danlos syndrome
2003	Zweers: haploinsufficiency of tenascin X is associated with Ehlers–Danlos syndrome hypermobility
2012	Symoens: presence of *COL5* mutations in over 90% of classic Ehlers–Danlos syndrome; enabled refining of Ehlers–Danlos syndrome classification

Box 10.2 A timeline of landmarks in Marfan syndrome

1875	Williams: Reports an association between arachnodactyly and ocular pathology
1896	Antoine Marfan: the first description of a Marfanoid habitus in a 5-year-old girl
1902	Mery and Babonneix: describe 'malalignment of the spine' in Marfan's paediatric case
1902	Achard: reports the presence of arachnodactyly, joint hypermobility, and familial nature of condition in patient with Marfanoid habitus
1909	MacCallum: publishes a drawing of a specimen with a chronic aortic dissection, now recognized as being typical of the type seen in Marfan syndrome
1914	Boerger: publishes case reports of an association between arachnodactyly and ocular pathology
1918	Bronson and Sutherland: describe a 6-year-old patient with phenotypic features typical for Marfan syndrome and an aortic aneurysm which ruptured into the pericardium
1923	Poynton and Maurice: publish a case report of a patient with arachnodactyly and organic heart disease
1926	Piper and Irwine Jones: first report of a patient in America with arachnodactyly and a Marfan phenotype—the patient also had congenital heart disease
1929	Ormond: first draws attention to the frequent association between skeletal abnormalities and congenital dislocation of the lens
1931	Weve: first attributes the term 'Marfan syndrome' to a patient with typical musculoskeletal deformities and demonstrates its transmission as an autosomal dominant trait
1936	Burch: documents the association between skeletal abnormalities and congenital dislocation of the lens, based on a detailed review of the case report literature
1943	Baer et al.: describe aneurysmal dilation and rupture in a patient with arachnodactyly
1943	Etter and Glover: describe aneurysmal dilation and rupture in a patient with arachnodactyly and ectopia lentis
1955	McKusick: detailed review of the cardiac involvement in Marfan syndrome based on observations in 105 cases within 50 families—suggested that abnormalities in connective tissue, possibly elastin, may be involved in patho-aetiology
1956	McLeod and Williams: review of the cardiovascular lesions in Marfan syndrome

Box 10.2 A timeline of landmarks in Marfan syndrome *(continued)*

1965	Schmick, McKusick et al.: large observational study in over 700 families which confirmed the association between Marfan syndrome and upward dislocation of the lens
1968	Bentall and de Bono: describe a technique for complete replacement of the aortic valve and ascending aorta in aortic valve ectasia
1972	Murdoch: review of 257 patients with Marfan syndrome demonstrating reduced survival due to associated complications: average life expectancy was 32 years
1981	Maumenee: detailed review of the eye pathologies associated with Marfan syndrome and their underlying mechanisms
1983	Crawford et al.: demonstrated that prophylactic grafting and aortic repair in Marfan syndrome resulted in reduction in hospital mortality and improvement in overall survival
1986	Gott et al.: landmark paper on using the Bentall technique for life-saving surgical treatment in Marfan syndrome and in establishing ongoing vascular management for Marfan syndrome patients
1986	Sakai et al.: isolate fibrillin, a component of extracellular microfibrils
1988	Beighton et al.: diagnostic criteria for the Marfan syndrome first published—this would be revised in 1996 and then again in 2010
1990	Hollister et al.: demonstrate that fibrillin is defective or deficient in the skin and fibroblasts of patients with Marfan syndrome
1990	Kainulanen et al.: map gene defect in Marfan syndrome to Chromosome 15
1991	Maslen et al.: clone and partially sequence DNA related to fibrillin and map it to Chromosome 15
1991	Lee at al.: demonstrate polymorphisms of the gene for fibrillin-1 and its linkage to Marfan syndrome
1991	Dietz et al.: demonstrate point mutations in the fibrillin gene are associated with Marfan syndrome
1994	Kainulanen et al.: demonstrate that mutations in fibrillin-1 gene (*FBN-1*) are linked to ectopia lentis
1994	Random controlled trial of propranolol in Marfan syndrome shows that it slows the rate of aortic dilation and that it reduces the rate of complications
1995	Silverman et al.: showed that survival in Marfan syndrome had increased after the introduction of medical and surgical treatment of complications
1996	De Paepe et al.: revised diagnostic criteria for Marfan syndrome

Box 10.2 A timeline of landmarks in Marfan syndrome *(continued)*

1997	Pereira et al.: gene targeting experiment in mice; mutating the fibrillin-1 gene led to a change in tissue's ability to withstand haemodynamic stress, suggesting that elastin disruption was a secondary rather than a primary event
1999	Pereira et al.: suggested that mice with reduced (rather than complete) deficiency of fibrillin-1 still had an Marfan syndrome phenotype and that there was a correlation between the quantity of fibrillin protein and the degree of vascular complications
2002	Yamazaki et al.: reviewed their surgical experience to try to identify indications for surgery and the optical surgical management
2002	Gott et al.: reports on 24 years of surgical experience performing aortic valve replacement on 271 patients—confirmed that elective repair should occur before valve diameter >6 cm
2003	Neptune et al.: mice deficient in fibrillin-1 have marked dysregulation of transforming growth factor β activation and signalling, resulting in apoptosis in the developing lung
2004	Ng et al.: increased transforming growth factor β associated with fibrillin-1 deficiency in mouse models of Marfan syndrome are involved in the pathogenesis of mitral valve prolapse and can be reversed by transforming growth factor β antagonists
2006	Habashi et al.: in mouse models of Marfan syndrome, aortic aneurysms are associated with increased transforming growth factor β and can be reversed with angiotensin II receptor blockade (e.g. losartan)
2008	Brooke et al.: cohort study demonstrating that angiotensin receptor blockade in paediatric patients with Marfan syndrome slows the rate of progression of aortic root dilation
2010	Loeys et al.: revised Ghent nosology for Marfan syndrome (2nd revision)

Paper 10.1: The clinical and genetic description of Ehlers–Danlos syndrome as an inherited trait

Reference

Johnson SA, Falls HF. Ehlers–Danlos syndrome—a clinical and genetic study. *Arch Derm Syphilol* 1949;60(1):82–95.

Purpose

An analysis of the published literature on the clinical, pathologic, radiographic, and familial aspects of Ehlers–Danlos syndrome, and a pedigree analysis of a large extended family.

Patients

The first part of the report brought together the literature describing the phenotypes that constitute Ehlers–Danlos syndrome and included a review of 15 previous pedigree studies. The second part of the report presented a family of six generations, comprising 123 persons and in which there were 32 affected individuals.

Study design

The report contained a literature review and analysis, and a pedigree study.

Results

The severity of characteristics varied among different persons and within sibships, and also to the degree that some members of a family had features of a forme fruste state of Ehlers–Danlos syndrome and might otherwise have been considered 'normal' without more detailed enquiry.

Normal individuals transmit the trait to affected offspring, and the pattern of inheritance was predominantly one of dominance, showing that Ehlers–Danlos syndrome was congenital and not an acquired condition.

The presence of Ehlers–Danlos syndrome in the affected offspring or unaffected parents might likely arise by any of three other genetic mechanisms: autosomal recessive genes, sex-linked genes, and the phenomenon of spontaneous mutation.

Significance and importance

Finkelstein and Key were among the early researchers to recognize a familial predisposition to lax or hypermobile joints [1, 2]. However, the paper by Johnson and Falls is seminal in concluding that Ehlers–Danlos syndrome is an inherited disorder with an autosomal dominant trait and set a foundation for future clinical genetic studies. Their observations also cemented the view first suggested by Stuart and Goldsmith that normal individuals can transmit the trait to affected offspring [3, 4].

This was the largest and most extensive family observational study of the time and also the first to detail the spectrum of phenotypes present in Ehlers–Danlos syndrome, based on the breadth of published literature. By comparison, most previous pedigree studies had involved only two to three generations, with the largest having 22 members, of which 11 had the disorder.

The clinical discussion in the paper is testimony not only to the powers of observation but also foresight. Two remarks stand out as true today as much as then: first, that all clinicians, and in particular those practising musculoskeletal medicine, should be more aware of the disorder and its presentations; and, second, that although the complete penetrance of Ehlers–Danlos syndrome is rare, a forme fruste or mild variant of Ehlers–Danlos syndrome can be recognized. The presence of this latter group would later be echoed in the description of Ehlers–Danlos syndrome type III (or hypermobility type) in the Villefranche 1997 classification [5] and the 1998 Brighton Criteria for Benign Joint Hypermobility Syndrome [6].

Also in contributions to the discussion, Tobias raised the topic of connective tissue properties in Ehlers–Danlos syndrome, noting that heterogeneity lay here too. He remarked that, in Ehlers–Danlos syndrome patients, dermatological tissue might be normal histologically or present with differing amounts of cutaneous elasticity versus ligament laxity, versus fragility. He also noted that electronic microscopic evaluation of collagen in skin of patients with Ehlers–Danlos syndrome had been found to be normal, increased, or decreased. He concluded that, in some cases of Ehlers–Danlos syndrome, both elastic and collagenous fibres were involved in the patho-aetiology, while in others only the collagenous fibres were involved, suggesting some heterogeneity in aetiology that might explain the different phenotypic presentations. That abnormalities of collagen were the likely explanation for Ehlers–Danlos syndrome would be further supported by the work of Jansen, McKusick, and Jackson and Bentley [7–9].

References

1 Finkelstein H. Joint hypotonia. *NY Med J* 1916;**104**:942–3.

2 Key JA. Hypermobility of joints as a sex-linked hereditary characteristic. *JAMA* 1927;**88**(22):1710–12.

3 Stuart AM. Three cases exhibiting the Ehlers–Danlos syndrome. *Proc R Soc Med* 1937;**30**(8):984–6.

4 Goldsmith WN. Ehlers–Danlos syndrome. *Proc Roy Soc Med* 1939;**32**(9):1027.

5 Beighton P, De Paepe A, Steimann B, et al. (1998) Ehlers–Danlos syndrome: revised nosology. *Am J Med Genet* **1997**;77(1):31–7.

6 Grahame R, Bird H, Child C. The revised (Brighton 1998) criteria for the diagnosis of benign joint hypermobility syndrome (BJHS). *J Rheumatol* 2000;**27**(7):1777–9.

7 Jansen LH. The structure of the connective tissue, an explanation of the symptoms of the Ehlers–Danlos syndrome. *Dermatologica* 1955;**110**(2):108–20.

8 McKusick VA. Heritable disorders of connective tissue, 1st edn. St. Louis, MO: CV Mosby; 1956.

9 Jackson DS, Bentley JP. On the significance of the extractable collagens. *J Biophys Biochem Cytol* 1960;**7**(1):31–42.

Paper 10.2: Heterogeneity and the classification of Ehlers–Danlos syndrome

Reference

Beighton P, Price A, Lord A, et al. Variants of the Ehlers–Danlos syndrome. Clinical, biochemical, haematological and chromosomal features of 100 patients. *Ann Rheum Dis* 1969;28(3):228–35.

Purpose

To observe and classify the associations between clinical and laboratory phenotypes and karyotype in Ehlers–Danlos syndrome, with the hypothesis that Ehlers–Danlos syndrome is not a heterogenic disorder but a condition comprised of distinct subgroups with a common pathogenesis.

Patients

This study examined a cohort of 100 clinic patients with Ehlers–Danlos syndrome.

Study design

This was a clinical and laboratory observation study and review of the literature on connective tissue biochemistry in Ehlers–Danlos syndrome.

Results

Literature on connective tissue biochemistry, haematology, and genetics in Ehlers–Danlos syndrome was found to show conflicting results, possibly because a mixed group of Ehlers–Danlos syndrome subtypes was being analysed.

Although stigmata were very similar in members of the same family, there was a very wide variation between families to the extent that the syndrome manifests as more than one entity.

Five well-defined types of Ehlers–Danlos syndrome emerged clinically and were named gravis, mitis, benign hypermobile, ecchymotic, and X-linked.

Ehlers–Danlos syndrome subgroup analysis of four markers of connective tissue turnover (urinary hydroxyproline excretion, plasma elastase inhibitor, urinary chondroitin and heparin sulphates (mucopolysaccharides), and urinary amino-acid chromatography) demonstrated normal levels of collagen activity and no identifiable and consistent haematological abnormalities of clotting. Multiple cells analyses from cases did not identify any consistent chromosomal abnormalities.

Significance and importance

It was the work of McKusick, Jackson and Bentley, Barabas, and Beighton et al. spanning a decade and a half from the mid-1950s to end of the 1960s that would lay the foundation for the modern classification of Ehlers–Danlos syndrome [1–6].

However, three ground-breaking observations arose from the work by Beighton, Price, Lord, and Dickinson. The first was the five-subtype classification that would continue to be recognized in later iterations that would also include molecular genetics [5].

Second, and profound in its observation, the authors in their discussion considered the complications of the different presentations observed and noted these to be clinically predictable in behaviour. In giving reasons for distinguishing between the types on medical grounds, four areas of concern were highlighted and remain valid to the present day:

+ prognosis—that death in youth or early adulthood arose in the ecchymotic variety and as a result of rupture or dissection of arteries;

+ operative risk—friable tissues and abnormal bleeding in the gravis and ecchymotic types increased the intra-operative risks of excessive blood loss and of poor wound healing;

+ obstetrics—that premature delivery arose in the gravis type; and

+ genetic counselling—given the autosomal dominant and X-linked patterns, the likelihood of passing on these conditions became clearer.

Third, the absence of identifiable biochemical and karyotype abnormalities suggested that other pathological mechanisms apart from collagen turnover or chromosomal abnormalities were in play. This would set the scene for future studies on connective tissue biology and molecular genetics. Recognition of the different types of collagen in skin, cartilage, and bone in humans arose. By the mid-1970s, the structural and biological characteristics of collagen were better understood, as was their relationship with disease [7–9].

References

1 **McKusick, VA**. Heritable disorders of connective tissue, 1st edn. St. Louis, MO: CV Mosby; 1956.

2 **Jackson DS, Bentley JP**. On the significance of the extractable collagens. *J Biophys Biochem Cytol* 1960;**7**(1):31–42.

3 **Barabas AP**. Heterogeneity of the Ehlers–Danlos Syndrome: description of three clinical types and a hypothesis to explain the basic defect(s). *BMJ* 1967;**2**(5552):612–6.

4 **Beighton P, Price A, Lord A, et al**. Variants of the Ehlers–Danlos syndrome. Clinical, biochemical, haematological and chromosomal features of 100 patients. *Ann Rheum Dis* 1969;**28**(3):228–35.

5 **Beighton P, De Paepe A, Steimann B, et al**. (1998) Ehlers–Danlos syndrome: revised nosology. *Am J Med Genet* 1997;**77**(1):31–7.

6 **Beighton, P**. The Ehlers-Danlos syndrome. London: William Heinemann Medical Books Ltd; 1970.

7 **Stark M, Miller EJ, Kühn K**. Comparative electron-microscope studies on the collagens extracted from cartilage, bone and skin. *Eur J Biochem* 1972;**27**(1):192–6.

8 **Miller EJ, Epstein EH Jr, Piez KA**. Identification of three genetically distinct collagens by cyanogen bromide cleavage of insoluble human skin and cartilage collagen. *Biochem Biophys Res Commun* 1971;**42**(6):1024–9.

9 **Nimni ME**. Collagen: its structure and function in normal and pathological connective tissues. *Semin Arth Rheum* 1974;**4**(2):95–150.

Paper 10.3: Collagen defects, and genetic linkage in Ehlers–Danlos syndrome

Reference

Pope FM, Martin GR, Lichtenstein JR, et al. Patients with Ehlers–Danlos syndrome type IV lack type III collagen. *Proc Natl Acad Sci U S A* 1975;72(4):1314–16.

Purpose

In two rare variants of Ehlers–Danlos syndrome, studies showed that hydroxylysine and lysyl hydroxylase levels were deficient or low, leading to fragile and hyperextensible connective tissues [1, 2]. However the Type IV (vascular) variant of Ehlers–Danlos syndrome, which is associated with arterial and bowel rupture, was not associated with hyperextensible connective tissues. The purpose of the study was to explore whether other pathologies arise in Ehlers–Danlos syndrome IV.

Patients

This study examined five patients with clinically diagnosed Ehlers–Danlos syndrome type IV.

Study design

Skin biopsies were taken from four patients with clinically diagnosed Type IV. Post-mortem samples of skin, aorta, bowel, and bone were collected from a fifth patient. Skin samples were obtained from age–sex matched controls.

Biochemical (including amino-acid electrophoresis) and histological analysis was undertaken of disease and normal tissue.

Results

Hydroxyproline and hydroxylisine levels were reduced compared to library data on normal samples, indicating biochemically that collagen levels were low.

Valine levels were raised compared to normal, indicating higher volumes of elastin.

Histological studies demonstrated reduced amounts of collagen in the dermis and also reduced size of collagen bundles.

Skin fibroblasts from normal individuals synthesize both Type I and Type III collagen. Ehlers–Danlos syndrome IV cells synthesized only Type I collagen.

Significance and importance

These results were the first to suggest that the fragile skin, blood vessels, and intestine of Ehlers–Danlos syndrome IV patients result from an absence or reduction of Type III collagen. Two years later Pope et al. linked the genotype to the molecular phenotype in Ehlers–Danlos syndrome IV and concluded that the inheritance was autosomal recessive [3].

In the ensuing two decades, linkage studies of encoding genes, molecular defects, and disease subgroups would be published. The gene encoding COL3A1 was first associated with the clinical phenotype of Ehlers–Danlos syndrome Type IV in reports by Tsipouras et al. and Nicholls et al. and with molecular abnormalities by Superti-Furga et al. [4–6]. Many genetic and molecular studies of individuals and families with Ehlers–Danlos syndrome Type IV followed and are best summarized in a review by Pepin et al. [7], in which defects in *COL3A1* were identified in 135 of 220 index cases [7].

References

1 **Pinnell SR, Krane SM, Kenzora JE, et al**. A heritable disorder of connective tissue: hydroxylysine-deficient collagen disease. *N Engl J Med* 1972;**286**(19):1013–20.

2 **Lichtenstein J, Nigra TP, Sussman MD, et al**. Molecular defect in a form of the Ehlers–Danlos syndrome: hydroxylysine deficient collagen (abstract). *Am J Hum Genet* 1972;**24**(6 Part 1):27a.

3 **Pope FM, Martin GR, McKusick VA**. Inheritance of Ehlers-Danlos type IV syndrome. *J Med Genet* 1977;**14**(3):200–4.

4 **Tsipouras P, Byers PH, Schwartz RC, et al**. Ehlers-Danlos syndrome type IV: cosegregation of the phenotype to a COL3A1 allele of type III procollagen. *Hum Genet* 1986;**74**(1):41–6.

5 **Nicholls AC, De Paepe A, Narcisi P, et al**. Linkage of a polymorphic marker for the type III collagen gene (*COL3A1*) to atypical autosomal dominant Ehlers–Danlos syndrome type IV in a large Belgian pedigree. *Hum Genet* 1988;**78**(3):276–81.

6 **Superti-Furga A, Steinmann B, Ramirez F, et al**. Molecular defects of type III procollagen in Ehlers–Danlos syndrome type IV. *Hum Genet* 1989;**82**(2):104–8.

7 **Pepin M, Schwarze U, Superti-Furga A, et al**. Clinical and genetic features of Ehlers–Danlos syndrome type IV, the vascular type. *N Engl J Med* 2000;**342**(10):673–80.

Paper 10.4: Genetic linkage in classical Ehlers–Danlos syndrome

Reference

Greenspan DS, Byers MG, Eddy RI, et al. Human collagen gene *COL5A1* maps to the q34.2–34.3 region of chromosome 9, near the locus for nail-patella syndrome. *Genomics* 1992;12(4):836–7.

Purpose

By the early 1990s, it was known that Type V collagen defects, and in particular those related to abnormalities in *COL5A1*, appeared to both define and explain the phenotype in the majority of cases of Type I/II (classical) Ehlers–Danlos syndrome. It was also recognized that Type V collagen is a minor constituent of connective tissue and typically co-expressed with Type 1 collagen [1, 2]. Its low representation in tissues and cell cultures limited biochemical analysis to the extent that involvement of Type V collagen genes in human disease had not been explored.

The purpose of this study was to map the *COL5A1* locus in order to facilitate linkage analysis.

Study design and results

The group had previously isolated cDNA and genomic clones from human and hamster libraries and had constructed the entire collagen α-1(V) coding sequence of both species [3]. These were used as probes for hybridization to filter-bound DNA from a panel of human-mouse hybrid cell lines and for in situ hybridization to metaphase chromosomes.

The studies established the chromosomal location of *COL5A1*, which encodes the collagen α-1(V) chain, within segment 9q34.2–q34.3, adding to the previously characterized dispersion of collagen genes in the human genome and demonstrating the first example of a collagen locus on chromosome nine.

Significance and importance

The group's publication is a humble, two-page, short communication that almost belies its translational importance. Following on from the 1991 work, Greenspan and colleagues undertook intron–exon boundary sequencing of *COL5A1*, paving the way for linkage analysis [4].

Linkage was first identified between *COL5A1* and Ehlers–Danlos syndrome Type II by Loughlin et al. in 1995 [5]. By carrying out similar linkage studies in two large British families with Ehlers–Danlos syndrome Type I/II and Type II, Burrows et al. also explored the role of *COL5A1* further as a candidate gene in mixed Ehlers–Danlos syndrome (Type I/II) [6, 7]. But it is ultimately in the findings of Symoens et al. that one sees the importance of the work by Greenspan and colleagues [8]. Symoens et al. explored *COL5A1* and *COL5A2* associations in over 100 patients fulfilling the Villefranche criteria for classical Ehlers–Danlos syndrome. In the overwhelming majority of cases (over 90%), a Type V collagen defect (due to either a null allele or a structural mutation) was found, and for the vast majority this related to *COL5A1*, which encodes collagen α-1(V). The reduced avail-ability of Type V collagen appeared to be the major disease-causing mechanism.

References

1 **Fessler JH, Fessler LI.** 'Type V collagen' in Structure and function of collagen types (Mayne R, Burgeson RE, eds); Orlando, FL: Academic Press; 1987; pp. 81–103.

2 **Emanuel BS, Cannizzaro LA, Seyer JM, et al.** Human alpha 1(III) and alpha 2(V) procollagen genes are located on the long arm of chromosome 2. *Proc Natl Acad Sci U S A* 1985;**82**(10):3385–9.

3 **Greenspan DS, Cheng W, Hoffman GG.** The pro-alpha 1(V) collagen chain. Complete primary structure, distribution of expression, and comparison with the pro-alpha 1(XI) collagen chain. *J Biol Chem* 1991;**266**(36):24727–33.

4 **Nicholls AC, Oliver JE, McCarron S, et al**. An exon skipping mutation of a type V collagen gene (*COL5A1*) in Ehlers–Danlos syndrome. *J Med Genet* 1996;**33**(11):940–6. Erratum in *J Med Genet* 1997;334(1):87.

5 **Loughlin J, Irven C, Hardwick LJ, et al**. Linkage of the gene that encodes the alpha 1 chain of type V collagen (COL5A1) to type II Ehlers–Danlos syndrome. *Hum Mol Genet* 1995;**4**(9):1649–51.

6 **Burrows NP, Nicholls AC, Yates JR, et al**. The gene encoding collagen alpha1(V)(COL5A1) is linked to mixed Ehlers–Danlos syndrome type I/II. *J Invest Dermatol* 1996;**106**(6):1273–6.

7 **Burrows NP, Nicholls AC, Yates JR, et al**. Genetic linkage to the collagen alpha 1 (v) gene (*COL5A1*) in two British Ehlers–Danlos syndrome families with variable type I and II phenotypes. *Clin Exp Dermatol* 1997;**22**(4):174–6.

8 **Symoens S, Syx D, Malfait F, et al**. Comprehensive molecular analysis demonstrates type V collagen mutations in over 90% of patients with classic EDS and allows to refine diagnostic criteria. *Hum Mutat* 2012;**33**(10):1485–93.

Paper 10.5: Cardiovascular pathology and Marfan syndrome

Reference

McKusick VA. The cardiovascular aspects of Marfan's syndrome: a heritable disorder of connective tissue. *Circulation* 1955;11(3):321–42.

Purpose

To describe the extent and nature of cardiac, pulmonary artery, and aortic involvement in Marfan syndrome.

Patients

A cohort of 105 cases of Marfan syndrome from within 50 families, was obtained from three sources: clinic databases of known families with ectopia lentis (specific but not pathognomonic of the syndrome), the post-mortem records of patients who died by aneurysmal rupture, and medical notes reporting arachnodactyly or a diagnosis of Marfan syndrome (Johns Hopkins Hospital, Baltimore, MD, USA).

Study design

This was a clinical observational study.

Results

Multiple identifiable cardiac pathologies from early and asymptomatic aortic root dilatation to major aortic valve regurgitation and aneurysms of the aortic root, arch, and descending aorta arise in Marfan syndrome.

Cardiac dysfunction was observed as associated with severe pectus deformities of the sternum.

On quarter of cases developed aortic aneurysm (in the absence of any other risk such as hypertension) before the age of 40. No patient with major valve or vascular disease lived beyond the age of 50 in this cohort.

Fifteen percent of cases arose de novo as probable new genetic mutations, and Marfan syndrome is inherited as a dominant trait.

Significance and importance

Up until the 1940s, the phenotype of Marfan syndrome only included musculoskeletal and ocular pathology. Now, among the complications of Marfan syndrome, aortic dilatation and rupture are understood to be the causes of early death.

Baer et al. and Etter and Glover described aneurysmal dilatation and rupture following aortic dissection in cases of Marfan syndrome [1, 2], and Macleod and Williams undertook a literature review on the subject, published within the same year [3]. However, McKusick's paper is rich in its clinical, radiological, and outcome observation of individuals and kinships. The mortality statistics were to be re-affirmed in a 1972 review by Murdoch et al., prior to a new era in the 1980s when surgical and medical interventions would begin to influence outcome [4].

In studying families of over three to four generations, McKusick was able to make several other profoundly important observations that would have implications for future research in Marfan syndrome and would lead to our current understanding of the management and surveillance of the condition.

McKusick also made the point that the principal cardiovascular component of Marfan syndrome, the abnormality of the aorta, was not in the true sense 'congenital heart disease' or a 'congenital malformation'. He compared it to the amyotrophies in neurology; that is, that the weakness is present at birth, perhaps not recognizable by ordinary histologic technique, and expresses itself from infancy on, and often much later.

That cardiovascular pathologies in Marfan syndrome are most often acquired over time from a congenital risk is now a fundamental principle and the basis for current practice of life-long observation.

McKusick observed that, in cardiac cases whose skeletal proportions were consistent with Marfan syndrome, it would be virtually impossible to be completely certain clinically whether Marfan syndrome was actually present unless '1—ectopia lentis, the least equivocal component of the syndrome, was also present or 2—unequivocal instances of the syndrome were represented by other members of the family'. This observation regarding the potential criteria for Marfan syndrome was to be integral the 1988 Berlin first classification criteria of Marfan syndrome, retained in its revision as the Ghent 1998 criteria, and remain a guiding principle within the 2010 revision of the Ghent criteria [5].

References

1 **Baer RW, Taussig HB, Oppenheimer EH**. Congenital aneurysmal dilatation of the aorta associated with arachnodactyly. *Bull Hopkins Hosp* 1943;**72**:309–31.

2 **Etter LE, Glover LP**. Arachnodactyly complicated by dislocated lens and death from rupture of a dissecting aneurysm of the aorta. *JAMA* 1943;**123**(2):88–9.

3 **Macleod M, Williams AW**. The cardiovascular lesions in Marfan's syndrome. *AMA Arch Pathol* 1956;**61**(2):143–8.

4 **Murdoch JL, Walker BA, Halpern BL, et al**. Life expectancy and causes of death in the Marfan syndrome. *N Engl J Med* 1972;**286**(15):804–8.

5 **Loeys BL, Dietz HC, Braverman AC, et al**. The revised Ghent nosology for the Marfan syndrome. *J Med Genet* 2010;**47**(7):476–85.

Paper 10.6: Vascular surgery in Marfan syndrome

Reference

Gott VL, Pyeritz RE, Magovern GJ Jr, et al. Surgical treatment of aneurysms of the ascending aorta in the Marfan syndrome. Results of composite-graft repair in 50 patients. *N Engl J Med* 1986;314(17):1070–4.

Background

Surgical mortality was high in Marfan syndrome and commonly due to uncontrollable haemorrhage, valve dehiscence, or further dissection. The more common surgical techniques at the time were patch repairs. Techniques for complete aortic root and arch replacement pioneered by Bentall and De Bono were applied anticipating reduction in morbidity and mortality [1].

Patients

Fifty consecutive patients with Marfan syndrome (38 males and 12 females; 44 electives and 6 emergencies) had operative repair of an aneurysm of the ascending aorta in the period 1976 to 1984. At surgery, the average age was 32 years, with a range from 9 to 52 years.

Study design

This was an eight-year clinical observational outcome study.

Results

There were no hospital deaths among the 44 patients who underwent elective repair, and only one death among the six requiring emergency surgery. The overall hospital mortality rate was therefore only 2% and therefore much lower than the mortality of 60% prior to these techniques.

Patients were followed up for eight years. During the first four years of the study, 4 deaths occurred among 11 patients. However in the subsequent four years of the study, there were no late deaths from surgical complications among the other 38 patients. Survival was 87% at both two and five years after surgery.

Significance and importance

Prior to Gott's report on the effectiveness of this type of surgical intervention, mortality from vascular pathology accounted for 90% of premature deaths, and the mortality at aneurysmal repair was approximately 50% [2].

Gott's paper is a landmark not only in demonstrating life-saving surgical treatment in Marfan syndrome but also in establishing ongoing management of vascular patients. Postoperatively, the team treated with β-blockade, conducted clinical evaluations of patients twice a year, and assessed the entire aorta with computer tomography once a year.

Gott expanded on his team's experience in further reports in 1999 and 2002 [3, 4], the latter amassing 24 years of experience in 271 cases of Marfan syndrome. Development of surgical techniques and exploration of their use alongside conservative interventions remains a fundamental area of clinical research in Marfan syndrome [5].

References

1 **Bentall HH, De Bono A**. A technique for complete replacement of the ascending aorta. *Thorax* 1968;**23**(4):338–9.

2 **Crawford ES**. Marfan's syndrome: broad spectral surgical treatment cardiovascular manifestations. *Ann Surg* 1983;**198**(4):487–505.

3 **Gott VL, Greene PS, Alejo DE, et al**. Replacement of the aortic root in patients with Marfan's syndrome. *N Engl J Med* 1999;**340**(17):1307–13.

4 **Gott VL, Cameron DE, Alejo DE, et al**. Aortic root replacement in 271 Marfan patients: a 24-year experience. *Ann Thorac Surg* 2002;**73**(2):438–43.

5 **Di Eusanio M, Berretta P, Folesani G, et al**. Aortic disease in Marfan syndrome: current role of surgery and thoracic endovascular aortic repair. *G Ital Cardiol (Rome)* 2013;**14**(7–8):538–47.

Paper 10.7: Connective tissue fragility—clinical evidence of the role of transforming growth factor β in Marfan syndrome

Reference

Neptune ER, Frischmeyer PA, Arking DE, et al. Dysregulation of TGF-beta activation contributes to pathogenesis in Marfan syndrome. *Nat Genet* 2003;33(3):407–11.

Purpose

The consensus view up to this point was that pathology in Marfan syndrome arose due to 'weakness', that is, fragility in connective tissues as a direct consequence of reduced quantities of fibrillin. This, however, did not explain the bone dysplasia and osteopenia, emphysema, body habitus, myopathy, and reduced levels of adipose tissue seen in Marfan syndrome. In 1997 Pereira et al. reported a gene-targeting experiment in mice that indicated that fibrillin-1 microfibrils are predominantly engaged in tissue homeostasis rather than elastic matrix assembly, suggesting that disruption of the elastic connective tissue was a secondary rather than a primary event [1]. Fibrillin-1 directly binds to a latent form of the cytokine transforming growth factor β, keeping it sequestered and unable to exert its biological activity. It was in this finding that the hypothesized aetiology for connective tissue dysfunction in Marfan syndrome moved from being structural and mechanical to more functional and metabolic [2].

A distinct subgroup of individuals with Marfan syndrome have distal airspace enlargement, historically described as emphysema, which frequently results in spontaneous lung rupture.

The aim of the study was to investigate the role of fibrillin and transforming growth factor defects in the pathogenesis of emphysema in a mouse model of Marfan syndrome.

Study design

This was a histological and biochemical analysis of lung phenotype of normal versus mice deficient in fibrillin-1 (an accepted model of Marfan syndrome) exploring the regulation of transforming growth factor β.

Results

Lung abnormalities were evident in the immediate postnatal period and manifest as a developmental impairment of distal alveolar septation.

Aged mice deficient in fibrillin-1 developed destructive emphysema, consistent with the view that early developmental perturbations can predispose to late-onset, seemingly acquired phenotypes.

The study showed that mice deficient in fibrillin-1 had marked dysregulation of transforming growth factor β activation and signalling, resulting in apoptosis in the developing lung.

Perinatal antagonism of transforming growth factor β attenuated apoptosis and rescued alveolar septation in vivo.

Significance and importance

The 1990s were the era of genetics and molecular biology in Marfan syndrome. Fibrillin had become the target protein. Studies documented consistent, relatively specific abnormalities of microfibrillar fibres in Marfan syndrome [3], specifically, mutations in fibrillin-1 leading to an autosomal dominant pattern of inheritance [4–6]. The discoveries of fibrillin and of the fibrillin gene defect in Marfan syndrome are clear landmarks. However, the data in the Neptune paper indicated that matrix sequestration of cytokines was crucial to their regulated activation and signalling and that perturbation of this cytokine function contributed to the pathogenesis of lung disease in Marfan syndrome. A similar observation with regard to mitral valve disease was made a year later [7].

The accepted treatment up to this point was geared towards physically re-strengthening weakened tissues, in particular aortic grafting, or utilizing beta blockers to slow disease progression. Consideration had also been given to correcting the defective gene. However, with the discovery of transforming growth factor β-mediated molecular pathways, the possibility arose to explore the impact of modulating molecular pathways and potentially preventing vascular disease [8–12], an area of therapeutics in Marfan syndrome that is at the forefront of clinical and molecular research today.

References

1 Pereira L, Andrikopoulos K, Tian J, et al. Targeting of the gene encoding fibrillin-1 recapitulates the vascular aspect of Marfan syndrome. *Nat Genet* 1997;**17**(2):218–22.

2 Pereira L, Lee SY, Gayraud B, et al. Pathogenetic sequence for aneurysm revealed in mice underexpressing fibrillin-1. *Proc Natl Acad Sci U S A* 1999;**96**(7):3819–23.

3 Hollister DW, Godfrey M, Sakai LY, et al. Immunohistologic abnormalities of the microfibrillar-fiber system in the Marfan syndrome. *New Engl J Med* 1990; **323**(3):152–9.

4 Dietz HC, Cutting GR, Pyeritz RE, et al. Marfan syndrome caused by a recurrent *de novo* missense mutation in the fibrillin gene. *Nature* 1991;**352**(6333):337–9.

5 Lee B, Godfrey M, Vitale E, et al. Linkage of Marfan syndrome and a phenotypically related disorder to two different fibrillin genes. *Nature* 1991;**352**(6333):330–4.

6 Pereira L, Lee SY, Gayraud B, et al. Pathogenetic sequence for aneurysm revealed in mice underexpressing fibrillin-1. *Proc Natl Acad Sci U S A* 1999;**96**(7):3819–23.

7 Ng CM, Cheng A, Myers LA, et al. TGF-beta-dependent pathogenesis of mitral valve prolapse in a mouse model of Marfan syndrome. *J Clin Invest* 2004;**114**(11):1586–92.

8 Igondjo-Tchen S, Pagès N, Bac P, et al. Marfan syndrome, magnesium status and medical prevention of cardiovascular complications by hemodynamic treatments and antisense gene therapy. *Magnes Res* 2003;**16**(1):59–64.

9 Habashi JP, Judge DP, Holm TM, et al. Losartan, an AT1 antagonist, prevents aortic aneurysm in a mouse model of Marfan syndrome. *Science* 2006;**312**(5770):117–21.

10 Kalluri R, Han Y. Targeting. Targeting TGF-beta and the extracellular matrix in Marfan's syndrome. *Dev Cell* 2008;**15**(1):1–2.

11 Lacro RV, Dietz HC, Wruck LM, et al. Rationale and design of a randomized clinical trial of beta blocker therapy (atenolol) versus angiotensin II receptor blocker therapy (losartan) in individuals with Marfan syndrome. *Am Heart J* 2007;**154**(4):624–31.

12 Brooke BS, Habashi JP, Judge DP, et al. Angiotensin II blockade and aortic-root dilation in Marfan's syndrome. *N Engl J Med* 2008;**358**(26):2787–95.

Summary

The work of Johnson and Falls in the 1940s elevated insight in to the inheritance of Ehlers–Danlos syndrome. They took the opportunity to explore in detail the phenotypes and heterogeneity of Ehlers–Danlos syndrome and the pedigree literature to date. Their observations and conclusions were to stand the test of time.

Sense of the ability to subgroup and classify cases of Ehlers–Danlos syndrome came in the 1960s. Barabas and Beighton et al. took the then knowledge of histological, biochemical, and inheritance patterns, together with clinical phenotypes, applied it to their substantial cohorts of patients and families, and established the basis for the modern classification of Ehlers–Danlos syndrome.

Molecular genetics came to the fore in the 1980s with the identification of the *COL1*, *COLIII*, and *COLV* genes. Greenspan and his group, alongside several other international research teams laid the foundation for ensuing linkage studies of the more common classic variant of Ehlers–Danlos syndrome.

The current Villefranche classification recognizes six subtypes, most of which are now linked to mutations in genes encoding fibrillar collagens or enzymes involved in post-translational modification of these proteins. Establishing the correct Ehlers–Danlos syndrome subtype has had important implications for genetic counselling and clinical management. Also, over the last few years, new variants of Ehlers–Danlos syndrome have been characterized, bringing insights into molecular pathogenesis by implicating genetic defects in the biosynthesis of extracellular matrix molecules such as tenascin-x.

It will no doubt not be too long before the Villefranche classification is refined to take account of this data, while very much reflecting the heterogeneity of the disorder as first observed over a century ago.

Marfan syndrome manifests as a triad of musculoskeletal pathology, ocular pathology, and cardiovascular pathologies, including aortic root dilatation, aortic dissection and rupture, and cardiac valve problems.

Over the twentieth century, from the earliest descriptions of the musculoskeletal phenomena through to the identification of genetic mutations of fibrillin and associated molecular aberrations of transforming growth factor β, a wealth of clinical and genetic knowledge has amassed, leading to detailed and specific classification of Marfan syndrome and the conditions that constitute the differential diagnosis.

McKusick's collation in the 1950s of the vascular pathologies in Marfan syndrome was fundamental in defining the breadth and complications of these associations. McKusick's observations were to also play a major role in defining clinical criteria for the diagnosis of Marfan syndrome.

Given the high mortality rates from vascular disease, surgical interventions were to herald a major breakthrough in improving life expectancy. The pioneering work of Crawford and Gott established surgical intervention and ongoing review at the centre of management in Marfan syndrome.

As molecular genetics came to the fore in the late 1980s, so the role of fibrillin gained clarity. However, it is the discovery of the role of transforming growth factor β in connective tissue homeostasis and in the aetiology of Marfan syndrome that led to a paradigm change. Thinking moved from a mechanical to a molecular view of the pathogenesis of tissue fragility in Marfan syndrome. Most profoundly, the discovery of the transforming growth factor β-mediated molecular pathways brought opportunities to explore potentially preventive interventions in the management of vascular disease.

Index

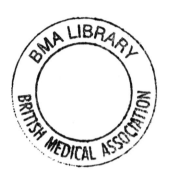